T0229127

Prostate Cancer Imaging and Therapy

Editors

RICHARD P. BAUM
CRISTINA NANNI

PET CLINICS

www.pet.theclinics.com

Consulting Editor
ABASS ALAVI

April 2017 • Volume 12 • Number 2

ELSEVIER

1600 John F. Kennedy Boulevard • Suite 1800 • Philadelphia, Pennsylvania, 19103-2899

http://www.pet.theclinics.com

PET CLINICS Volume 12, Number 2
April 2017 ISSN 1556-8598, ISBN-13: 978-0-323-52423-0

Editor: John Vassallo (j.vassallo@elsevier.com)
Developmental Editor: Meredith Madeira

PET Clinics (ISSN 1556-8598) is published quarterly by Elsevier Inc., 360 Park Avenue South, New York, NY 10010-1710. Months of issue are January, April, July, and October. Periodicals postage paid at New York, NY, and additional mailing offices. Subscription prices per year are $232.00 (US individuals), $381.00 (US institutions), $100.00 (US students), $263.00 (Canadian individuals), $428.00 (Canadian institutions), $140.00 (Canadian students), $268.00 (foreign individuals), $428.00 (foreign institutions), and $140.00 (foreign students). To receive student and resident rate, orders must be accompanied by name of affiliated institution, date of term, and the signature of program/residency coordinator on institution letterhead. Orders will be billed at individual rate until proof of status is received. Foreign air speed delivery is included in all Clinics subscription prices. All prices are subject to change without notice. POSTMASTER: Send address changes to PET Clinics, Elsevier Health Sciences Division, Subscription Customer Service, 3251 Riverport Lane, Maryland Heights, MO 63043. **Customer Service: 1-800-654-2452 (U.S. and Canada); 314-447-8871 (outside U.S. and Canada). Fax: 314-447-8029. E-mail: journalscustomerservice-usa@elsevier.com (for print support); journalsonlinesupport-usa@elsevier.com (for online support).**

Reprints. For copies of 100 or more of articles in this publication, please contact the Commercial Reprints Department, Elsevier Inc., 360 Park Avenue South, New York, NY 10010-1710. Tel.: 212-633-3874; Fax: 212-633-3820; E-mail: reprints@elsevier.com.

PET Clinics is covered in MEDLINE/PubMed (Index Medicus).

Contributors

CONSULTING EDITOR

ABASS ALAVI, MD, MD (Hon), PhD (Hon), DSc (Hon)
Professor, Division of Nuclear Medicine, Department of Radiology, Hospital of the University of Pennsylvania, University of Pennsylvania Perelman School of Medicine, Philadelphia, Pennsylvania

EDITORS

RICHARD P. BAUM, MD, PhD
Professor, Chairman and Clinical Director, THERANOSTICS Center for Molecular Radiotherapy and Molecular Imaging (PET/CT), ENETS Center of Excellence, Zentralklinik Bad Berka, Bad Berka, Germany

CRISTINA NANNI, MD
Consultant, Nuclear Medicine Unit, AOU di Bologna, Policlinico S.Orsola-Malpighi, Bologna, Italy

AUTHORS

LUCIA BARATTO, MD
Division of Nuclear Medicine and Molecular Imaging, Department of Radiology, Stanford University, Stanford, California

RICHARD P. BAUM, MD, PhD
Professor, Chairman and Clinical Director, THERANOSTICS Center for Molecular Radiotherapy and Molecular Imaging (PET/CT), ENETS Center of Excellence, Zentralklinik Bad Berka, Bad Berka, Germany

PAOLO CASTELLUCCI, MD
Service of Nuclear Medicine, S. Orsola-Malpighi University Hospital, University of Bologna, Bologna, Italy

FRANCESCO CECI, MD
Service of Nuclear Medicine, S. Orsola-Malpighi University Hospital, University of Bologna, Bologna, Italy

SAMUEL R. DENMEADE, MD
The Sidney Kimmel Comprehensive Cancer Center at Johns Hopkins, Johns Hopkins University School of Medicine, Baltimore, Maryland

ALEXANDER DRZEZGA, MD
Department of Nuclear Medicine, University Hospital of Cologne, Cologne, Germany

STEFANO FANTI, MD
Service of Nuclear Medicine, S. Orsola-Malpighi University Hospital, University of Bologna, Bologna, Italy

MICHAEL A. GORIN, MD
The James Buchanan Brady Urological Institute and Department of Urology, Johns Hopkins University School of Medicine, Baltimore, Maryland

MARINA HODOLIČ, MD, PhD
Nuclear Medicine Physician; Clinical Research Supervisor, Nuclear Medicine Research Department, Iason, Graz, Austria; Assistant Professor, Department of Nuclear Medicine, Palack University Olomouc, Olomouc, Czech Republic

MICHAEL S. HOFMAN, MBBS, FRACP, FAANMS
Associate Professor, Department of Cancer Imaging, Centre for Molecular Imaging, Peter MacCallum Cancer Centre; University of Melbourne, Melbourne, Victoria, Australia

ANDREI IAGARU, MD, FACNM
Associate Professor of Radiology – Nuclear Medicine, Division of Nuclear Medicine and Molecular Imaging, Department of Radiology, Stanford University, Stanford, California

AMIR IRAVANI, MD, FRACP
Nuclear Medicine Physician, Department of Cancer Imaging, Centre for Molecular Imaging, Peter MacCallum Cancer Centre, Melbourne, Victoria, Australia

KALEVI J.A. KAIREMO, MD, PhD, MSc (Eng)
Chief Physician and Professor, Departments of Molecular Radiotherapy and Nuclear Medicine, Docrates Cancer Center, Helsinki, Finland; Visiting Professor, Department of Nuclear Medicine, The University of Texas MD Anderson Cancer Center, Houston, Texas

ANDREAS KJAER, MD, PhD, DMSc
Professor, Department of Clinical Physiology, Nuclear Medicine & PET and Cluster for Molecular Imaging, Rigshospitalet and University of Copenhagen, Copenhagen, Denmark

HARSHAD R. KULKARNI, MD
THERANOSTICS Center for Molecular Radiotherapy and Molecular Imaging (PET/CT), ENETS Center of Excellence, Zentralklinik Bad Berka, Bad Berka, Germany

THEODOSIA MAINA, PhD
Molecular Radiopharmacy, INRASTES, NCSR "Demokritos", Attikis, Athens, Greece

BERTHOLD A. NOCK, PhD
Molecular Radiopharmacy, INRASTES, NCSR "Demokritos", Attikis, Athens, Greece

MORTEN PERSSON, MSc, PhD
CEO, Curasight Aps, Copenhagen, Denmark

MARTIN G. POMPER, MD, PhD
The Russell H. Morgan Department of Radiology and Radiological Science, Johns Hopkins University School of Medicine, Baltimore, Maryland

STEVEN P. ROWE, MD, PhD
The Russell H. Morgan Department of Radiology and Radiological Science, Johns Hopkins University School of Medicine, Baltimore, Maryland

ROBERTO A. SALAS FRAGOMENI, MD
The Russell H. Morgan Department of Radiology and Radiological Science, Johns Hopkins University School of Medicine, Baltimore, Maryland

BITAL SAVIR-BARUCH, MD
Assistant Professor, Department of Radiology, Loyola University Medical Center, Maywood, Illinois

DAVID M. SCHUSTER, MD
Associate Professor, Department of Radiology and Imaging Sciences, Emory University Hospital, Emory University, Atlanta, Georgia

AVIRAL SINGH, MD, MSc
THERANOSTICS Center for Molecular Radiotherapy and Molecular Imaging (PET/CT), ENETS Center of Excellence, Zentralklinik Bad Berka, Bad Berka, Germany

DORTHE SKOVGAARD, MD, PhD
Department of Clinical Physiology, Nuclear Medicine & PET and Cluster for Molecular Imaging, Rigshospitalet and University of Copenhagen, Copenhagen, Denmark

IDA SONNI, MD
Division of Nuclear Medicine and Molecular Imaging, Department of Radiology, Stanford University, Stanford, California

LUCIA ZANONI, MD
Department of Nuclear Medicine, Policlinico Sant'Orsola-Malpighi, Azienda Ospedaliero-Universitaria di Bologna, Bologna, Italy

Contents

Preface: Prostate Cancer Imaging in the Era of Molecular Medicine xi

Richard P. Baum and Cristina Nanni

Imaging of Prostate Cancer Using ^{11}C-Choline PET/Computed Tomography 137

Paolo Castellucci, Francesco Ceci, and Stefano Fanti

This article reviews the role of ^{11}C-choline-PET/computed tomography (CT) in patients with prostate cancer for diagnosis, staging, and restaging the disease in case of biochemical recurrence after primary treatment. The main application of this imaging procedure is restaging of the disease in case of biochemical recurrence. ^{11}C-Choline-PET/CT proved its value for metastases-directed salvage therapies and for monitoring therapy response in castration-resistant patients. Prostate-specific antigen and prostate-specific antigen kinetics values confirmed their correlation with ^{11}C-choline PET/CT sensitivity. ^{11}C-CholinePET/CT, despite low sensitivity to stage disease or in case of biochemical failure with low PSA levels, has an important impact on the management of patients with prostate cancer.

Imaging of Prostate Cancer Using Fluciclovine 145

Bital Savir-Baruch, Lucia Zanoni, and David M. Schuster

Prostate cancer is the most common cancer and the second leading cause of cancer death in men in the United States. Despite high disease prevalence, diagnosis and surveillance of the disease with conventional imaging are limited typically because of indolent biology. Functional imaging with advanced molecular techniques improves the ability to detect disease. Amino acids are building blocks of proteins, and intracellular transport of amino acids is upregulated in prostate cancer. This review provides a detailed overview of the use of F-18 fluciclovine PET in prostate cancer imaging.

Imaging of Prostate Cancer Using Gallium-68–Labeled Bombesin 159

Ida Sonni, Lucia Baratto, and Andrei Iagaru

Nuclear medicine can play an important role in evaluating prostate cancer combining anatomical and functional information with hybrid techniques. Various PET radiopharmaceuticals have been used for targeting specific biological markers in prostate cancer. Research is ideally oriented towards the development of radiopharmaceuticals targeting antigens overexpressed in prostate cancer, as opposed to normal prostate tissue. In this regard, gastrin-releasing peptide receptors (GRPR) are excellent candidates. Bombesin analogues targeting the GRPR have been investigated. Gallium-68 (^{68}Ga) is an interesting PET radioisotope due to several advantages, such as availability, ease of radiochemistry, half-life, and costs. The focus of this review is on ^{68}Ga-labeled bombesin analogues in prostate cancer.

Imaging of Prostate Cancer Using ^{18}F-Choline PET/Computed Tomography 173

Marina Hodolič

^{18}F-fluorocholine (FCH) PET/computed tomography (CT) is a valuable imaging modality in prostate cancer disease. Probably, its main role is restaging of patients with

cancer (PCa). Despite the progress of conventional imaging strategies, significant limitations remain, including identification of small-volume disease and assessment of bone. Clinical studies have demonstrated that ^{68}Ga-PSMA is a promising tracer for detection of PCa metastases, even in patients with low prostate-specific antigen. To provide an accurate interpretation of ^{68}Ga-PSMA PET/computed tomography, nuclear medicine specialists and radiologists should be familiar with physiologic ^{68}Ga-PSMA uptake, common variants, patterns of locoregional and distant spread of PCa, and inherent pitfalls.

Clinical Experience with ^{18}F-Labeled Small Molecule Inhibitors of Prostate-Specific Membrane Antigen **235**

Steven P. Rowe, Michael A. Gorin, Roberto A. Salas Fragomeni, Alexander Drzezga, and Martin G. Pomper

Prostate cancer (PCa) is the most common noncutaneous malignancy diagnosed in men. Despite the large number of men who will suffer from PCa at some point during their lives, conventional imaging modalities for this important disease (contrast-enhanced computed tomography, bone scan, and MR imaging) have provided only marginal to moderate success in appropriately guiding patient management in certain clinical contexts. In this review, the authors discuss radiofluorinated small molecule radiotracers that have been developed to bind to the transmembrane glycoprotein prostate-specific membrane antigen, a target that is nearly universally overexpressed on PCa epithelial cells.

Imaging of Prostate Cancer Using Urokinase-Type Plasminogen Activator Receptor PET **243**

Dorthe Skovgaard, Morten Persson, and Andreas Kjaer

Urokinase-type plasminogen activator receptor (uPAR) overexpression is an important biomarker for aggressiveness in cancer including prostate cancer (PC) and provides independent clinical information in addition to prostate-specific antigen and Gleason score. This article focuses on uPAR PET as a new diagnostic and prognostic imaging biomarker in PC. Many preclinical uPAR-targeted PET imaging studies using AE105 in cancer models have been undertaken with promising results. A major breakthrough was obtained with the recent human translation of uPAR PET in using ^{64}Cu- and ^{68}Ga-labelled versions of AE105, respectively. Clinical results from patients with PC included in these studies are encouraging and support continuation with large-scale clinical trials.

PET/Computed Tomography for Radiation Therapy Planning of Prostate Cancer **257**

Kalevi J.A. Kairemo

This article is a short review of PET tracers, which have been used in clinical routine in single institutions. Preliminary anecdotal research supports the use of PET techniques in therapy planning of prostate cancer. The existing literature is discussed. For external beam radiation therapy, the biological target volume definition can only be based on PET imaging. There are not yet any prospective and randomized trials available; therefore, single-institution experiences cannot yet be recommended as clinical routine.

PET CLINICS

FORTHCOMING ISSUES

July 2017
Novel PET Radiotracers with Potential Clinical Applications
Neil Vasdev and Abass Alavi, *Editors*

October 2017
Molecular Imaging and Precision Medicine, Part II
Rathan M. Subramaniam, *Editor*

January 2018
Lung Cancer
Gang Cheng and Timothy Akhurst, *Editors*

RECENT ISSUES

January 2017
Molecular Imaging and Precision Medicine, Part 1
Rathan M. Subramaniam, *Editor*

October 2016
PET/MRI: Clinical Applications
Drew A. Torigian, Andreas Kjær, Habib Zaidi, and Abass Alavi, *Editors*

July 2016
PET-Based Molecular Imaging in Evolving Personalized Management Design
Sandip Basu and Abass Alavi, *Editors*

RELATED INTEREST

Magnetic Resonance Imaging Clinics of North America,
February 2016 (Vol. 24, Issue 1)
Functional and Molecular Imaging in Oncology
Antonio Luna, *Editor*
Available at: http://www.mri.theclinics.com/

PROGRAM OBJECTIVE

The goal of the *PET Clinics* is to keep practicing radiologists and radiology residents up to date with current clinical practice in positron emission tomography by providing timely articles reviewing the state of the art in patient care.

TARGET AUDIENCE

Practicing radiologists, radiology residents, and other health care professionals who provide patient care utilizing radiologic findings.

LEARNING OBJECTIVES

Upon completion of this activity, participants will be able to:

1. Review clinical applications of molecular imaging in prostate cancer.
2. Discuss various methods of prostate cancer imaging and therapy.
3. Recognize the use of PET/CT scanning in the treatment of prostate cancer.

ACCREDITATION

The Elsevier Office of Continuing Medical Education (EOCME) is accredited by the Accreditation Council for Continuing Medical Education (ACCME) to provide continuing medical education for physicians.

The EOCME designates this enduring material for a maximum of 15 *AMA PRA Category 1 Credit*(s)™. Physicians should claim only the credit commensurate with the extent of their participation in the activity.

All other health care professionals requesting continuing education credit for this enduring material will be issued a certificate of participation.

DISCLOSURE OF CONFLICTS OF INTEREST

The EOCME assesses conflict of interest with its instructors, faculty, planners, and other individuals who are in a position to control the content of CME activities. All relevant conflicts of interest that are identified are thoroughly vetted by EOCME for fair balance, scientific objectivity, and patient care recommendations. EOCME is committed to providing its learners with CME activities that promote improvements or quality in healthcare and not a specific proprietary business or a commercial interest.

The planning committee, staff, authors and editors listed below have identified no financial relationships or relationships to products or devices they or their spouse/life partner have with commercial interest related to the content of this CME activity:
Abass Alavi, MD, MD (Hon), PhD (Hon), DSc (Hon); Lucia Baratto, MD; Richard P. Baum, MD, PhD; Paolo Castellucci, MD; Francesco Ceci, MD; Alexander Drzezga, MD; Stefano Fanti, MD; Anjali Fortna; Marina Hodolič, MD, PhD; Michael S. Hofman, MBBS, FRACP, FAANMS; Amir Iravani, MD, FRACP; Kalevi J.A. Kairemo, MD, PhD, MSc (Eng); Harshad R. Kulkarni, MD; Cristina Nanni, MD; Steven P. Rowe, MD, PhD; Roberto A. Salas Fragomeni, MD; Aviral Singh, MD, MSc; Ida Sonni, MD; John Vassallo; Rajakumar Venkatesan; Katie Widmeier; Amy Williams.

The planning committee, staff, authors and editors listed below have identified financial relationships or relationships to products or devices they or their spouse/life partner have with commercial interest related to the content of this CME activity:
Samuel R. Denmeade, MD is a consultant/advisor for Medicenna Therapeutics, Inc, and Sophiris Bio, Corp.
Michael A. Gorin, MD is a consultant/advisor for Progenics Pharmaceuticals, Inc.
Andrei Iagaru, MD, FACNM has research support form General Electric; Bayer AG; and Piramal Imaging, a division of the Piramal Group.
Andreas Kjaer, MD, PhD, DMSc has stock ownership in Curasight.
Theodosia Maina, PhD has research support from, and she and her spouse receive royalties/patents from, Advanced Accelerator Applications.
Berthold A. Nock, PhD has research support from, and he and his spouse receive royalties/patents from, Advanced Accelerator Applications.
Morten Persson, MSc, PhD has stock ownership in Curasight.
Martin G. Pomper, MD, PhD receives royalties/patents from Progenics Pharmaceuticals, Inc.
Bital Savir-Baruch, MD grant support by Blue Earth Diagnostics Limited.
David M. Schuster, MD has research support from Blue Earth Diagnostics Limited and Nihon Medi-Physics Co., Ltd, and is on the speakers' bureau for PETNET Solutions Inc, a subsidiary of Siemens Medical Solutions USA, Inc.
Dorthe Skovgaard, MD, PhD has research support from Curasight.
Lucia Zanoni, MD has research support from The Bologna University Hospital Authority St. Orsola-Malpighi.

UNAPPROVED/OFF-LABEL USE DISCLOSURE

The EOCME requires CME faculty to disclose to the participants:

1. When products or procedures being discussed are off-label, unlabelled, experimental, and/or investigational (not US Food and Drug Administration [FDA] approved); and
2. Any limitations on the information presented, such as data that are preliminary or that represent ongoing research, interim analyses, and/or unsupported opinions. Faculty may discuss information about pharmaceutical agents that is outside of

FDA-approved labelling. This information is intended solely for CME and is not intended to promote off-label use of these medications. If you have any questions, contact the medical affairs department of the manufacturer for the most recent prescribing information.

TO ENROLL

To enroll in the PET Clinics Continuing Medical Education program, call customer service at 1-800-654-2452 or sign up online at http://www.theclinics.com/home/cme. The CME program is available to subscribers for an additional annual fee of USD $235.

METHOD OF PARTICIPATION

In order to claim credit, participants must complete the following:

1. Complete enrolment as indicated above.
2. Read the activity.
3. Complete the CME Test and Evaluation. Participants must achieve a score of 70% on the test. All CME Tests and Evaluations must be completed online.

CME INQUIRIES/SPECIAL NEEDS

For all CME inquiries or special needs, please contact elsevierCME@elsevier.com.

Preface
Prostate Cancer Imaging in the Era of Molecular Medicine

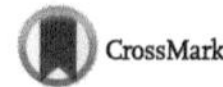

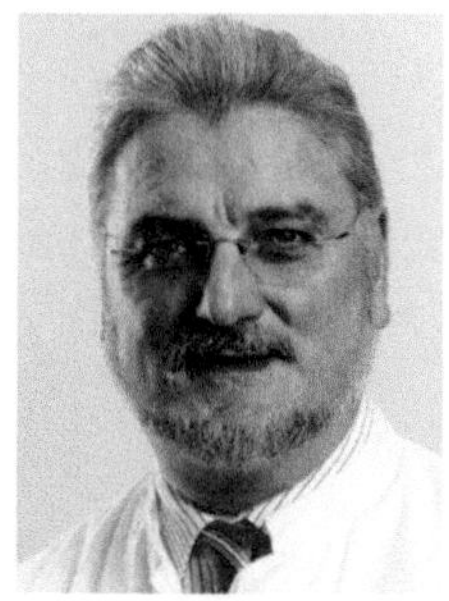

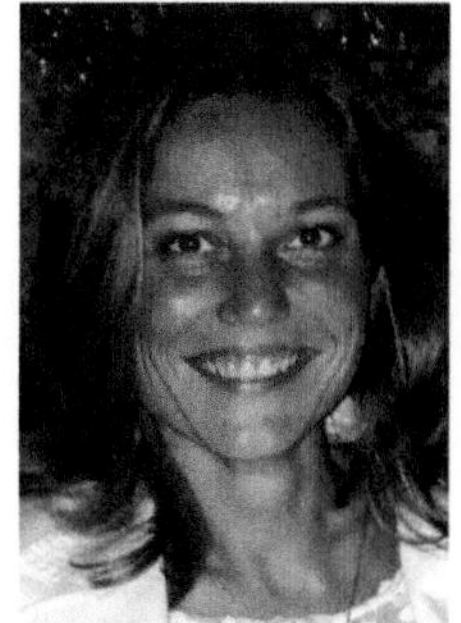

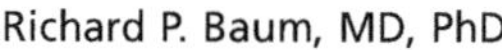

Richard P. Baum, MD, PhD

Cristina Nanni, MD

Editors

Prostate-specific antigen (PSA) is currently the most widely used biomarker of prostate cancer (PCa). PSA suggests the presence of primary tumor and disease relapse after treatment, but it is not able to provide information on the site of disease. To that aim, molecular and functional imaging is a reliable tool for primary tumor detection and disease extension assessment, in both staging and restaging. ^{11}C and ^{18}F-Choline PET/CT are well established procedures that are currently used especially for restaging after radical treatment. However, those procedures are known to provide an insufficient detection rate in the case of low PSA values. That's why new compounds have been tested clinically, and some of them recently found a routine application in the workup of patients with PCa. Ga-PSMA, for example, is a tracer targeting a type II transmembrane protein with an extensive extracellular domain, a transmembrane segment, and an intracellular domain that is overexpressed in PCa, including androgen-independent, advanced, and metastatic disease. ^{68}Ga-PSMA PET/CT was proved to have a higher positivity rate as compared with Choline in the case of PCa relapse with low PSA values. Furthermore, by substituting the imaging isotope (Gallium) with a therapeutic one (such as Lutetium-177), it is possible to conjugate a molecular-targeted therapy that was proved to be effective in preliminary cases. Better results as compared with Choline were obtained also with ^{18}F-FACBC, a recently FDA-approved synthetic amino acid analogue PET radiotracer for the evaluation of recurrent PCa. ^{18}F-FACBC has a more favorable distribution (low background) and provides a higher target-to-background signal as well as a higher specificity.

Other promising PET tracers are currently under evaluation. To this group belong to this group of compounds, ^{68}Ga-PSMA-labeled Bombesin, ^{64}Cu-PSMA, ^{18}F-labeled small molecular inhibitors of PSMA, and the uPAR-PET: future research will define the role and value of those compounds in the clinical management of patients with PCa.

Richard P. Baum, MD, PhD
THERANOSTICS Center for Molecular Radiotherapy
and Molecular Imaging (PET/CT)
ENETS Center of Excellence
Zentralklinik Bad Berka
Robert-Koch-Allee 9
99437 Bad Berka, Germany

Cristina Nanni, MD
Nuclear Medicine Unit, Building 30
AOU di Bologna
Policlinico S.Orsola-Malpighi
Via Massarenti 9
40138 Bologna, Italy

E-mail addresses:
richard.baum@zentralklinik.de (R.P. Baum)
cristina.nanni@aosp.bo.it (C. Nanni)

PET Clin 12 (2017) xi
http://dx.doi.org/10.1016/j.cpet.2017.01.001
1556-8598/17/© 2017 Published by Elsevier Inc.

Imaging of Prostate Cancer Using ^{11}C-Choline PET/Computed Tomography

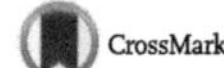

Paolo Castellucci, MD, Francesco Ceci, MD*, Stefano Fanti, MD

KEYWORDS

• Prostate cancer • Choline PET/CT • Diagnosis • Staging

KEY POINTS

- ^{11}C-Choline PET/CT has a limited role in the diagnosis of prostate cancer, whereas for nodal staging, choline PET/CT showed low sensitivity but a high specificity.
- The main application of this imaging procedure is the restaging of the disease in case of biochemical recurrence.
- ^{11}C-Choline-PET/CT proved its value for metastases-directed salvage therapies and for monitoring therapy response in castration-resistant patients.
- PSA and PSA kinetics values confirmed their correlation with ^{11}C-choline PET/CT sensitivity.

INTRODUCTION

Prostate cancer (PCa) is the most common solid cancer in men.[1] The evidence of PCa is generally assessed by digital rectal examination, serum levels of prostate-specific antigen (PSA), and transrectal ultrasound.[1] Many different imaging procedures, such as transrectal ultrasound, MR imaging, computerized tomography (CT), and bone scintigraphy, are used for local staging (to evaluate the tumor extension) and to assess the presence of distant metastasis.[1] Although primary treatment with radical intent (radical prostatectomy associated with lymph node dissection or radiation therapy) is associated with excellent oncologic results, many patients experience relapse after primary treatment.

This article reviews the role of ^{11}C-choline PET/CT in patients with PCa for staging and restaging the disease in case of biochemical recurrence (BCR) after primary treatment and for therapy monitoring in patients with castration-resistant PCa (CRPC) treated with systemic therapy.

^{11}C-CHOLINE PET/COMPUTED TOMOGRAPHY IN PROSTATE CANCER DIAGNOSIS

Multiparametric MR imaging represents the standard of reference for the detection of intraprostatic cancer.[2] The role of ^{11}C-choline PET/CT for the initial diagnosis of PCa has been extensively evaluated over the last decade. The first study performed on a sextant-basis in comparison with histology was by Farsad and colleagues.[3] The authors investigated 36 patients scheduled for surgery. ^{11}C-Choline PET/CT showed a sensitivity of 66%, a specificity of 81%, an accuracy of 71%, a positive predictive value (PPV) of 87%, and a low negative predictive value of 55%. In the following years other authors confirmed these findings.[4–6] Other results confirming the lack of accuracy for ^{11}C-choline PET/CT in this field were recently published. Bundschuh and colleagues[7] correlated the uptake of ^{11}C-choline PET/CT in the prostate gland with histopathology. The assessed sensitivity was poor because only 46% of lesions evaluated by histology showed an

The authors have nothing to disclose.

Service of Nuclear Medicine, S. Orsola-Malpighi University Hospital, University of Bologna, Bologna, Italy
* Corresponding author: UO Medicina Nucleare PAD. 30, Azienda Ospedaliero-Universitaria di Bologna, Policlinico S. Orsola-Malpighi, Via Massarenti 9, Bologna 40138, Italy.
E-mail address: francesco.ceci@studio.unibo.it

PET Clin 12 (2017) 137–143
http://dx.doi.org/10.1016/j.cpet.2016.11.002

increased choline uptake. In a study proposed by Grosu and colleagues,[8] ^{11}C-choline-increased uptake has been found in neoplastic and nonneoplastic tissue. Moreover in some cases the intensity of the uptake was even higher in nonneoplastic tissue. Van den Bergh and colleagues[9] compared ^{11}C-choline PET/CT and MR imaging, showing that sensitivity increased, but specificity decreased combining both modalities. In conclusion, the suboptimal sensitivity of ^{11}C-choline PET/CT is mainly caused by the presence of small foci of cancer, whereas the suboptimal specificity is mainly caused by the frequent presence of nonneoplastic conditions within the prostate gland that may show increased choline uptake, such as benign prostatic hyperplasia or prostatitis.

PET/COMPUTED TOMOGRAPHY IN PROSTATE CANCER STAGING

Over the last decade many authors have evaluated the role of ^{11}C-choline PET/CT for lymph nodal or bone staging before primary treatment. The detection of nodal or distant metastases assessed by ^{11}C-choline PET/CT should help clinicians provide patients a tailored treatment strategy.[1] Schiavina and colleagues[10] showed that ^{11}C-choline PET/CT has low sensitivity (60%) but high specificity (98%) in a population of 57 with intermediate and high risk PCa. Contractor and colleagues[11] showed a sensitivity of 40% and a specificity of 98% in nodal staging using ^{11}C-choline PET/CT before surgery in 28 patients with PCa. Van Den Bergh and colleagues[12] prospectively used ^{11}C-choline PET/CT and diffusion weighted (DW)-MR imaging for nodal staging in patients with high risk for nodal involvement. Seventy-five patients N0 at CT were enrolled. A total of 37 of 75 patients (49%) were positive at histology. On a patient-based analysis ^{11}C-choline PET/CT showed a sensitivity of 18.9% and a PPV of 63.6%, whereas DW-MR imaging showed a sensitivity of 36.1% and a PPV of 86.7%. On a region-based analysis, ^{11}C-choline PET/CT showed a sensitivity of 8.2% and a PPV of 50.0%, whereas DW-MR imaging showed a sensitivity of 9.5% and a PPV of 40.0%. The poor results obtained by both these imaging modalities should remind clinicians that even in patients at high risk for positive lymph nodes at presentation and even in highly selected patient populations, poor sensitivity and poor PPV may occur either on a patient or lymph node based analysis. Finally, Evangelista and colleagues[13] evaluated by a systematic review the role of ^{18}F or ^{11}C-choline PET/CT for staging PCa. Most of the papers analyzed confirmed preliminary findings showing a lack of sensitivity but high specificity for nodal staging. Pooled sensitivity and specificity were, respectively, 49% and 95% on a patient basis. ^{11}C-Choline PET/CT low sensitivity could be explained by the presence of micrometastasis and thus by the size of nodal metastatic deposit, because it is unlikely that ^{11}C-choline PET/CT may detect lesions smaller than 5 mm. On the contrary, the main reason for false-positive findings is the presence of reactive lymph nodes that may show increased choline uptake.

In conclusion, the use of ^{11}C-choline PET/CT for lymph nodal staging should be reserved to high-risk and very-high-risk patients (according to the most accepted nomograms) to reduce the incidence of false-negative scans and to optimize the number of positive ^{11}C-choline PET/CT.

PET/COMPUTED TOMOGRAPHY IN PROSTATE CANCER RESTAGING

BCR after radical treatment is a frequent event, involving up to 50% of patients treated.[14] The role of any imaging procedure is to differentiate between the presence of a local and/or distant relapse.[14] Imaging should select patients with single or oligometastatic disease (potentially treatable with salvage treatments) from patients affected by metastatic disease treatable with systemic therapies. In the last years ^{11}C-cholinePET/CT demonstrated a significant clinical impact on patient management. In three papers recently published from three different patient series, ^{11}C-choline PET/CT demonstrated a change in the decision-making process in approximately 50% of cases.[15–17]

Prostate-Specific Antigen Values and ^{11}C-Choline PET/Computed Tomography

^{11}C-Choline PET/CT has been widely used in case of BCR. Nevertheless, despite the large number of data available, there is still no consensus about the optimal timing to perform the scan. Recently, the European Association of Urology guidelines[14] suggested the use of choline PET/CT in patients with BCR and PSA levels greater than 1 ng/mL, preferably with PSA values between 1 and 2 ng/mL. At this stage of the disease, differentiating between the presence of single, oligo, or multi metastatic disease would have a major impact on clinical management. In a recent meta-analysis Fanti and colleagues[18] analyzed 29 studies with a total of 2686 patients enrolled. The authors reported for ^{11}C-choline PET/CT a detection rate for any site of relapse of 62% (95% confidence interval, 53%–71%). In a single-institution patient series, analyzing 4426 scans in 3203 patients with BCR,

Graziani and colleagues[19] assessed overall sensitivity for ^{11}C-choline PET/CT of 52.8%. It is interesting to point out that in 995 scans that were performed in patients with PSA levels between 1 and 2 ng/mL the sensitivity for ^{11}C-choline PET/CT was not as low (44.7%) if compared with the sensitivity assessed in the whole population. In the receiver operating characteristic curve analysis, PSA value of 1.16 ng/mL was the optimal cutoff value able to predict a positive scan.

Sites of Relapse and Choline PET

MR imaging is the standard of reference for the detection of prostate bed recurrence.[20] ^{11}C-Choline PET/CT showed low sensitivity in the detection of local relapse in comparison with MR imaging.[20–22] The assessed sensitivity for local recurrence (either using ^{18}F or ^{11}C-choline PET/CT)[20–22] was 50% to 60%. Kitajima and colleagues[23] confirmed these data in a population of 115 patients showing a sensitivity, specificity, and accuracy of 54%, 92%, and 65% for ^{11}C-choline PET/CT in the detection of local relapse, in comparison with a sensitivity, specificity, and accuracy of 88%, 84%, and 87% showed by MR imaging. However, in the same study, the authors showed a better accuracy for ^{11}C-choline PET/CT compared with MR imaging (92% vs 70%) in pelvic lymph node metastasis detection, regardless of PSA values.[23] The performance of ^{11}C-choline PET/CT in the detection of bone lesions has been compared with bone scan by Picchio and colleagues[24] in 78 patients with BCR. The authors showed lower sensitivity values for ^{11}C-choline PET/CT compared with bone scan (89% vs 100%), but a significant higher specificity (98% vs 75%). Fuccio and colleagues[25] showed the presence of multiple sites of relapse at ^{11}C-choline PET/CT in almost half of the 25 patients who showed only one single lesion at bone scan. The authors confirmed the high sensitivity and the high specificity for ^{11}C-choline PET/CT (86% and 100%, respectively) in the detection of bone metastatic lesions. Choline uptake in bone lesions changes and may vary in the different type of bone lesions. Ceci and colleagues[26] analyzed 304 bone lesions (184 osteoblastic, 99 osteolytic, and 21 bone marrow lesions) in a cohort of 140 patients with PCa with BCR. They demonstrated a significant difference for SUVmax values between osteoblastic (lower values) and osteolytic (higher values) lesions.

Salvage Therapies and Choline PET

One of the most promising applications for PET/CT imaging is to select and differentiate those patients who can benefit from tailored PET-guided treatment from patients who should be addressed by systemic therapies. However, before performing aggressive treatment, such as metastasis-directed salvage radiation therapy (S-RT) or salvage lymph node dissection (S-LND), all efforts should made to exclude the presence of metastasis already present at the time of salvage treatments and not included in the planned target volume or that could not be removed by an S-LND. In this regard, Castellucci and colleagues[27] studied with ^{11}C-choline PET/CT a cohort 605 recurrent patients showing low PSA values (PSA range, 0.2–2 ng/mL) after radical prostatectomy (RP) and listed for S-RT in the prostatic bed. ^{11}C-Choline PET/CT detected a disease limited to the pelvis in 13.7% of patients, whereas the presence of an extrapelvic disease was observed in 14.7%. The authors observed that ^{11}C-choline PET/CT detection rate increased dramatically in patients with fast PSA doubling time (^{11}C-choline PET/CT detection rate 47% with PSA doubling time <6 months). The authors concluded that ^{11}C-choline PET/CT should be performed before salvage therapies especially in those patients showing fast PSA kinetics to exclude the presence of distant lesions that could not be removed with SLND or included in the planned target volume.

The first prospective study aimed to assess the role of ^{11}C-choline PET/CT in guiding aggressive treatments has been published by Rigatti and colleagues.[28] The authors studied a cohort of 79 patients showing BCR after RP. Patients who showed no more than two positive lymph nodes on ^{11}C-choline PET/CT received S-PLND. Biochemical relapse-free survival rates at 3 years of 27.5% and at 5 years of 10.3% were reported. Five-year clinical recurrence-free survival was lower for patients with positive retroperitoneal lymph nodes at ^{11}C-choline PET/CT versus patients with only pelvic ^{11}C-choline PET/CT-positive nodes (11% vs 53%; $P < .001$). Karnes and colleagues[29] enrolled a group of 52 patients treated with S-LND according to ^{11}C-choline PET/CT results. After a median follow-up of 20 months, 30 out of 52 patients (57.7%) were biochemical relapse-free and 50 of 52 patients (96.2%) were alive. Suardi and colleagues[30] studied 56 patients and demonstrated clinical relapse-free and cancer-specific mortality-free survival rates at 8 years of 38% and 81%, respectively. Multivariate analysis showed that PSA higher than 2 ng/mL at the time of ^{11}C-choline PET/CT and the presence of retroperitoneal positive lymph nodes on ^{11}C-choline PET/CT were predictors of clinical relapse. PET/CT-guided S-RT can be performed in patients showing single or oligometastatic disease.[31,32] Würschmidt and colleagues[33]

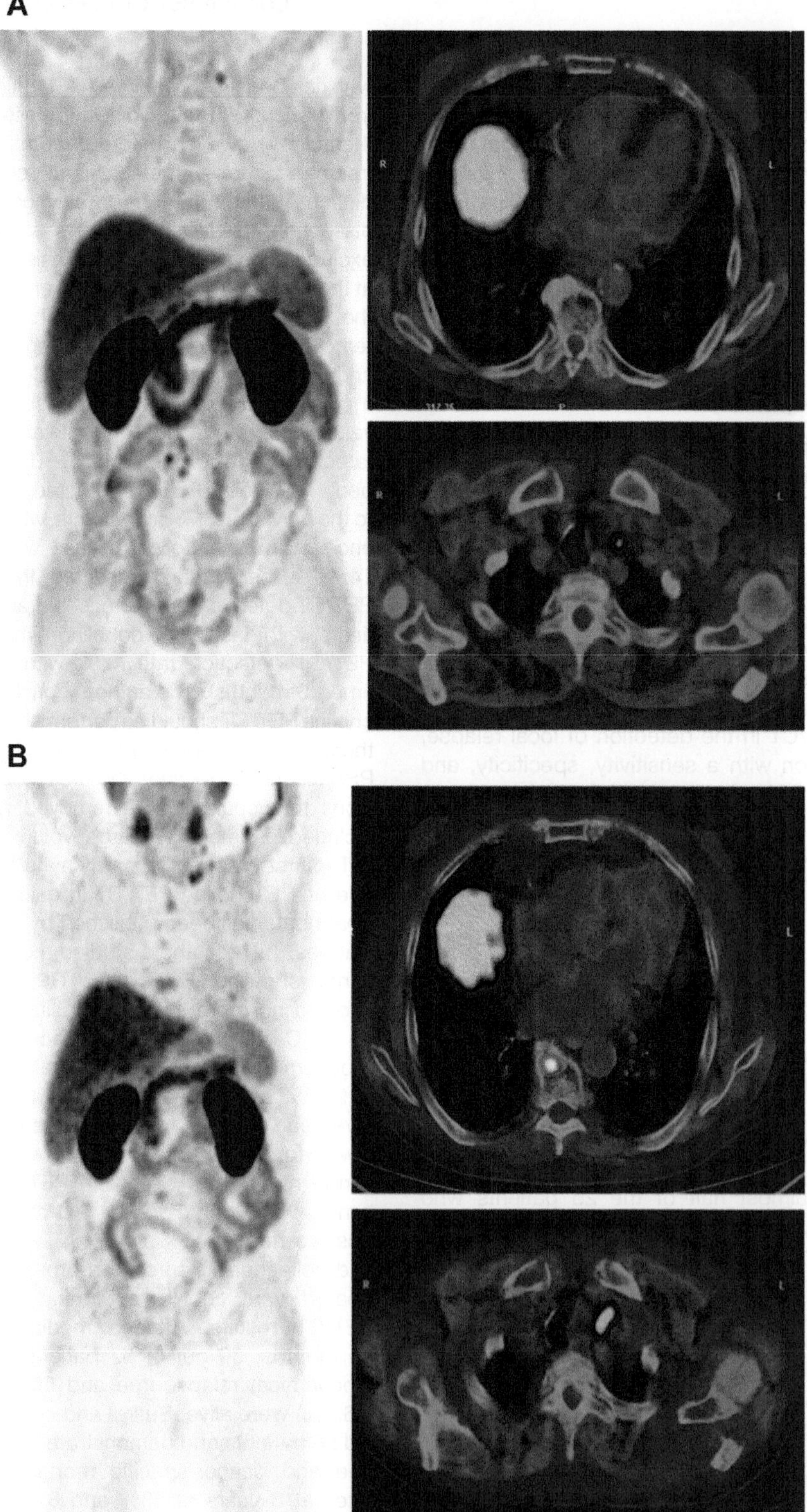

Fig. 1. A 64-year-old man (Gleason score 4 + 4; T3N1Mx; presentation PSA, 9 ng/mL) treated with radical prostatectomy and pelvic lymph node dissection as primary treatment. BCR occurred 20 months after surgery. Patient was subsequently treated continuously with androgen-deprivation therapy for 27 months with good PSA response, once showed resistance to androgen-deprivation therapy. (*A*) With increasing PSA levels (PSA, 8.73 ng/mL) ^{11}C-choline PET/CT has been performed assessing the presence of multiple sites of disease. The patient was addressed with abiraterone acetate + prednisone. The PSA levels decreased up to 5.35 ng/mL after 4 months of treatment and the patient was referred to a further ^{11}C-choline PET/CT to restage the disease. (*B*) ^{11}C-Choline PET/CT demonstrated progression of the disease with the appearance of new active lesions. Progression of the disease was confirmed with clinical follow-up.

performed ^{11}C-choline PET/CT-guided S-RT in 19 patients showing BCR. Almost half of the patients were biochemical relapse-free after 28 months of follow-up. Picchio and colleagues[34] used ^{11}C-choline PET/CT to guide helical tomotherapy in 83 patients showing lymph node relapse after primary treatment. The authors achieved an early biochemical response in 70% of cases. The same research group published a study[35] in which 68 patients showing ^{11}C-choline PET/CT-positive lymph nodes were enrolled. After PET-guided helical tomotherapy 2-year overall survival, locoregional relapse-free survival, clinical relapse-free survival, and biochemical-free survival were 87%, 91%, 51%, and 40%, respectively.

Early detection of the site relapse in patients with PCa with BCR is crucial, because it leads to a more favorable patient outcome. The detection of oligometastatic disease on ^{11}C-choline PET/CT gives clinicians the chance to plan a dedicated and personalized treatment strategy.

PET/COMPUTED TOMOGRAPHY IN CASTRATION-RESISTANT PROSTATE CANCER

CRPC is a frequent condition in advanced disease and is related to a high mortality rate, with an overall survival of 2 to 3 years. In this condition, palliation is the goal of treatment.[14] Many different therapies can be used, such as docetaxel and cabazitaxel, or new novel androgen receptor targeted therapies, such as abiraterone and enzalutamide.[14] The assessment of PSA levels over time is routinely used to evaluate therapy response and outcome prediction. However, this is not a reliable marker because it can be impaired by flare phenomena, tumor cells heterogeneity, and active visceral metastases not producing PSA. Conventional imaging methods, including CT, MR imaging, and bone scan, are late indicators of treatment efficacy, whereas PET/CT has the potential to identify the response to therapy early. The evaluation of changes provided by PET/CT, rather than morphologic changes during therapy, may be an early and reliable alternative to other indicators of treatment benefit, such as radiologic progression-free survival and PSA.

In a few preliminary studies[9,10] the role of choline-PET/CT was investigated. De Giorgi and colleagues[36] used ^{18}F-choline PET/CT for evaluating the early response to treatment with abiraterone in 43 patients with metastatic CRPC (mCRPC). The authors confirmed that the response assessed with ^{18}F-choline PET/CT was associated with a more favorable overall survival than a PSA response of greater than or equal to 50%. Maines and colleagues[37] confirmed these data in 30 patients with mCRPC treated with enzalutamide. The authors observed that SUVmax values measured at ^{18}F-choline PET/CT performed before enzalutamide were significantly related with biochemical, radiologic, and overall survival. Ceci and colleagues[38] studied a cohort of 61 patients with mCRPC with ^{11}C-choline PET/CT performed before and after treatment with docetaxel. A comparison between the response to docetaxel assessed by ^{11}C-choline PET/CT and the PSA response has been performed. ^{11}C-Choline PET/CT showed progression of the disease in the 44% of patients who showed a PSA response after docetaxel. The tumor burden, expressed as more than 10 PET-positive bone lesions measured before docetaxel, was also significantly associated with an increased probability of progression after treatment.

Prospective future trials should better investigate this potential application of choline PET/CT. It could be interesting to assess if PET/CT imaging could identify progression versus nonprogression of the disease earlier and more accurately than PSA and conventional imaging (**Fig. 1**). In particular, the more relevant clinical contribution of PET/CT will occur when decreasing PSA is associated with radiologic progression. The availability of a procedure to accurately and early assess the response to systemic therapies will have an important impact on CRPC management. It could lead to a more tailored therapy, especially for those patients presenting with decreasing PSA levels during treatment, whereas imaging could show progression. These patients could switch to a second line of chemotherapy and/or new antiandorgen therapies and radiotherapy on the not-responding lesions or ^{223}radium. As a consequence, besides an improvement in life expectancy, the collateral effects/toxicity and costs of futile therapy will be reduced.

REFERENCES

1. Heidenreich A, Bastian PJ, Bellmunt J, et al. EAU guidelines on prostate cancer. Part 1: screening, diagnosis, and local treatment with curative intent-update 2013. Eur Urol 2014;65(1):124–37.
2. Metzger GJ, Kalavagunta C, Spilseth B, et al. Detection of prostate cancer: quantitative multiparametric MR imaging models developed using registered correlative histopathology. Radiology 2016;279(3):805–16.
3. Farsad M, Schiavina R, Castellucci P, et al. Detection and localization of prostate cancer: correlation of (11)C-choline PET/CT with histopathologic step-section analysis. J Nucl Med 2005;46:1642–9.

4. Giovacchini G, Picchio M, Coradeschi E, et al. [(11) C]Choline uptake with PET/CT for the initial diagnosis of prostate cancer: relation to PSA levels, tumour stage and anti-androgenic therapy. Eur J Nucl Med Mol Imaging 2008;35:1065–73.
5. Martorana G, Schiavina R, Corti B, et al. 11C-Choline positron emission tomography/computerized tomography for tumor localization of primary prostate cancer in comparison with 12-core biopsy. J Urol 2006;176:954–60.
6. Testa C, Schiavina R, Lodi R, et al. Prostate cancer: sextant localization with MR imaging, MR spectroscopy, and 11C-choline PET/CT. Radiology 2007; 244(3):797–806.
7. Bundschuh RA, Wendl CM, Weirich G, et al. Tumour volume delineation in prostate cancer assessed by [11C]choline PET/CT: validation with surgical specimens. Eur J Nucl Med Mol Imaging 2013;40:824–31.
8. Grosu AL, Weirich G, Wendl C, et al. 11C-Choline PET/pathology image coregistration in primary localized prostate cancer. Eur J Nucl Med Mol Imaging 2014;41:2242–8.
9. Van den Bergh L, Koole M, Isebaert S, et al. Is there an additional value of (11)C choline PET-CT to T2-weighted MRI images in the localization of intraprostatic tumor nodules? Int J Radiat Oncol Biol Phys 2012;83:1486–92.
10. Schiavina R, Scattoni V, Castellucci P, et al. 11C-Choline positron emission tomography/computerized tomography for preoperative lymph-node staging in intermediate-risk and high-risk prostate cancer: comparison with clinical staging nomograms. Eur Urol 2008;54:392–401.
11. Contractor K, Challapalli A, Barwick T, et al. Use of [11C]choline PET-CT as a noninvasive method for detecting pelvic lymph node status from prostate cancer and relationship with choline kinase expression. Clin Cancer Res 2011;17:7673–83.
12. Van den Bergh L, Lerut E, Haustermans K, et al. Final analysis of a prospective trial on functional imaging for nodal staging in patients with prostate cancer at high risk for lymph node involvement. Urol Oncol 2015;33(3):109.e23-31.
13. Evangelista L, Guttilla A, Zattoni F, et al. Utility of choline positron emission tomography/computed tomography for lymph node involvement identification in intermediate- to high-risk prostate cancer: a systematic literature review and metaanalysis. Eur Urol 2013;63:1040–8.
14. Heidenreich A, Bastian PJ, Bellmunt J, et al. EAU guidelines on prostate cancer. Part II: treatment of advanced, relapsing, and castration-resistant prostate cancer. European Association of Urology. Eur Urol 2014;65(2):467–79.
15. Ceci F, Herrmann K, Castellucci P, et al. Impact of 11C-choline PET/CT on clinical decision making in recurrent prostate cancer: results from a retrospective two-centre trial. Eur J Nucl Med Mol Imaging 2014;41(12):2222–31 [Erratum in Eur J Nucl Med Mol Imaging 2014;41(12):2359].
16. Soyka JD, Muster MA, Schmid DT, et al. Clinical impact of 18F-choline PET/CT in patients with recurrent prostate cancer. Eur J Nucl Med Mol Imaging 2012;39(6):936–43.
17. Goldstein J, Even-Sapir E, Ben-Haim S, et al. Does choline PET/CT change the management of prostate cancer patients with biochemical failure? Am J Clin Oncol 2014. [Epub ahead of print].
18. Fanti S, Minozzi S, Castellucci P, et al. PET/CT with (11)C-choline for evaluation of prostate cancer patients with biochemical recurrence: meta-analysis and critical review of available data. Eur J Nucl Med Mol Imaging 2016;43(1):55–69.
19. Graziani T, Ceci F, Castellucci P, et al. (11)C-Choline PET/CT for restaging prostate cancer. Results from 4,426 scans in a single-centre patient series. Eur J Nucl Med Mol Imaging 2016;43(11):1971–9.
20. Panebianco V, Sciarra A, Lisi D, et al. Prostate cancer: 1HMRS-DCEMR at 3T versus [(18)F]choline PET/CT in the detection of local prostate cancer recurrence in men with biochemical progression after radical retropubic prostatectomy (RRP). Eur J Radiol 2012;81(4):700–8.
21. Castellucci P, Fuccio C, Rubello D, et al. Is there a role for ^{11}C-choline PET/CT in the early detection of metastatic disease in surgically treated prostate cancer patients with a mild PSA increase of 1.5 ng/ml? Eur J Nucl Med Mol Imaging 2011;38(1): 55–63.
22. Mamede M, Ceci F, Castellucci P, et al. The role of 11C-choline PET imaging in the early detection of recurrence in surgically treated prostate cancer patients with very low PSA level <0.5 ng/mL. Clin Nucl Med 2013;38(9):e342–5.
23. Kitajima K, Murphy RC, Nathan MA, et al. Detection of recurrent prostate cancer after radical prostatectomy: comparison of 11C-choline PET/CT with pelvic multiparametric MR imaging with endorectal coil. J Nucl Med 2014;55(2):223–32.
24. Picchio M, Spinapolice EG, Fallanca F, et al. [11C] Choline PET/CT detection of bone metastases in patients with PSA progression after primary treatment for prostate cancer: comparison with bone scintigraphy. Eur J Nucl Med Mol Imaging 2012 Jan; 39(1):13–26.
25. Fuccio C, Castellucci P, Schiavina R, et al. Role of 11C-choline PET/CT in the re-staging of prostate cancer patients with biochemical relapse and negative results at bone scintigraphy. Eur J Radiol 2012; 81(8):e893–6.
26. Ceci F, Castellucci P, Graziani T, et al. 11C-Choline PET/CT identifies osteoblastic and osteolytic lesions in patients with metastatic prostate cancer. Clin Nucl Med 2015;40(5):e265–70.

27. Castellucci P, Ceci F, Graziani T, et al. Early biochemical relapse after radical prostatectomy: which prostate cancer patients may benefit from a restaging 11C-choline PET/CT scan before salvage radiation therapy? J Nucl Med 2014;55(9):1424–9.
28. Rigatti P, Suardi N, Briganti A, et al. Pelvic/retroperitoneal salvage lymph node dissection for patients treated with radical prostatectomy with biochemical recurrence and nodal recurrence detected by [11C] choline positron emission tomography/computed tomography. Eur Urol 2011;60(5):935–43.
29. Karnes RJ, Murphy CR, Bergstralh EJ, et al. Salvage lymph node dissection for prostate cancer nodal recurrence detected by 11C-choline positron emission tomography/computerized tomography. J Urol 2015;193(1):111–6.
30. Suardi N, Gandaglia G, Gallina A, et al. Long-term outcomes of salvage lymph node dissection for clinically recurrent prostate cancer: results of a single-institution series with a minimum follow-up of 5 years. Eur Urol 2015;67(2):299–309.
31. Bolla M, Van Tienhoven G, Warde P, et al. External irradiation with or without long-term androgen suppression for prostate cancer with high metastatic risk: 10-year results of an EORTC randomised study. Lancet Oncol 2010;11:1066–73.
32. Stephenson AJ, Bolla M, Briganti A, et al. Postoperative radiation therapy for pathologically advanced prostate cancer after radical prostatectomy. Eur Urol 2012;61(3):443–51.
33. Wurschmidt F, Petersen C, Wahl A, et al. [18F]Fluoroethylcholine-PET/CT imaging for radiation treatment planning of recurrent and primary prostate cancer with dose escalation to PET/CT-positive lymph nodes. Radiat Oncol 2011;6:44.
34. Picchio M, Berardi G, Fodor A, et al. 11C-Choline PET/CT as a guide to radiation treatment planning of lymph-node relapses in prostate cancer patients. Eur J Nucl Med Mol Imaging 2014;41(7):1270–9.
35. Incerti E, Fodor A, Mapelli P, et al. Radiation treatment of lymph node recurrence from prostate cancer: is 11C-choline PET/CT predictive of survival outcomes? J Nucl Med 2015;56(12):1836–42.
36. De Giorgi U, Caroli P, Burgio SL, et al. Early outcome prediction on 18F-fluorocholine PET/CT in metastatic castration-resistant prostate cancer patients treated with abiraterone. Oncotarget 2014;5(23):12448–58.
37. Maines F, Caffo O, Donner D, et al. Serial (18)F-choline-PET imaging in patients receiving enzalutamide for metastatic castration-resistant prostate cancer: response assessment and imaging biomarkers. Future Oncol 2016;12(3):333–42.
38. Ceci F, Castellucci P, Graziani T, et al. 11C-Choline PET/CT in castration-resistant prostate cancer patients treated with docetaxel. Eur J Nucl Med Mol Imaging 2016;43(1):84–91.

Imaging of Prostate Cancer Using Fluciclovine

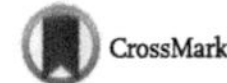

Bital Savir-Baruch, MD[a,*], Lucia Zanoni, MD[b], David M. Schuster, MD[c]

KEYWORDS

• FACBC • Fluciclovine • Axumin • CT • PET • Prostate

KEY POINTS

- Functional molecular imaging with PET improves the ability to detect prostate cancer.
- Fluciclovine is beneficial for the localization of recurrent prostate disease when conventional imaging is negative.
- When interpreted with knowledge of radiotracer biodistribution and normal variants, fluciclovine PET is highly specific for extraprostatic metastasis but has lower specificity for disease within intact or treated prostate.
- Less data are available on the performance of fluciclovine in bone metastases; therefore, skeletal-specific imaging is recommended for suspected bone involvement if fluciclovine PET is unrevealing.

RADIOLABELED AMINO ACIDS AS PET RADIOTRACERS FOR PROSTATE CANCER IMAGING

Amino acids play a central role in cell metabolism and are the building blocks of proteins. Transmembrane amino acid transporters are upregulated in cancer cells to provide nutrients for tumor cell growth.[1,2] Certain amino acids such as leucine and glutamine are key components in the mammalian target of rapamycin cancer signaling pathway.[3] Because this upregulation of amino acid transport also occurs in prostate cancer cells, using an amino acid–based radiotracer can localize prostate cancer as well.[4]

Many amino acid transporter systems are overexpressed in prostate cancer, predominantly large neutral amino acid transporters (systems L: LAT1, LAT3, and LAT4) and alanine-serine-cysteine transporters (systems ASC: ASCT1, ASCT2).[1,3,5–14] Of these transporters, LAT1 and ASCT2 are particularly associated with more aggressive tumor behavior.[7,15–17] Both ASCT2 and LAT3 expression are stimulated by androgen signaling in androgen-dependent prostate cancer cells.[18]

Prostate cancer may be imaged using both radiolabeled natural and synthetic amino acids. Naturally occurring amino acids such as C-11-methionine are not optimal for imaging because

Disclosures: B. Savir-Baruch has participated in sponsored research involving fluciclovine through the Emory University Office of Sponsored Projects (R01CA129356, P50 CA 128301), including funding from Blue Earth Diagnostics, Ltd and Nihon Medi-Physics Co, Ltd, scientific relationship with the company "Blue Earth Diagnostics, Ltd" as principal investigator of a sponsored study BED003 (LOCATE, NCT02680041). No financial relationship. L. Zanoni has a scientific relationship with the company "Blue Earth Diagnostics, Ltd" as Medical Staff of the Sponsored Study BED001 (118/2014/O/Oss). No financial relationship. No compensation received. D. M. Schuster has participated in sponsored research involving fluciclovine through the Emory University Office of Sponsored Projects, including funding from Blue Earth Diagnostics, Ltd and Nihon Medi-Physics Co, Ltd (R01CA129356; P50 CA 128301, R01 CA169188, RO1 CA156755; R21 CA176684-01). Emory University and Dr Mark Goodman are eligible to receive royalties from fluciclovine.

[a] Department of Radiology, Loyola University Medical Center, 2160 South 1st Avenue, Maywood, IL 60153, USA; [b] Department of Nuclear Medicine, Policlinico Sant'Orsola-Malpighi, Azienda Ospedaliero-Universitaria di Bologna, via Massarenti 9, Bologna 40138, Italy; [c] Department of Radiology and Imaging Sciences, Emory University Hospital, Emory University, 1364 Clifton Road, Atlanta, GA 30322, USA

* Corresponding author.

E-mail address: bital.savir-baruch@lumc.edu

PET Clin 12 (2017) 145–157
http://dx.doi.org/10.1016/j.cpet.2016.11.005

pet.theclinics.com

of accumulation of metabolites in nontarget organs, whereas radiolabeled synthetic, nonmetabolized amino acid analogues are preferred due to simpler kinetics and the ability to radiolabel with longer-lived radionuclides.[1]

Anti-1-amino-3-F-18-fluorocyclobutane-1-carboxylic acid (FACBC or fluciclovine) is a nonnaturally occurring amino acid analogue for which the most comprehensive clinical studies for prostate cancer have been performed to date.[10,17,19–26] Fluciclovine is predominantly transported via ASCT2 and LAT1. Because these transporters mediate both influx and efflux of amino acids, peak uptake in tumors occurs at 5 to 20 minutes after injection with variable washout.[17,22,27]

FLUCICLOVINE FROM DEVELOPMENT TO US FOOD AND DRUG ADMINISTRATION APPROVAL

The development of C-11 aminocyclobutane arboxylic acid (ACBC) was first described in 1978 by Washburn and colleagues.[28] ACBC was structurally modified from 1-aminocyclopentanecarboxylic acid. Subsequently, ACBC was radiolabeled with Carbon-11 and found to have potential for imaging soft tissue tumors in humans.[29] However, C-11 has a half-life of 20 minutes, which requires an on-site cyclotron for production. In 1995, Dr Mark Goodman and coworkers described the synthesis of fluorine-18 (half-life 109.8 minutes) labeled anti-1-amino-3-fluorocyclobutane-1-carboxylic acid, 3-FACBC. In 1999, they reported the evaluation of 3-FACBC in gliomas.[30] In 2002, the synthesis of the 3-FACBC labeling precursor and 3-FACBC were improved for routine production for clinical use.[31,32]

Early work suggested that fluciclovine was transported into the cell most like leucine via system L, especially LAT1.[31,33] Subsequent in vitro studies found that the ASC transporter system, specifically ASCT2, plays the largest role in fluciclovine transport, whereas LAT1 transport may become elevated in an acidic tumor environment or with castration-resistant cells.[10,16–18] Thus, it is currently thought that fluciclovine transport more closely mirrors that of glutamine rather than leucine.[34] When compared with methionine, glutamine, choline, and acetate, uptake of fluciclovine in prostate cancer cell lines has also been noted to be higher.[17] Experiments with a rat orthotopic prostate cancer model compared the uptake of fluciclovine with that of fludeoxyglucose (FDG). It was found that target-to-background ratio was higher for fluciclovine with only minimal bladder accumulation.[33]

In human clinical studies, fluciclovine was initially developed for the evaluation of cerebral gliomas.[30] Further evaluation in human dosimetry studies demonstrated physiologic highest tracer uptake by the liver and pancreas, with less intense heterogeneous uptake within the marrow, salivary glands, lymphoid tissue, and pituitary gland, and only minimal brain and kidney uptake. Variable activity was noted in the bowel[27] (**Fig. 1**). When compared with FDG, fluciclovine is only minimally eliminated by the kidneys during the typical imaging time course. Hence, evaluation of fluciclovine for imaging of renal and pelvic malignancies seemed promising.

Fluciclovine was next evaluated for staging of patients with renal cancer. Although no highly promising data from renal mass evaluation were observed, an important incidental finding was reported in a patient with intense uptake within retroperitoneal lymphadenopathy and subsequent biopsy-proven metastatic prostate cancer.[35] Evaluation of fluciclovine for prostate cancer imaging took priority, and in 2007, Schuster and colleagues[22] described the first experience with fluciclovine for the evaluation of 9 patients with primary and 6 patients with recurrent prostate cancer. Early results reported promising correlation between biopsy-proven disease and fluciclovine uptake. Further human studies with fluciclovine, which will be detailed in later discussion, demonstrated the potential to detect local and distant recurrent prostate cancer.

A New Drug Application was subsequently accepted in December 2015 by the US Food and Drug Administration (FDA) as filed by Blue Earth Diagnostics, Ltd for priority review based on data collected from 877 subjects, including 797 patients with prostate cancer in the United States and Europe, and approval was granted to fluciclovine (trade name: Axumin) on May 2016 for the clinical indication of suspected prostate cancer recurrence based on elevated prostate-specific antigen levels following prior treatment.[36]

FLUCICLOVINE IN THE EVALUATION OF PATIENTS WITH SUSPECTED RECURRENCE OF PROSTATE CANCER

Fluciclovine has been most extensively studied in relation to recurrent prostate cancer. Fluciclovine diagnostic performance has been reported to be significantly higher than that of In-111-capromab pendetide and computed tomography (CT) in the diagnosis of patients with suspected disease relapse.[21,24,37] A single-center study with 115

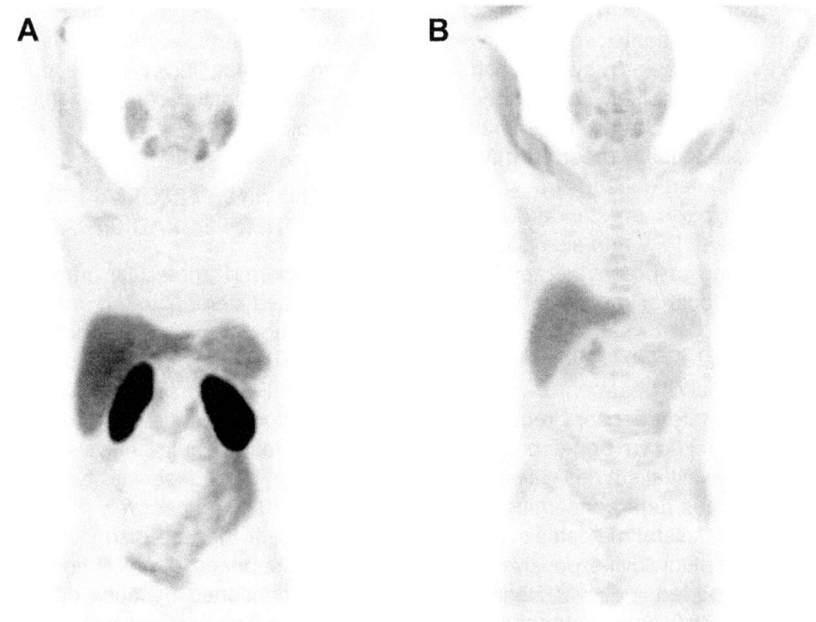

Fig. 1. Comparison of 11C choline and 18F fluciclovine physiologic biodistribution. 18F fluciclovine (*B*, MIP) is physiologically found in pancreas, liver, bone marrow, and muscle, with negligible uptake in kidneys, bowel, and delayed urinary excretion, thus leading to a more favorable distribution in the abdomen and pelvis, compared with 11C choline (*A*, MIP), for evaluating prostate cancer. (*Courtesy of* Dr Cristina Nanni, Programma di ricerca Regione-Università 2010-2012 Regione Emilia Romagna-Bando Giovani Ricercatori, Bologna, Italy.)

patients who underwent definitive treatment of prostate cancer and presented with biochemical failure by the American Urological Association (AUA) and American Society of Radiation Oncology (ASTRO) criteria was completed.[38] In a subset analysis of 93 patients with negative bone scan and In-111-capromab pendetide, single-photon emission computed tomography–computed tomography (SPECT-CT) within 90 days of the fluciclovine PET/CT, overall positive scans (positivity rate) was 82.8%. Biopsy was the primary reference standard. One hundred percent of true positive prostate/prostate bed lesions and 86.4% of true positive extraprostatic lesions were confirmed histologically. For prostate/prostate bed recurrence, fluciclovine had 90.2% sensitivity, 40.0% specificity, 73.6% accuracy, 75.3% positive predictive value (PPV), and 66.7% negative predictive value (NPV); the respective values for In-111-capromab pendetide were 67.2%, 56.7%, 63.7%, 75.9%, and 45.9%. For extraprostatic recurrence, fluciclovine had 55.0% sensitivity, 96.7% specificity, 72.9% accuracy, 95.7% PPV, and 61.7% NPV; the respective values for In-111-capromab pendetide were10.0%, 86.7%, 42.9%, 50.0%, and 41.9%. Fluciclovine identified 14 more positive prostate/prostate bed recurrences (55 vs 41) and 18 more patients with extraprostatic involvement (22 vs 4), and a 25.7% change in stage was reported by use of fluciclovine PET.

Similar patterns were reported when fluciclovine imaging was compared with the performance of CT (n = 53) in another subanalysis from this trial.[21] For the prostate/prostate bed, fluciclovine had 88.6% sensitivity, 56.3% specificity, 78.4% accuracy, 81.6% PPV, and 69.2% NPV; the respective values for CT were 11.4%, 87.5%, 35.3%, 66.7%, and 31.1%. For extraprostatic regions, fluciclovine had 46.2% sensitivity, 100% specificity, 65.9% accuracy, 100% PPV, and 51.7% NPV; the respective values for CT were 11.5%, 100%, 43.9%, 100%, and 39.5%. Positivity rates with fluciclovine PET/CT varied with prostate-specific antigen (PSA) levels, PSA doubling times, and original Gleason scores, but were higher than positivity rates for CT. For PSA (ng/mL) levels of less than 1, 1 to 2, greater than 2 to 5, and greater than 5, 37.5%, 77.8%, 91.7%, and 83.3% fluciclovine scans were positive, respectively.

Although fluciclovine demonstrates high PPV for extraprostatic disease, fluciclovine utility for the evaluation of local recurrence within the prostate may be challenging with relatively higher false positive results compared with extraprostatic locations. In particular, patients who underwent prostate-sparing initial therapies may demonstrate nonspecific uptake patterns likely confounded by prostatic hypertrophy and chronic inflammation. Savir-Baruch and colleagues[39] reported that the fluciclovine pattern of heterogeneous tracer distribution exhibits lower maximum standard uptake value (SUV_{max}) and lower PPV and also is associated with the presence of brachytherapy seeds when compared with focal or multifocal distribution patterns.

Evaluation of potential skeletal lesions is essential for proper staging and treatment of patients with suspected prostate cancer recurrence. Because patients with known bone metastasis were excluded from the initial studies via negative bone scan, there are less data concerning accuracy of fluciclovine for skeletal metastasis. Nevertheless, patients with fluciclovine-positive bone lesions have been reported.[20,21,37,40] Nanni and colleagues[20] reported 7/89 patients in their study with bone lesions in which 5 were positive with fluciclovine (**Fig. 2**). Schuster and colleagues[37] reported 3/93 patients with uptake within skeletal lesions enrolled after negative bone scan. A phase 2a clinical trial by Inoue and colleagues[41] of 10 patients reported 7 patients with abnormal increased fluciclovine uptake within metastatic bone lesions, similar to that of conventional imaging. In the authors' experience, fluciclovine demonstrates intense focal uptake in lytic prostate cancer lesions, and moderate uptake within mixed sclerotic lesions, but there may be absent uptake in dense sclerotic lesions. Thus, it is recommended that fluciclovine should not replace the use of dedicated bone scintigraphy when clinically indicated.

FLUCICLOVINE PERFORMANCE COMPARED WITH OTHER PET RADIOTRACERS

Other reported molecular imaging PET radiotracers have demonstrated promising results in the detection of prostate cancer, including C-11 choline, F-18 choline, C-11 acetate (**Fig. 3**), and Ga-68 or F-18–labeled prostate-specific membrane antigen ligands (PSMA).[40,42–49] For C-11 choline, a recent meta-analysis with 1270 patients reported a pooled sensitivity and specificity of 89% and 89%, respectively.[40] Although these results suggest that the diagnostic performance of choline is superior to that of fluciclovine, exercise must be cautioned because differences in study design, interpretative criteria, and reference standards may bias results. In fact, a single-center study by Nanni and colleagues[20] found fluciclovine to be slightly superior to the performance of C-11 choline for patients radically treated for prostate cancer with biochemical relapse when a single patient underwent both scans within 1 week (n = 89). With C-11 choline versus fluciclovine, sensitivity was 32% and 37%, specificity was 40% and 67%, PPV was 90% and 97%, NPV was 3% and 4%, and accuracy was 32% and 38%, respectively.[20] Overall, it was concluded that

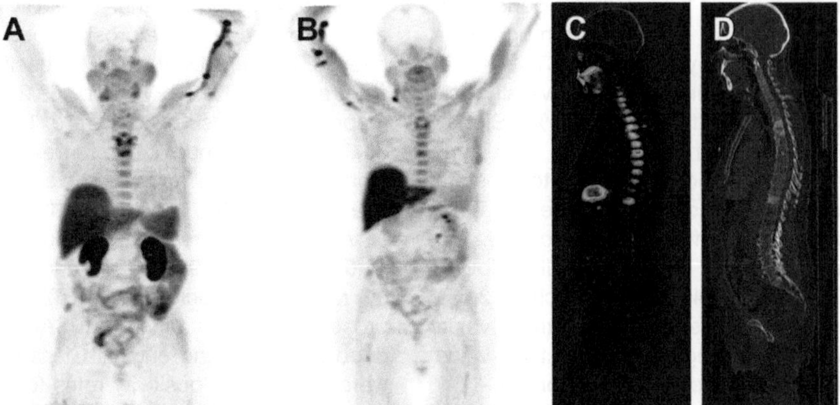

Fig. 2. 11C choline and 18F fluciclovine PET/CT detects multiple bone metastases in biochemically recurrent prostate cancer. Patient with prostate cancer treated with radical surgery and hormonal therapy, now presenting with high and rapidly increasing PSA (PSA-Trigger = 14.80 ng/mL; PSA-DT = 2.8 months; A-Vel = 33.5 ng/mL/y) underwent PET imaging. Both 11C choline (*A*, MIP) and 18F fluciclovine PET/CT (*B*, MIP; *C*, sagittal fused) identified multiple avid bone lesions in right femur, right iliac bone, left pubis, multiple vertebra, sternum and left scapula, corresponding to small osteosclerotic lesions on low-dose CT images (*D*, sagittal). Positive findings were concordant with the 2 tracers, although showing different uptake pattern. (*Courtesy of* Dr Cristina Nanni, Programma di ricerca Regione-Università 2010-2012 Regione Emilia Romagna-Bando Giovani Ricercatori, Bologna, Italy.)

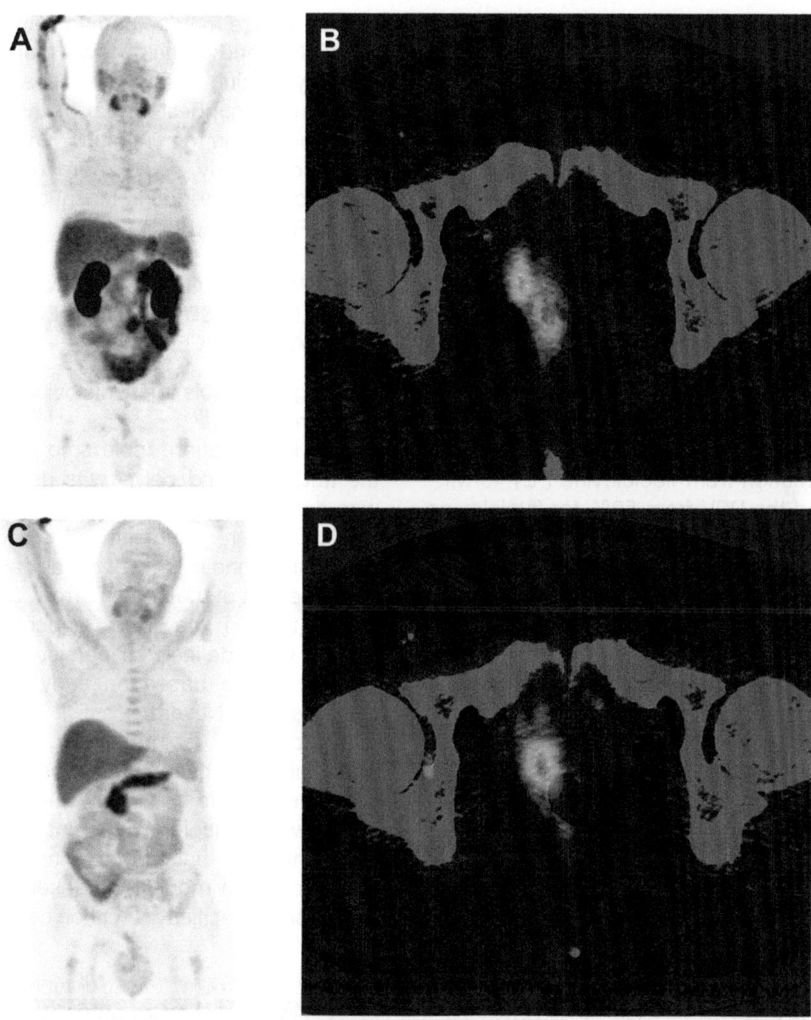

Fig. 3. 11C choline and 18F fluciclovine PET/CT detect local relapse in biochemically recurrent patient with prostate cancer. Patient with prostate cancer treated with radical surgery, salvage radiation, and hormonal therapy, now presenting with rapidly increasing PSA (PSA-Trigger 4.8 ng/mL, PSA-DT = 0.8 months, PSA-Vel = 24.8 ng/mL/y) and inconclusive findings at conventional 18F choline PET/CT and MR imaging. 11C choline PET/CT (*A*, *B*, MIP and transaxial fused) and 18F fluciclovine (*C*, *D*) performed within 1 week demonstrated focal uptake in the right prostate bed, more evident with the amino-acidic compound. A subsequent transrectal ultrasound (TRUS) biopsy reported a 7- to 10-mm nodule of adenocarcinoma GS 4 + 4 thus confirming local relapse. (*Courtesy of* Dr Cristina Nanni, Programma di ricerca Regione-Università 2010-2012 Regione Emilia Romagna-Bando Giovani Ricercatori, Bologna, Italy.)

fluciclovine as an imaging radiotracer also demonstrates other advantages, including ease of production, longer half-life, and lower physiologic background activity.

Ga-68 PSMA as well has demonstrated promising results for the imaging of patients with suspected prostate cancer relapse.[46–48,50] PSMA is overexpressed in prostate cancer cells. Targeting of PSMA expression was previously used in imaging with In-111-capromab pendetide directed to the intracellular epitope of the PSMA receptor, which significantly limits its diagnostic performance. Ga-68–labeled PSMA ligands have been structured to attach to the extracellular domain, significantly increasing sensitivity.[51,52] When Ga-68 PSMA performance was compared with F-18 choline within the same patients, Ga-68 PSMA was found to be superior to choline with significantly higher SUV_{max}. Ga-68 PSMA detected 56 lesions versus 26 with F-18 choline.[45] Similar results may well occur in comparison to PSMA-based radiotracers to fluciclovine, and direct comparison possibly will be the subject of future research.

FLUCICLOVINE EVALUATION OF PRIMARY PROSTATE CANCER

Multiparametric MR imaging (MP-MR) is considered the most useful single modality for the characterization of primary prostate cancer, although there are limitations including that of specificity.[43,53] Turkbey and colleagues[54] investigated the use of fluciclovine PET with MP-MR imaging for 22 patients with primary prostate cancer scheduled to undergo prostatectomy and whole-mount histologic analysis. Although mean SUV_{max} of the tumor was significantly higher than that of normal prostate tissue, there was a significant overlap of fluciclovine uptake between tumor foci and benign prostate hyperplasia. Adding the information from fluciclovine PET to MP-MR increased the PPV from 50% for fluciclovine alone and 76% for MP-MR alone to 82% for a combination of all methods. The limitations of fluciclovine for primary prostate cancer had also been reported previously by Schuster and colleagues[25] in a 10-patient study correlating fluciclovine uptake with MR imaging and histologic sextant analysis.[25] Although the study reported a correlation between SUV_{max} and Gleason score and statistically significant differences in SUV_{max} between malignant and benign sextants, overlap was noted. No correlation was found between uptake (SUV_{max}) and Ki-67. Both studies concluded that fluciclovine imaging for the evaluation of primary prostate cancers was limited, although there may be some utility as an adjunct to MP-MR and to help guide biopsy as well as possibly staging of high-risk disease. In addition, both studies suggested that delayed imaging, 15 to 20 minutes in the first study and 28 minutes in the second study, could improve diagnostic performance for the characterization of primary lesions (**Figs. 4** and **5**).

IMAGING PROTOCOL AND INTERPRETATIVE CRITERIA FOR SUSPECTED RECURRENT PROSTATE CANCER

Differing protocols of fluciclovine imaging have been reported.[19,22,24,25,35,37,40,55] During early clinical investigation, triple time point imaging of the abdomen and pelvis was used, and uptake was defined as mild, moderate, or intense when activity in the region of interest was visually below that of the bone marrow (typically at L3), equal to or above that of the bone marrow, and equal to or above that in the liver, respectively. Positive lesions were defined as persistent moderate or intense uptake based on early to delayed sequences.[24,37] Nevertheless, it was recognized that triple time point imaging is not clinically practical. A subsequent retrospective analysis compared results from early single time point imaging with multiple time point interpretation. It was concluded that early imaging with fluciclovine is feasible with modest increased sensitivity and decreased specificity.[56] Other centers have also

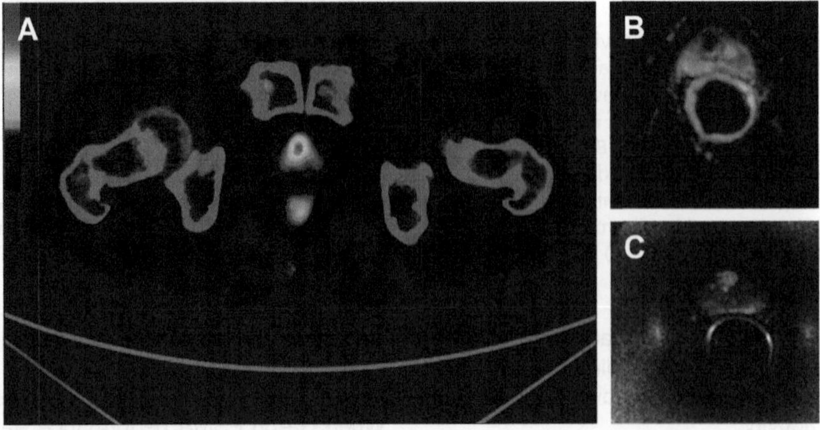

Fig. 4. Pretreatment staging 18F fluciclovine PET/CT identifies the most predominant aggressive intraprostatic lesion in primary prostate cancer (in agreement with 11C choline and MP-MR imaging). A 71-year-old patient affected by high-risk prostate cancer (PSA 8 ng/mL, GS 4 + 4, cT2) underwent MP-MR imaging (*B*, axT2; *C*, axDWI) and 11C choline PET/CT, as part of the normal staging workflow before radical surgery, and an additional 18F fluciclovine scan (*A*, transaxial fused), as part of an ongoing clinical trial. The procedures detected a focal right intermediate prostate lesion, corresponding to a 19-mm, GS 4 + 5 nodule of acinar adenocarcinoma. On the contrary, a smaller and less aggressive focus of GS 3 + 3 was under the limit of lesion detectability in all cases. (*Courtesy of* Dr Lucia Zanoni, Programma di ricerca Regione-Università Area 1-Bando Giovani ricercatori "Alessandro Liberati" 2013, Bologna, Italy.)

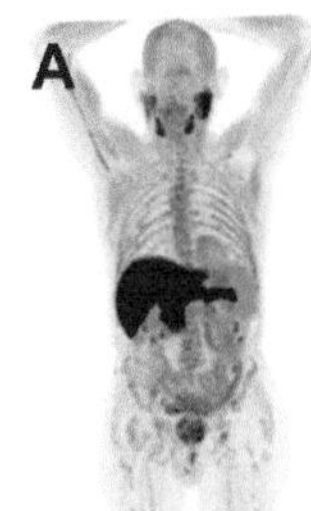

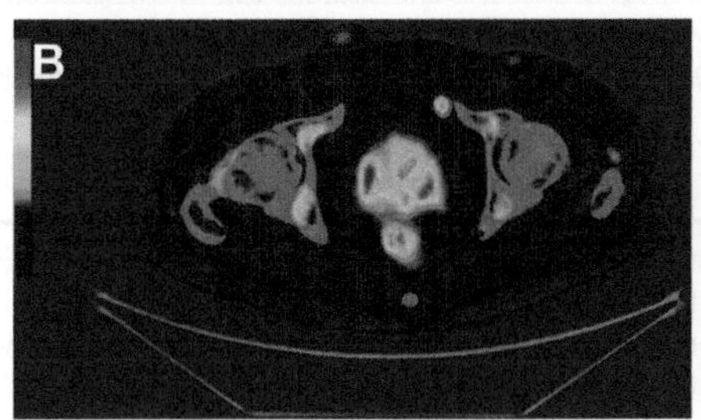

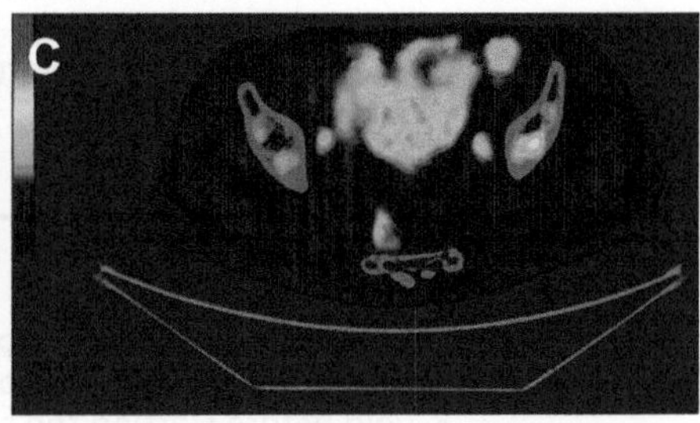

Fig. 5. Pretreatment staging 18F fluciclovine PET/CT in a patient with primary prostate cancer, scheduled for radical surgery, detects multiple nodal and bone metastases leading to a change in treatment management. Patient with high-risk prostate cancer (PSA 18,65, GS 4 + 5, 50% positive core biopsy) was scheduled for radical surgery and lymphadenectomy according to pelvic MR imaging and 11C choline PET/CT standard staging. The experimental tracer 18F fluciclovine detected multiple avid pelvic lymphadenopathies (*B* and *C*, transaxial fused) and inhomogeneous and diffuse uptake throughout the skeleton (*A*, MIP). Considering the disease extent, the patient was finally excluded from surgery. (*Courtesy of* Dr Lucia Zanoni, Programma di ricerca Regione-Università Area 1-Bando Giovani ricercatori "Alessandro Liberati" 2013, Bologna, Italy.)

used whole-body single time point imaging with success.[20] With the knowledge of efflux of radiotracer with a generally downsloping time activity curve, early imaging within the first 30 minutes after injection is therefore recommended. A protocol for imaging and study interpretation as adapted from the FDA package insert and the Axumin (fluciclovine F18) Imaging and Interpretation Manual is provided in **Table 1**, and it is recommended that the full documents be reviewed by the reader.[57]

As with other radiotracers, knowledge of normal physiologic distribution and variants as well as typical patterns of cancer recurrence is important for proper interpretation of fluciclovine PET. A comprehensive review paper describing radiotracer uptake patterns, incidental findings, and variants that may simulate disease is available.[23] Uptake may not only occur in prostate cancer but also in other malignancies (**Fig. 6**). Uptake may also be present in benign conditions such as inflammation and infection and other metabolically active benign lesions such as meningioma and osteoid osteoma (**Fig. 7**)

For patients who have undergone nonprostatectomy therapy, nonspecific elevation of fluciclovine uptake in remaining prostate likely due to underlying hyperplastic prostate tissue or inflammation may be present.[54] Moderate focal asymmetric uptake, visually equal to or greater than bone marrow, is considered suspicious for cancer recurrence. Ongoing studies are exploring the use of fluciclovine for biopsy planning for recurrent disease.[58] For patients with history of prostatectomy, any focal uptake within the prostate bed or seminal vesicles may be considered abnormal especially if greater than bone marrow, although small lesions (<1 cm) subject to the partial volume effect may be suspicious if visually greater than blood pool. Review of sagittal images is especially useful for evaluation of the urethral anastomosis. Uptake within lymph nodes at sites of typical prostate cancer spread is highly specific for neoplastic involvement with a low false positives rate, and understanding the common patterns of lymph node metastasis in prostate cancer is essential to minimize false positive interpretation.[20,24,37,55] Uptake visually equal to or above that of lumbar marrow should be considered abnormal, although with nodes less than 1 cm, uptake may be suspicious if in a typical pattern of spread and greater than blood pool. Nevertheless, for example, inguinal lymph nodes may demonstrate nonspecific moderate symmetric inflammatory uptake. For bone lesions to be considered positive, focal uptake should be clearly seen on maximum intensity projection (MIP) images. Densely sclerotic lesions may not be fluciclovine avid. In contradistinction to FDG-PET, degenerative uptake is not a common variant. Skeletal metastases resembling Schmorl nodes but with fluciclovine uptake have been described. **Table 1** provides more detailed interpretative guidelines as well as pearls, pitfalls, and variants.

GUIDELINES FOR THE USE OF FLUCICLOVINE IMAGING IN PATIENTS WITH RECURRENT PROSTATE CANCER

Fluciclovine PET is highly useful in the detection of recurrent prostate cancer even in the presence of negative or equivocal conventional imaging. The current FDA-approved indication is for men with suspected prostate cancer recurrence based on elevated blood PSA levels following

Table 1
Axumin (fluciclovine F18) imaging and interpretation manual

Fluciclovine PET/CT	Description
Imaging protocol	Patient preparation: • Avoid significant exercise for at least 1 d before PET imaging. • Nothing to eat or drink for at least 4 h (other than small amounts of water for taking medications) before radiotracer administration. • Void before starting the scanning procedure. Dose and injection: • 10 mCi/370 MBq as an intravenous bolus injection while the patient is positioned in the PET/CT scanner with arms down. • Injection into the right arm is suggested to avoid misinterpretation of stasis in left axillary vein as Virchow node. • Subsequently, administer an intravenous flush of sterile sodium chloride injection, 0.9%, to ensure full delivery of the dose. Image acquisition: • Position the patient supine with arms above the head if possible. • High-quality CT acquisition for anatomic correlation and attenuation correction. • Begin PET 3–5 min after injection (goal of 4 min). • Image from the mid thighs to base of skull. • Imaging guidelines recommend 5 min per bed position acquisition in the pelvis and 3 min per bed position in the remainder of the body, but these suggestions are scanner dependent. Image reconstruction: • The highest-quality scanner at an institution should be used. • If a scanner has time of flight, iterative reconstruction and/or a reconstruction algorithm using recovery resolution should be used. • Gaussian smoothing filter (if applicable) should not exceed 5 mm.
Diagnostic criteria	Generally defined as: Localization of prostate cancer recurrence in sites typical for prostate cancer recurrence in comparison with tissue background. Prostate/bed Prostatectomy • Focal uptake, visually equal to or greater than bone marrow, in sites typical for prostate cancer recurrence suspicious for cancer. ◦ However, if a focus of uptake is small (<1 cm), it may be considered suspicious if the uptake is visually greater than blood pool. Nonprostatectomy • Moderate focal asymmetric uptake, visually equal to or greater than bone marrow, is suspicious for cancer recurrence. ◦ However, if a focus of uptake is small (<1 cm) and in a site typical for recurrence, it may still be considered suspicious if the uptake is visually greater than blood pool. Lymph nodes Typical sites for prostate cancer recurrence • Uptake, visually equal to or greater than bone marrow, is considered suspicious for cancer. ◦ However, if a node is small (<1 cm) and in a site typical for recurrence, it may still be considered suspicious if visually greater than blood pool. Atypical sites for recurrence (inguinal, distal external iliac, hilar, and axillary nodes) • Mild, symmetric uptake is typically considered physiologic uptake, but if uptake is present within the context of other clear malignant disease, it may be considered suspicious for cancer recurrence. Bone • Focal uptake clearly visualized on MIP or PET-only images is considered suspicious for cancer. ◦ A bone abnormality visualized on CT (eg, dense sclerosis without uptake) does not exclude the presence of metastasis. Alternative imaging, for example, MR, NaF PET-CT, or SPECT-CT bone scan, should be considered.

(*continued on next page*)

Table 1
(continued)

Fluciclovine PET/CT	Description
Differential diagnosis	Prostate • Cancer, inflammatory changes, benign prostatic hypertrophy. Extraprostate • Typical locations for nodal spread of prostate cancer: metastatic prostate cancer • Uptake may occur in other cancers • Nodal inflammation, especially if mild and symmetric and in atypical locations for prostate cancer spread such as inguinal or distal external iliac. • Uptake may also occur from benign processes such as infection, and metabolically active benign bone lesions such as osteoid osteoma.

Pearls, pitfalls, variants	• Performance affected by PSA levels. Less likely to be positive with PSA <1 ng/mL unless doubling time is rapid.
	• Read from the "inside out." That is, be aware of typical locations for prostate cancer spread (eg, deep pelvic vs peripheral inguinal or distal external iliac nodes).
	  ○ Mild benign symmetric uptake within the inguinal lymph nodes may be seen and should not be called positive unless "disease pattern marching out of pelvis."
	• Higher false positive rate within intact or treated prostate.
	• Abnormal activity in postprostatectomy bed is more specific.
	  ○ Sagittal images helpful with identification of disease at urethral anastomosis.
	• Uptake in lytic skeletal lesions is typically intense, moderate in mixed lesions, but may be absent in densely sclerotic lesions.
	  ○ If skeletal lesion is seen on CT, consider skeletal-specific imaging.
	• Degenerative uptake in bone is not a common variant in fluciclovine as it is with FDG and should be further evaluated for the presence of metastatic bone lesions. Skeletal metastases that resemble Schmorl nodes but with fluciclovine uptake within them have been described.
	• Fluciclovine may be taken up by other cancer cells with upregulated amino acid transport. Be familiar with normal physiologic patterns of activity. In these instances, further correlation with clinical presentation and/or other imaging may be helpful.
	• In a small percentage of patients, fluciclovine may demonstrate moderate early bladder activity, interfering with evaluation of the prostate bed.

What the referring physician needs to know	• Fluciclovine PET/CT demonstrates utility in the localization of recurrent prostate cancer disease (FDA-approved indication). • Fluciclovine PET can identify true positive prostate cancer foci even when conventional imaging, such as CT, MR, and bone scan, is negative. • No absolute PSA threshold is recommended. However, positivity is more likely with PSA >1 ng/mL or if PSA <1 ng/mL with rapid PSA kinetics. • Fluciclovine PET/CT scan should be considered before salvage therapy, for accurate treatment planning.

prior treatment. There is no absolute threshold for PSA level in the recommendation of when to obtain fluciclovine PET, yet clearly, diagnostic performance varies with PSA level and kinetics. Fluciclovine PET positivity rate will increase with increasing PSA and with more rapid doubling times.[20,21,59] Based on logistic regression analysis in one study, a PSA of 1 ng/mL equated to a 71.8% probability of a positive fluciclovine scan.[37] One group has reported that functional imaging with choline or fluciclovine PET/CT together with MP-MR to be the most valuable imaging techniques in the detection of prostate cancer relapse and should be highly considered before treatment planning.[60] The group acknowledged the limitation of these PET radiotracers with underlying low PSA levels of less than 1 ng/mL. They suggested that functional images may be cost-effective when PSA velocity is high and PSA doubling time is short. Therefore, until more data are available, an elevated PSA or a concerning PSA velocity or doubling time, which clinically triggers salvage therapy in patients, may be a useful reference as to when a fluciclovine PET study should be obtained in suspected recurrent prostate cancer.

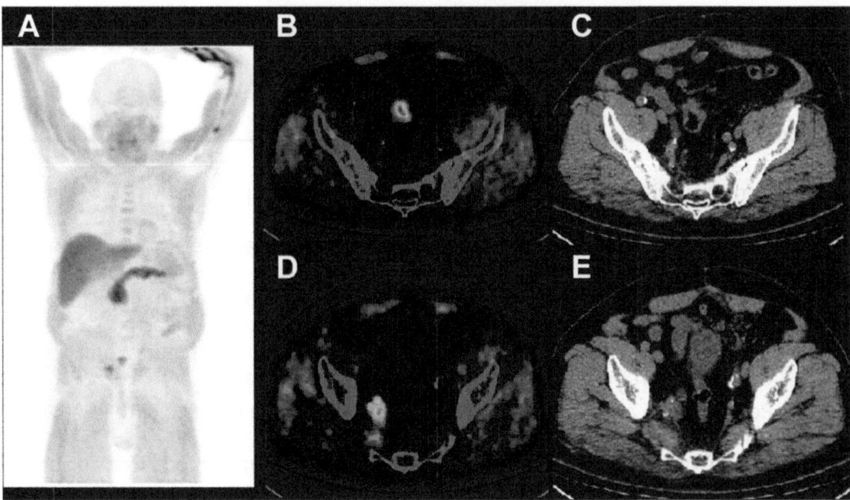

Fig. 6. 18F fluciclovine PET/CT detects nodal metastasis in biochemically recurrent prostate cancer and incidental sigmoid cancer. Patient with prostate cancer treated with radical surgery, salvage radiation, and hormonal therapy, now presenting with low but rapidly increasing PSA (PSA-Trigger = 0.94 ng/mL; PSA-DT = 5.9 months; PSA-Vel = 1.1 ng/mL/y) and negative TRUS. 18F fluciclovine showed 2 focal lesions in MIP images (*A*) corresponding with right internal iliac tissue (*D, E* transaxial fused and low-dose CT), causing grade II hydroureteronephrosis, and sigmoid wall thickening (*B, C*). Urologic contrast-enhanced CT and bowel endoscopy confirmed the findings, in keeping with secondary nodal lesions from prostate cancer and new sigmoid cancer. The patient was treated with ureteral stenting, hormonal therapy, and bowel resection, achieving PSA response. (*Courtesy of* Dr Cristina Nanni, Programma di ricerca Regione-Università 2010-2012 Regione Emilia Romagna-Bando giovani Ricercatori, Bologna, Italy.)

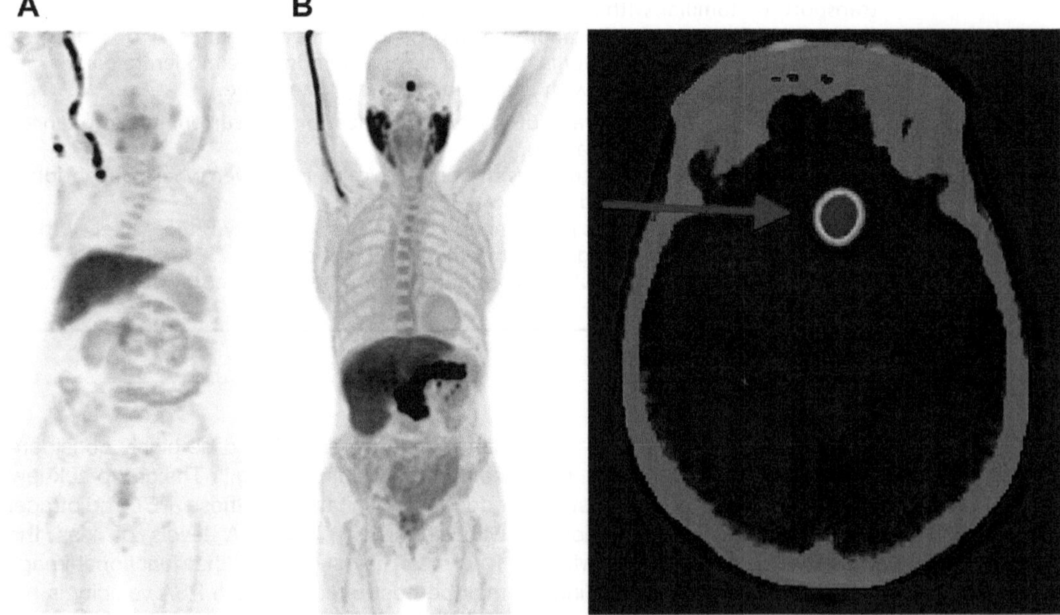

Fig. 7. Variants and pitfalls. (*A*) 18F fluciclovine uptake along the vessel of intravenous administration. (*B*) 18F fluciclovine avid meningioma. It is well established that physiologic tracer biodistribution in normal brain is very low or absent. In this case, PET/CT images showed intense and focal brain uptake (SUV_{max} = 17, MIP and transaxial fused; *red arrow*) in keeping with known meningioma. (*Courtesy of* [*A*] Dr Cristina Nanni, Programma di ricerca Regione-Università 2010-2012 Regione Emilia Romagna-Bando Giovani Ricercatori, Bologna, Italy; and [*B*] Dr Lucia Zanoni, Programma di ricerca Regione-Università Area 1-Bando Giovani ricercatori "Alessandro Liberati" 2013, Bologna, Italy.)

SUMMARY

Fluciclovine is currently FDA approved for the localization of recurrent prostate cancer in a patient with elevated PSA. Based on comprehensive clinical data, fluciclovine is beneficial in the identification of disease even when other conventional imaging is negative. Knowledge of normal physiologic distribution and variants as well as typical patterns of prostate cancer spread is important for proper interpretation of fluciclovine PET.

REFERENCES

1. Huang C, McConathy J. Radiolabeled amino acids for oncologic imaging. J Nucl Med 2013;54(7):1007–10.
2. Jager PL, Vaalburg W, Pruim J, et al. Radiolabeled amino acids: basic aspects and clinical applications in oncology. J Nucl Med 2001;42(3):432–45.
3. Morgan TM, Koreckij TD, Corey E. Targeted therapy for advanced prostate cancer: inhibition of the PI3K/Akt/mTOR pathway. Curr Cancer Drug Targets 2009;9(2):237–49.
4. Wibmer AG, Burger IA, Sala E, et al. Molecular imaging of prostate cancer. Radiographics 2016;36(1):142–59.
5. Chuaqui RF, Englert CR, Strup SE, et al. Identification of a novel transcript up-regulated in a clinically aggressive prostate carcinoma. Urology 1997;50(2):302–7.
6. Cole KA, Chuaqui RF, Katz K, et al. cDNA sequencing and analysis of POV1 (PB39): a novel gene up-regulated in prostate cancer. Genomics 1998;51(2):282–7.
7. Fuchs BC, Bode BP. Amino acid transporters ASCT2 and LAT1 in cancer: partners in crime? Semin Cancer Biol 2005;15(4):254–66.
8. Heublein S, Kazi S, Ogmundsdottir MH, et al. Proton-assisted amino-acid transporters are conserved regulators of proliferation and amino-acid-dependent mTORC1 activation. Oncogene 2010;29(28):4068–79.
9. Muller A, Chiotellis A, Keller C, et al. Imaging tumour ATB0,+ transport activity by PET with the cationic amino acid O-2((2-[18F]fluoroethyl)methyl-amino)ethyltyrosine. Mol Imaging Biol 2014;16(3):412–20.
10. Okudaira H, Shikano N, Nishii R, et al. Putative transport mechanism and intracellular fate of trans-1-amino-3-18F-fluorocyclobutanecarboxylic acid in human prostate cancer. J Nucl Med 2011;52(5):822–9.
11. Sakata T, Ferdous G, Tsuruta T, et al. L-type amino-acid transporter 1 as a novel biomarker for high-grade malignancy in prostate cancer. Pathol Int 2009;59(1):7–18.
12. Segawa A, Nagamori S, Kanai Y, et al. L-type amino acid transporter 1 expression is highly correlated with Gleason score in prostate cancer. Mol Clin Oncol 2013;1(2):274–80.
13. Smolarz K, Krause BJ, Graner FP, et al. (S)-4-(3-18F-fluoropropyl)-L-glutamic acid: an 18F-labeled tumor-specific probe for PET/CT imaging–dosimetry. J Nucl Med 2013;54(6):861–6.
14. Wang Q, Tiffen J, Bailey CG, et al. Targeting amino acid transport in metastatic castration-resistant prostate cancer: effects on cell cycle, cell growth, and tumor development. J Natl Cancer Inst 2013;105(19):1463–73.
15. McConathy J, Yu W, Jarkas N, et al. Radiohalogenated nonnatural amino acids as PET and SPECT tumor imaging agents. Med Res Rev 2012;32(4):868–905.
16. Oka S, Okudaira H, Yoshida Y, et al. Transport mechanisms of trans-1-amino-3-fluoro[1-(14)C]cyclobutanecarboxylic acid in prostate cancer cells. Nucl Med Biol 2012;39(1):109–19.
17. Okudaira H, Oka S, Ono M, et al. Accumulation of trans-1-amino-3-[(18)F]fluorocyclobutanecarboxylic acid in prostate cancer due to androgen-induced expression of amino acid transporters. Mol Imaging Biol 2014;16(6):756–64.
18. Ono M, Oka S, Okudaira H, et al. [(14)C]Fluciclovine (alias anti-[(14)C]FACBC) uptake and ASCT2 expression in castration-resistant prostate cancer cells. Nucl Med Biol 2015;42(11):887–92.
19. Nanni C, Schiavina R, Boschi S, et al. Comparison of 18F-FACBC and 11C-choline PET/CT in patients with radically treated prostate cancer and biochemical relapse: preliminary results. Eur J Nucl Med Mol Imaging 2013;40(Suppl 1):S11–7.
20. Nanni C, Zanoni L, Pultrone C, et al. (18)F-FACBC (anti1-amino-3-(18)F-fluorocyclobutane-1-carboxylic acid) versus (11)C-choline PET/CT in prostate cancer relapse: results of a prospective trial. Eur J Nucl Med Mol Imaging 2016;43(9):1601–10.
21. Odewole OA, Tade FI, Nieh PT, et al. Recurrent prostate cancer detection with anti-3-[18F]FACBC PET/CT: comparison with CT. Eur J Nucl Med Mol Imaging 2016;43(10):1773–83.
22. Schuster DM, Votaw JR, Nieh PT, et al. Initial experience with the radiotracer anti-1-amino-3-F-18-fluorocyclobutane-1-carboxylic acid with PET/CT in prostate carcinoma. J Nucl Med 2007;48(1):56–63.
23. Schuster DM, Nanni C, Fanti S, et al. Anti-1-amino-3-18F-fluorocyclobutane-1-carboxylic acid: physiologic uptake patterns, incidental findings, and variants that may simulate disease. J Nucl Med 2014;55(12):1986–92.
24. Schuster DM, Savir-Baruch B, Nieh PT, et al. Detection of recurrent prostate carcinoma with anti-1-amino-3-18F-fluorocyclobutane-1-carboxylic acid PET/CT and 111In-capromab pendetide SPECT/CT. Radiology 2011;259(3):852–61.

25. Schuster DM, Taleghani PA, Nieh PT, et al. Characterization of primary prostate carcinoma by anti-1-amino-2-[(18)F] -fluorocyclobutane-1-carboxylic acid (anti-3-[(18)F] FACBC) uptake. Am J Nucl Med Mol Imaging 2013;3(1):85–96.
26. Sorensen J, Owenius R, Lax M, et al. Regional distribution and kinetics of [18F]fluciclovine (anti-[18F] FACBC), a tracer of amino acid transport, in subjects with primary prostate cancer. Eur J Nucl Med Mol Imaging 2013;40(3):394–402.
27. Nye JA, Schuster DM, Yu W, et al. Biodistribution and radiation dosimetry of the synthetic nonmetabolized amino acid analogue anti-18F-FACBC in humans. J Nucl Med 2007;48(6):1017–20.
28. Washburn LC, Sun TT, Anon JB, et al. Effect of structure on tumor specificity of alicyclic alpha-amino acids. Cancer Res 1978;38(8):2271–3.
29. Washburn LC, Sun TT, Byrd B, et al. 1-aminocyclobutane[11C]carboxylic acid, a potential tumor-seeking agent. J Nucl Med 1979;20(10):1055–61.
30. Shoup TM, Olson J, Hoffman JM, et al. Synthesis and evaluation of [18F]1-amino-3-fluorocyclobutane-1-carboxylic acid to image brain tumors. J Nucl Med 1999;40(2):331–8.
31. Martarello L, McConathy J, Camp VM, et al. Synthesis of syn- and anti-1-amino-3-[18F]fluoromethyl-cyclobutane-1-carboxylic acid (FMACBC), potential PET ligands for tumor detection. J Med Chem 2002;45(11):2250–9.
32. McConathy J, Voll RJ, Yu W, et al. Improved synthesis of anti-[18F]FACBC: improved preparation of labeling precursor and automated radiosynthesis. Appl Radiat Isot 2003;58(6):657–66.
33. Oka S, Hattori R, Kurosaki F, et al. A preliminary study of anti-1-amino-3-18F-fluorocyclobutyl-1-carboxylic acid for the detection of prostate cancer. J Nucl Med 2007;48(1):46–55.
34. Okudaira H, Nakanishi T, Oka S, et al. Kinetic analyses of trans-1-amino-3-[18F]fluorocyclobutanecarboxylic acid transport in Xenopus laevis oocytes expressing human ASCT2 and SNAT2. Nucl Med Biol 2013;40(5):670–5.
35. Schuster DM, Nye JA, Nieh PT, et al. Initial experience with the radiotracer anti-1-amino-3-[18F] Fluorocyclobutane-1-carboxylic acid (anti-[18F] FACBC) with PET in renal carcinoma. Mol Imaging Biol 2009;11(6):434–8.
36. Available at: http://www.blueearthdiagnostics.com/u-s-fda-approves-blue-earth-diagnostics-axumintm-fluciclovine-f-18-injection-priority-review-pet-imaging-recurrent-prostate-cancer. Accessed July 29, 2016.
37. Schuster DM, Nieh PT, Jani AB, et al. Anti-3-[(18)F] FACBC positron emission tomography-computerized tomography and (111)In-capromab pendetide single photon emission computerized tomography-computerized tomography for recurrent prostate carcinoma: results of a prospective clinical trial. J Urol 2014;191(5):1446–53.
38. Cookson MS, Aus G, Burnett AL, et al. Variation in the definition of biochemical recurrence in patients treated for localized prostate cancer: the American Urological Association Prostate Guidelines for Localized Prostate Cancer Update Panel report and recommendations for a standard in the reporting of surgical outcomes. J Urol 2007;177(2):540–5.
39. Savir-Baruch B, Odewole O, Alaei Taleghani P, et al. Anti-3-[F18] FACBC uptake pattern in the prostate affects positive predictive value and is associated with the presence of brachytherapy seeds. J Nucl Med 2013;54(2_MeetingAbstracts):346.
40. Fanti S, Minozzi S, Castellucci P, et al. PET/CT with (11)C-choline for evaluation of prostate cancer patients with biochemical recurrence: meta-analysis and critical review of available data. Eur J Nucl Med Mol Imaging 2016;43(1):55–69.
41. Inoue Y, Asano Y, Satoh T, et al. Phase IIa clinical trial of trans-1-amino-3-18F-fluoro-cyclobutyl-carboxylic acid in metastatic prostate cancer. Asia Ocean J Nucl Med Biol 2014;2(2):87–94.
42. Sandblom G, Sorensen J, Lundin N, et al. Positron emission tomography with C11-acetate for tumor detection and localization in patients with prostate-specific antigen relapse after radical prostatectomy. Urology 2006;67(5):996–1000.
43. Mena E, Turkbey B, Mani H, et al. 11C-Acetate PET/CT in localized prostate cancer: a study with MRI and histopathologic correlation. J Nucl Med 2012;53(4):538–45.
44. Brogsitter C, Zophel K, Kotzerke J. 18F-Choline, 11C-choline and 11C-acetate PET/CT: comparative analysis for imaging prostate cancer patients. Eur J Nucl Med Mol Imaging 2013;40(Suppl 1):S18–27.
45. Afshar-Oromieh A, Zechmann CM, Malcher A, et al. Comparison of PET imaging with a (68)Ga-labelled PSMA ligand and (18)F-choline-based PET/CT for the diagnosis of recurrent prostate cancer. Eur J Nucl Med Mol Imaging 2014;41(1):11–20.
46. Afshar-Oromieh A, Hetzheim H, Kubler W, et al. Radiation dosimetry of (68)Ga-PSMA-11 (HBED-CC) and preliminary evaluation of optimal imaging timing. Eur J Nucl Med Mol Imaging 2016;43(9):1611–20.
47. Afshar-Oromieh A, Haberkorn U, Schlemmer HP, et al. Comparison of PET/CT and PET/MRI hybrid systems using a 68Ga-labelled PSMA ligand for the diagnosis of recurrent prostate cancer: initial experience. Eur J Nucl Med Mol Imaging 2014;41(5):887–97.
48. Afshar-Oromieh A, Avtzi E, Giesel FL, et al. The diagnostic value of PET/CT imaging with the (68)Ga-labelled PSMA ligand HBED-CC in the diagnosis of recurrent prostate cancer. Eur J Nucl Med Mol Imaging 2015;42(2):197–209.

49. Ackerstaff E, Pflug BR, Nelson JB, et al. Detection of increased choline compounds with proton nuclear magnetic resonance spectroscopy subsequent to malignant transformation of human prostatic epithelial cells. Cancer Res 2001;61(9):3599–603.
50. Freitag MT, Radtke JP, Hadaschik BA, et al. Comparison of hybrid (68)Ga-PSMA PET/MRI and (68)Ga-PSMA PET/CT in the evaluation of lymph node and bone metastases of prostate cancer. Eur J Nucl Med Mol Imaging 2016;43(1):70–83.
51. Lutje S, Heskamp S, Cornelissen AS, et al. PSMA ligands for radionuclide imaging and therapy of prostate cancer: clinical status. Theranostics 2015;5(12):1388–401.
52. Lutje S, Rijpkema M, Franssen GM, et al. Dual-modality image-guided surgery of prostate cancer with a radiolabeled fluorescent anti-PSMA monoclonal antibody. J Nucl Med 2014;55(6):995–1001.
53. Turkbey B, Albert PS, Kurdziel K, et al. Imaging localized prostate cancer: current approaches and new developments. AJR Am J Roentgenol 2009;192(6):1471–80.
54. Turkbey B, Mena E, Shih J, et al. Localized prostate cancer detection with 18F FACBC PET/CT: comparison with MR imaging and histopathologic analysis. Radiology 2014;270(3):849–56.
55. Nanni C, Schiavina R, Brunocilla E, et al. 18F-fluciclovine PET/CT for the detection of prostate cancer relapse: a comparison to 11C-choline PET/CT. Clin Nucl Med 2015;40(8):e386–91.
56. Savir-Baruch B, Odewole O, Master V, et al. Diagnostic performance of synthetic amino acid anti-3-[18F] FACBC PET in recurrent prostate carcinoma utilizing single-time versus dual-time point criteria. J Nucl Med 2014;55(Suppl 1):21.
57. Available at: http://www.axumin.com/. Accessed July 30, 2016.
58. Fei B, Nieh PT, Schuster DM, et al. PET-directed, 3D Ultrasound-guided prostate biopsy. Diagn Imaging Eur 2013;29(1):12–5.
59. Kairemo K, Rasulova N, Partanen K, et al. Preliminary clinical experience of trans-1-amino-3-(18)F-fluorocyclobutanecarboxylic acid (anti-(18)F-FACBC) PET/CT imaging in prostate cancer patients. Biomed Res Int 2014;2014:305182.
60. Schiavina R, Brunocilla E, Borghesi M, et al. Diagnostic imaging work-up for disease relapse after radical treatment for prostate cancer: how to differentiate local from systemic disease? The urologist point of view. Rev Esp Med Nucl Imagen Mol 2013;32(5):310–3.

Imaging of Prostate Cancer Using Gallium-68–Labeled Bombesin

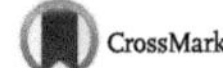

Ida Sonni, MD*, Lucia Baratto, MD, Andrei Iagaru, MD

KEYWORDS

• Prostate cancer • Bombesin • Gastrin-releasing peptide receptor • PET • Imaging • Gallium-68

KEY POINTS

- Gastrin-releasing peptide receptors (GRPRs) are overexpressed on the cell membranes of prostate cancer, unlike normal prostate tissue and benign prostate hyperplasia.
- Bombesin/gastrin-releasing peptide (GRP) analogs, targeting the GRPR, can be radiolabeled for imaging and therapeutic purposes of GRPR-overexpressing tumors, such as prostate cancer.
- Several bombesin-like peptides have been developed in recent years for prostate cancer imaging and theranostic applications.
- Gallium-68 (^{68}Ga) is one of the most interesting radioisotopes for PET imaging.

Prostate cancer is the most common malignancy in men.[1] According to the American Cancer Society, it was estimated that there would be 180,890 new cases of prostate cancer and 26,120 deaths from prostate cancer in 2016 in the United States and that it would be the second leading cause of cancer death after lung and bronchus tumors.[2] Large advances have been made in the treatment and understanding of the underlying biology. The 5-year relative survival rates for prostate cancer have increased from 83% in the late 1980s to 93% in the early 1990s and 99% since 2000, among all races.[2]

At the time of initial presentation, 80% of patients have local disease, 12% have regional disease, and 4% have metastatic disease, whereas the remaining 4% are classified as unknown.[3] Approximately 20% to 40% of men experience a rising prostate-specific antigen (PSA) (biochemical failure) within 10 years from the primary prostate cancer treatment.[4] Approximately 25% to 35% of men with an increasing serum PSA level develop locally recurrent disease, 20% to 25% develop metastatic disease, and 45% to 55% develop both local recurrence and metastatic disease.[3] A rise in PSA is also registered in many prostate cancer patients who develop progressive disease after castration. Risk assessment of prostate cancer patients takes into account many factors (patient age, clinical tumor stage, serum PSA, PSA density, Gleason score, number of positive prostate biopsies, amount of malignant tissue per core) and is key in defining patient management.[1] Over time, serum PSA became the most used biomarker of prostate cancer for screening and follow-up purposes. It is cost effective and widely diffused. It helps in detection of primary tumor and disease relapse after treatment, even though it cannot recognize local versus distant disease.[5] Furthermore, PSA screening has resulted in high overdiagnosis rates, estimated at 23% to 42% for screen-detected cancers,[6,7] which have inevitably led to early unnecessary therapy in many patients. For these reasons, routine

Disclosure Statement: A. Iagaru provides research support to GE Healthcare, Bayer Healthcare, Piramal Imaging, and GmbH. I. Sonni and L. Baratto have nothing to disclose.

Division of Nuclear Medicine and Molecular Imaging, Department of Radiology, Stanford University, 300 Pasteur Drive, Stanford, CA 94305, USA
* Corresponding author.
E-mail address: isonni@stanford.edu

PET Clin 12 (2017) 159–171
http://dx.doi.org/10.1016/j.cpet.2016.11.003

screening with the PSA test is no longer recommended, and consequently the number of prostate cancer diagnoses recently declined, even if it still remains the most frequent malignancy in men in the United States.[2] During the past decade much progress has been made in research of prostate cancer, from improvements in genetic knowledge that could lead to targeted screening of patients at risk to more efficient therapy.

Prostate cancer treatments range from active surveillance alone to multimodality treatments. Radical prostatectomy, external-beam radiotherapy, and brachytherapy are all standard local treatments for prostate cancer, even though they have never been compared in robust randomized trials.[8–13] Newer modalities, such as cryotherapy, high-intensity focal ultrasound, and photodynamic therapy, are also used. For physicians to prescribe the most appropriate treatment, it is essential to determine whether the cancer has spread out of the prostate or not. In summary, nuclear medicine imaging, using new accurate and cost-effective tracers, can play an important role in improving diagnoses, staging, and follow-up of prostate cancer.

PET RADIOPHARMACEUTICALS IN PROSTATE CANCER

Fluorine-18 Fluorodeoxyglucose

Characteristics of different radiopharmaceuticals used in prostate cancer are summarized in **Table 1**. Cancer detection with Fluorine-18 fluorodeoxyglucose (^{18}F-FDG) PET is a result of the increased glucose metabolism in malignant cells, in comparison to the normal tissues (Warburg effect).[14] In primary tumor diagnosis and staging, ^{18}F-FDG PET/CT has a low sensitivity. The main reasons for this are the physiologic excretion of ^{18}F-FDG through the urinary tract and its proximity to prostate,[15] which can impair the visualization of the pelvic area, and the possible overlap of tracer accumulation in normal gland, benign prostatic hyperplasia, and prostate cancer.[16] ^{18}F-FDG shows higher uptake in poorly differentiated primary tumors,[17] due to the higher glucose metabolism. The glucose analog can be useful in case of biochemical relapse without standard imaging evidence of disease[18] and in men with advanced prostate cancer[19] to identify metabolically active bone lesions.[20] Finally, it is a valid tool in metastatic prostate cancer treatment evaluation. Its accumulation at metastatic sites tends to decrease with successful chemohormonal therapy.[21,22]

Fluorine-18/Carbon-11 Choline

Radiolabeled choline accumulates in prostate cancer[23] via the incorporation in the tumor cell membranes in the form of phosphatidylcholine.[24] The use of PET with either carbon-11 (^{11}C)-labeled choline or Fluorine-18 (^{18}F)-labeled choline for the detection of primary prostate cancer is controversial. As for ^{18}F-FDG, choline is unable to clearly distinguish normal prostate tissue from benign prostatic hyperplasia and prostate cancer.[25] In biochemical failure and restaging, ^{11}C-choline PET/CT has an important role for the evaluation of lymph nodes metastasis and extension of disease, even though its sensitivity is correlated to serum PSA levels, with an increase of sensitivity for high PSA values.[26] PET/CT with ^{11}C-choline is a good imaging tool for assessment of bone lesions. Many studies reported a change in patient management based on choline PET/CT findings, performed either as a first imaging study, or after bone scan scintigraphy.[27–30]

Carbon-11 Acetate

Acetate participates in cytoplasmic lipid synthesis, which is increased in tumors.[31] Carbon-11 acetate (^{11}C-acetate) has little renal excretion,[32] giving it an advantage over ^{18}F-FDG and choline in prostate cancer imaging. The tracer's uptake generally is higher in the tumor than in normal prostatic tissue and benign prostatic hyperplasia, even though there can be a considerable overlap.[33] ^{11}C-acetate may be useful in the detection of tumor recurrence after prostatectomy or radiation therapy, with a reported lesion detectability of 75%.[34–36] The median ^{11}C-acetate uptake is higher than ^{18}F-FDG for local recurrence and regional lymph node metastases, whereas the opposite happens with distant metastases.[37] No significant difference has been found between the use of ^{11}C-acetate and ^{11}C-choline in the detection of local recurrence after radical prostatectomy.[34] Like choline, the sensitivity of ^{11}C-acetate seems to be related to serum PSA value.[35]

Prostate-Specific Membrane Antigen

Prostate-specific membrane antigen (PSMA) is a transmembrane protein expressed in all types of prostatic tissues, including carcinoma.[38–43] Data from multicentric prospective trials are not currently available, but many investigators demonstrated a higher diagnostic efficacy of ^{68}Ga-PSMA compounds compared with conventional imaging, including PET using other tracers (eg, ^{18}F-choline and ^{11}C-choline).[44–49] In particular, ^{68}Ga-PSMA PET/CT seems to be a promising tool for staging of primary prostate cancer and restaging after biochemical recurrence. In biochemical relapse, ^{68}Ga-PSMA PET imaging can increase detection of metastatic sites, even at low serum PSA

Table 1
Major PET radiopharmaceuticals used in prostate cancer

	^{18}F-FDG	^{11}C/^{18}F-choline	^{11}C-acetate	PSMA Compounds	^{18}F-FACBC
Mechanism of uptake	Glucose metabolism	Fatty acid metabolism	Fatty acid metabolism	PSMA	Transmembrane amino acid transport
Diagnosis and staging	• Low sensitivity ○ Overlap uptake in tumor/benign prostatic hyperplasia/normal tissue • Higher uptake in poorly differentiated tumors	• Low sensitivity ○ Overlap uptake in tumor/benign prostatic hyperplasia/normal tissue • Detection rate correlated to PSA levels	• Generally higher uptake in tumor than benign prostate hyperplasia/normal tissue	• High diagnostic and staging efficacy	• High sensitivity in diagnosis of primary tumor
Biochemical relapse and re-staging	• Distant metastasis • Assessment of treatment response	• Evaluation of lymph node metastasis and extension of disease • Sensitivity increases with higher values of PSA • Assessment of bone metastasis	• Detection of tumor recurrence after prostatectomy or radiation • Sensitivity increases with higher values of PSA	• High sensitivity with low PSA level • PMSA > bone scan in the detection of bone metastasis	• Improvement in the detection rate of recurrent disease compared to other radio tracers

Abbreviation: ^{18}F-FACBC, fluorine-18 fluciclovine.

values.[50] A recent study reported detection rates of 73% and 58% in patients with biochemical recurrence after radical prostatectomy in a PSA range of 0.5 ng/mL to 1.0 ng/mL and 0.2 ng/mL to 0.5 ng/mL, respectively.[51] In intermediate-risk–high-risk patients with primary prostate cancer, PSMA improves detection of metastatic disease.[50] Pyka and colleagues[52] indicate that the detection rate of ^{68}Ga-PSMA for bone metastases is superior to traditional bone scan. PSMA can be also used for targeted radiation treatment. Interesting preliminary results are reported from both clinical studies with lutetium-177 (^{177}Lu) and preclinical studies using different radioactive isotopes.[53–57]

Fluorine-18 Fluciclovine

Anti-1-amino-3-^{18}F-fluorocyclobutane-1-carboxylic acid (fluorine-18 fluciclovine [^{18}F-FACBC]) is a promising radiopharmaceutical for PET imaging. It is a synthetic amino acid analog that reflects transmembrane amino acid transport, which is typically up-regulated in prostate cancer.[58] ^{18}F-FACBC has little renal excretion and bladder activity, which makes this radiotracer favorable in imaging of the prostate. ^{18}F-FACBC has been successful in the assessment of primary and metastatic prostate cancer[59,60] with reported sensitivity of 90% in localization of dominant prostate cancer.[61] Nanni and colleagues[62] reported greater image quality obtained with ^{18}F-FACBC compared with ^{11}C-choline, in terms of sharpness and target-to-background ratio. Some investigators describe an improvement of 20% to 30% in the detection rate of recurrent disease in comparison with other imaging radiotracers.[62,63]

BOMBESIN AND GASTRIN-RELEASING PEPTIDE RECEPTORS

Discovered in the 1970s by the Italian pharmacologist Vittorio Erspamer, bombesin is a natural 14–amino acid peptide. The interesting name choice is due to the initial isolation of the peptide from the skin of the European amphibians *Bombina bombina* and *Bombina variegata variegata*.[64] Bombesin was later found present in many other species,[65] but it was named after the genus of the frog from which it was initially isolated and subsequently gave the name to the bigger family of peptides, called bombesin-like peptides. The mammalian GRP is another component of the family.[66–69] It is a 27–amino acid peptide originally isolated from porcine stomach. GRP and bombesin have a similar structure, sharing a sequence of 7 carboxyl-terminal amino acids, which are essential for receptor binding and biological activity (**Fig. 1**). GRP is widely distributed in both the peripheral nervous system and peripheral tissues, particularly in the gastrointestinal tract.[70] In addition to its known physiologic functions,[71] it has been shown that several cancer cell lines, as well as primary human tumors, can also synthesize it. GRP explicates its role through G protein–coupled receptors with 7 transmembrane domains.[70] Four subtypes of bombesin receptors have been described, 3 of which are mammalian: the neuromedin B receptor (BB_1), GRPR (BB_2), and bombesin receptor subtype 3 (BB_3).[72] GRPRs are characterized by a high affinity binding for bombesin and GRP,[73] and the interaction of GRP with the GRPRs is responsible for the mitogenic activity of the former, which is now known to induce cell growth in various tumors.[70]

The recent rise of interest toward bombesin-like peptides comes from the discovery that various tumors, such as prostate cancers, breast cancers, small cell lung carcinomas, non–small cell lung carcinomas, and renal cell carcinomas, highly express the GRPRs.[73–78] In prostate cancer in particular, Bologna and colleagues[65] demonstrated in 1989 that bombesin dose-dependently stimulates the growth rate of PC-3 cell lines, androgen-independent human prostatic cancer epithelial cell lines. Furthermore, tumor cell growth can be

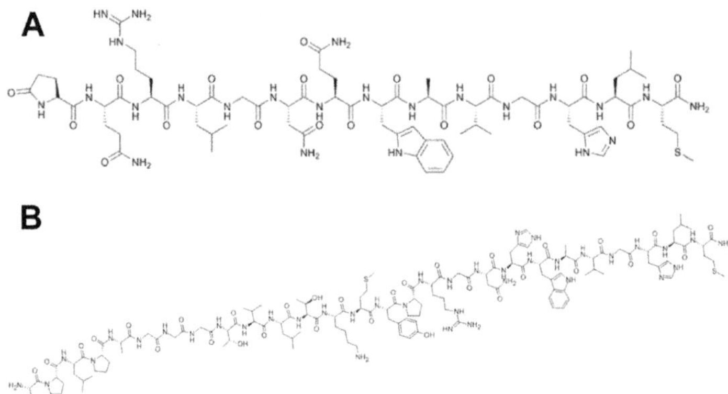

Fig. 1. Chemical structure and amino acid sequence of (*A*) bombesin and (*B*) GRP. Highlighted in bold is the amino acidic sequence shared between bombesin and GRP. (*A*) Bombesin: pGlu^1-Gly^2-Arg^3-Leu^4-Gly^5-Thr^6-Gln^7-Trp^8-Ala^9-Val^{10}-Gly^{11}-His^{12}-Leu^{13}-Met^{14}-NH_2. (*B*) GRP: H-Ala^1-Pro^2-Val^3-Ser^4-Val^5-Gly^6-Gly^7-Gly^8-Thr^9-Val^{10}-Leu^{11}-Ala^{12}-Lys^{13}-Met^{14}-Tyr^{15}-Pro^{16}-Arg^{17}-Gly^{18}-Asn^{19}-His^{20}-Trp^{21}-Ala^{22}-Val^{23}-Gly^{24}-His^{25}-Leu^{26}-Met^{27}-NH_2. ([*A*] *Courtesy of* Noel O'Boyle, PhD, Cambridge, United Kingdom.)

specifically inhibited by antibodies versus the GRP, due to a cross-reaction with bombesin. The action of bombesin on androgen-independent human prostate cancer cell lines (PC-3 and DU145) has been shown related to activation of nuclear factor κB and proangiogenic genes expression.[79] Levine and colleagues[79] demonstrated that this leads to up-regulation of interleukin-8 and vascular endothelial growth factor, key players in the process of neoangiogenesis and therefore crucial in conferring to prostate cancer cells the ability to proliferate and metastasize. In 1999, using autoradiography on human neoplastic and non-neoplastic prostatic tissues, Markwalder and Reubi[73] showed that GRPRs are overexpressed on the cell membranes of prostatic intraepithelial neoplasias and in primary prostate cancer, as opposed to normal prostate tissue and, in most cases, benign prostate hyperplasia. This important discovery spurred the interest of research toward the development of bombesin/GRP analogs, which could be used in therapeutic settings to inhibit tumor cell growth (GRPR antagonists with antiproliferative effect).[80] Another promising approach to bombesin analogs is radiolabeling for molecular imaging and peptide receptor radionuclide therapy (PRRT) of cancers.

Bombesin has recently emerged as an interesting nuclear medicine tool for tumor evaluation, in particular prostate cancer, for imaging and treatment purposes.

Gallium-68 Radiolabeling

Among all positron-emitting radioisotopes, ^{68}Ga is one of the most interesting due to several favorable characteristics. ^{68}Ga decays by β^+ emission for 89% (1.92 MeV, maximum energy of condition), and by orbital electron capture for 11%. It has a short half-life (67.71 minutes), compatible with the pharmacokinetics of most low-molecular-weight radiopharmaceuticals and convenient characteristics for PET imaging.[81] One of its most important advantages is the production from the long-lived parent germanium-68 (^{68}Ge) (half-life of 271 days) via an in-house ^{68}Ga/^{68}Ge generator, which allows an on-demand production of ^{68}Ga. Production of ^{68}Ga, therefore, does not require an onsite cyclotron, which represents a limiting factor for the widespread use of many radiopharmaceuticals and increases costs of cyclotron-produced radioisotopes. Some important progresses have been made since the first generation of ^{68}Ga/^{68}Ge generators developed in the 1960s,[82–84] which had some drawbacks limiting the extensive use of ^{68}Ga radiopharmaceuticals. Labeling yield of new commercially available generators is better than older ones but does not reach maximum levels yet. The short half-life of ^{68}Ga allows generator elution every 2 to 3 hours, and several applications in patients per day, but still not as many as for ^{18}F. New automated technologies, aimed at reducing the presence of metallic impurities and increasing specific radioactivity of the final product, are still a work in progress, and could potentially allow ^{68}Ga/^{68}Ge generators to become the workhorse of PET, just like molibdenum-99/technetium-99m (^{99}Mo/^{99m}Tc) is for single-photon emission CT (SPECT).[85]

Another advantage of ^{68}Ga-labeled radiopharmaceuticals is the ease of the radiolabeling procedure. ^{68}Ga can be labeled to chelator-conjugated biomolecules, with which it creates stable complexes, allowing kit production.[81,86] Different chelators can be used for ^{68}Ga radiolabeling, such as diethylenetriaminepentaacetic acid (DTPA) or the 1,4,7,10-tetraazacyclododecane-1,4,7,10-tetraacetic acid (DOTA). Different chelators, having different properties, give the molecule different kinetic properties and influence biodistribution of the radiolabeled molecule.[86]

^{68}Ga-labeled somatostatin analogs are successfully used for PET imaging neuroendocrine tumors (DOTATOC, DOTATATE, and DOTANOC). ^{68}Ga-labeled bombesin analogs are seen as promising emerging markers for different tumors, such as prostate cancer and breast cancer. The focus of this article is on bombesin analogs radiolabeled with ^{68}Ga for imaging of prostate cancer (**Table 2**), with the idea that these ^{68}Ga-labeled radiopharmaceuticals can have a significant clinical impact.

Gallium-68–Labeled Gastrin-Releasing Peptide Receptor Agonists

Initial research on bombesin analogs was aimed at finding molecules with good binding affinity and potency to the GRPR, for both imaging of and radionuclide therapy for GRPR-overexpressing cancers. The first category of bombesin analogs that has been explored is that of GRPR agonists, given their known ability to be internalized in GRPR-expressing cells. This was initially seen as a desirable characteristic, because it was considered essential for a prolonged retention in the targeted cell and therefore a prerequisite for high in vivo uptake. It was discovered, however, that GRPR agonists have a major drawback: a mitogenic effect.

^{68}Ga-AMBA is a potent ^{68}Ga-labeled GRPR agonist. The first clinical use of ^{68}Ga-AMBA was done by Baum and colleagues[87] in 2007 in 10 patients affected by different malignancies, including

Table 2
Gallium-68–bombesin analogs

Gastrin-Releasing Peptide Receptor Analogs	Radiopharmaceutical	Properties	Clinical Development	References
AMBA	^{68}Ga-AMBA	GRPR agonist	Clinical	Baum et al,[87] 2007
JMV594	^{68}Ga-NODAGA-JMV594	GRPR antagonist	Preclinical	Llinares et al,[92] 1999; Azay et al,[93] 1998; Tokita et al,[94] 2001; Sun et al,[103] 2016
RM1	^{68}Ga-DOTA-RM1	GRPR antagonist	Preclinical	Mansi et al,[96] 2009
RM2	^{68}Ga-RM2 (^{68}Ga-DOTA-RM2)	GRPR antagonist	Clinical	Kähkönen et al,[98] 2013; Roivanen et al,[99] 2013; Minamimoto et al,[100] 2016; Iagaru et al,[110] 2016
RM26	^{68}Ga-NOTA-P2-RM26	GRPR antagonist	Preclinical	Varasteh et al,[101] 2013
MJ9	^{68}Ga-NOTA-MJ9 ^{68}Ga-NODAGA-MJ9	GRPR antagonist	Preclinical	Gourni et al,[102] 2014
SB3	^{68}Ga-SB3	GRPR antagonist	Clinical	Maina et al,[104] 2016
SCH1	^{68}Ga-NODAGA-SCH1	GRPR antagonist	Preclinical	Sun et al,[103] 2016
NeoBOMB$_1$	^{68}Ga-NeoBOMB$_1$	GRPR antagonist	Clinical	Dalm et al,[107] 2016; Nock et al,[109] 2016
ZY1	^{68}Ga-NODAGA-ZY1	GRPR antagonist	Preclinical	Sun et al,[106] 2016
MATBBN	^{68}Ga-NOTA-MATBBN	GRPR antagonist	Preclinical	Pan et al,[105] 2014
DOTABOM	^{68}Ga-DOTABOM	GRPR antagonist	Clinical	Hofmann et al,[108] 2004

2 patients with prostate cancer. The radiopharmaceutical was well tolerated by patients, with only minor adverse effects and no significant uptake in other organs. ^{68}Ga-AMBA identified metastatic disease in 1 patient affected by prostate cancer and allowed following treatment with the same analog radiolabeled with ^{177}Lu (^{177}Lu-AMBA). The possibility of a theranostic application is an attractive feature of this molecule.[88–90]

The advent of many new GRPR antagonists, which showed similar if not better properties than agonists, including the absence of side effects and mitogenic activity, placed aside research on GRPR agonists.

Gallium-68–Gastrin-Releasing Peptide Receptor Antagonists

Interest of researchers toward GRPR antagonists increased after discovering that antagonists of somatostatin receptors were able to recognize more binding sites than agonists and had an even better uptake and retention in tumor cells in vivo compared with their corresponding radiolabeled agonist.[91] Furthermore, another important advantage of antagonists is their greater biosafety, due to the lacking internalization and therefore absence of mitogenic effect on the tumor cell, seen with agonists. The identification of a stable molecule with a high binding affinity to the GRPR, and which could possibly be radiolabeled with β^+ (for PET imaging) and β^- (for PRRT), is an important area of research. Several GRPR antagonists have been developed and are at different stages of clinical and preclinical development.

Statine-based GRPR antagonists are the most studied family of bombesin analogs. Different groups[92–94] developed, in the 1990s, several potent GRPR antagonists belonging to the family, including JMV641[95] and JMV594. The latter was obtained by modifying a bombesin agonist (D-Phe6-bombesin[6–14]) in the C-terminal part (Leu-13 and Leu-14) and was later radiolabeled with ^{68}Ga but, to the authors' knowledge, not yet used in clinical studies. JMV594 was modified by adding different spacers and chelators, and it was made suitable for labeling with different radiometals, for PET and SPECT imaging and for therapy. Mansi and colleagues[96] synthesized a new statine-based GRPR antagonist, RM1

(DOTA-Gly-aminobenzoic acid-D-Phe-Gln-Trp-Ala-Val-Gly-His-Sta-Leu-NH_2), by adding glycine-4-aminobenzoyl and the chelator DOTA to JMV594. ^{68}Ga–DOTA-RM1 was used in PC-3 tumor-bearing mice and confirmed high and specific accumulation in the tumor. In 2011, Mansi and colleagues[97] developed another molecule, RM2, formerly also known as BAY86-7548 (DOTA-4-amino-1-carboxymethyl-piperidine-D-Phe-Gln-Trp-Ala-Val-Gly-His-Sta-Leu-NH_2), that was radiolabeled with ^{68}Ga and studied in preclinical prostate cancer tumor models in healthy men and prostate cancer patients.[98–100] In 2013, Varasteh and colleagues[101] developed a new ^{68}Ga-labeled imaging agent based on a 9–amino acid bombesin analog, RM26 (D-Phe-Gln-Trp-Ala-Val-Gly-His-Sta-Leu-NH_2), using 1,4,7-triazacyclononane-1,4,7-triacetic acid (NOTA) and the synthetic polymer, diethylene glycol (PEG2). The radiopharmaceutical showed high and specific uptake in PC-3 xenografts and high tumor-to-background ratios and, therefore, could potentially be used in clinical studies.

In 2014, Gourni and colleagues[102] reported results obtained with a new peptide-chelator conjugate, MJ9 (H-4-amino-1-carboxymethyl-piperidine-D-Phe-Gln-Trp-Ala-Val-Gly-His-Sta-Leu-NH_2), which was radiolabeled with ^{68}Ga using 2 different chelators, that is, NOTA (^{68}Ga–NOTA-MJ9) and NODAGA (^{68}Ga–NOTA-MJ9). MJ9 came after the discovery of the excellent pharmacokinetic performances of the previously developed statine-based bombesine analogs (ie, RM1 and RM2) and was synthesized with the intent to improve, even more, binding affinity and pharmacokinetics of radiolabeled GRPR antagonists. Of the 2 ^{68}Ga-labeled MJ9 conjugates, NODAGA-MJ9 showed some advantages and is currently in some phase I clinical studies. In 2011, Sun and colleagues[102] developed a novel bombesin analog, SCH1, modifying the original peptide JMV594 and adding NODAGA as chelator for ^{68}Ga radiolabeling. ^{68}Ga–NODAGA-SCH1 was compared with ^{68}Ga–NODAGA-JMV594 and showed excellent properties on PC-3 tumor-bearing nude mice, such as high tumor uptake and high tumor-to-background ratio, representing a good candidate for translation into clinical PET studies.

Recently, Maina and colleagues[104] introduced a new ^{68}Ga-labeled bombesin analog belonging to a different class (the C-terminal amide derivative), ^{68}Ga-SB3, which is a mimic of ^{99m}Tc-DB1. The study describes results from preclinical (on mice bearing PC-3 xenografts) and first clinical experience with the PET imaging agent. Results of the clinical study is discussed later.

Other ^{68}Ga-labeled radiopharmaceuticals that showed favorable properties and pharmacokinetics are ^{68}Ga–NOTA-MATBBN, developed by Pan and colleagues,[105] and, more recently ^{68}Ga–NODAGA-ZY1, by Sun and colleagues,[106] and ^{68}Ga-NeoBOMB1, by Dalm and colleagues.[107] ^{68}Ga-NeoBOMB1 was developed together with the ^{177}Lu-labeled analog for theranostics purposes.[107]

Clinical Use of Bombesin Analogs

Despite the number of ^{68}Ga-labeled bombesin analogs developed for PET imaging/PRRT therapy continuously growing, at present, few of the radiopharmaceuticals have made it to the next step in clinical settings. Among those that made it are ^{68}Ga-AMBA[87] (GRPR agonist), ^{68}Ga-DOTABOM, ^{68}Ga-SB3, and ^{68}Ga-RM2 (GRPR antagonists). The clinical experience with the GRPR agonist AMBA is discussed previously.

Among GRPR antagonists translated clinically and studied in prostate cancer patients, there is ^{68}Ga-DOTABOM. Hofmann and colleagues[108] evaluated ^{68}Ga-DOTABOM in 11 patients, finding rapid renal excretion and early, 12-minute to 25-minute peak tumor uptake. ^{68}Ga-DOTABOM was able to identify tumor sites in lesions subsequently proved pathologic with histology. Results with this radiopharmaceutical were promising in primary tumor and locoregional metastasis detection.

Maina and colleagues[104] used ^{68}Ga-SB3 in a study of 17 patients, 9 men with prostate cancer and 8 women with breast cancer. All patients included in the clinical study had disseminated recurrent disease, and many of them had a history of previous therapies (including antihormonal therapy), which could potentially reduce expression of GRPR on tumor cells. Despite this aspect, ^{68}Ga–SB3 PET/CT was positive in 55% of prostate cancer patients (5 patients of 9).

Nock and colleagues[109] recently studied an antagonist, NeoBOMB1, in patients with prostate cancer. The investigators reported that independent of the radiometal applied, this GRPR antagonist has shown comparable behavior in prostate cancer models, in favor of future theranostic use in GRPR-positive cancer patients.

The most widely used ^{68}Ga-labeled bombesin analog in clinical settings is ^{68}Ga-RM2 (**Fig. 2**). In 2013, Roivainen and colleagues[99] published the first study conducted on 5 healthy men using ^{68}Ga–RM2 PET/CT. The investigators investigated plasma pharmacokinetics, whole-body distribution, metabolism, and radiation dosimetry of the bombesin antagonists. The study demonstrated fast blood and renal clearance, with rapid

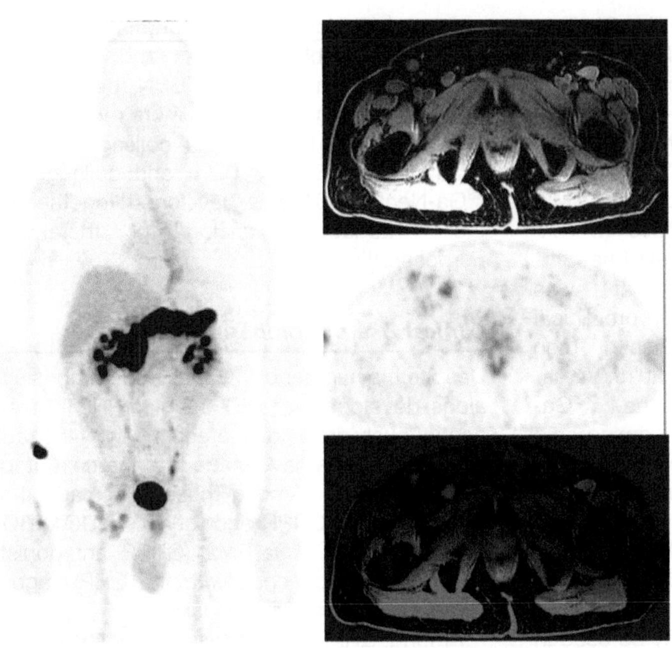

Fig. 2. A 72-year-old man with Gleason score 4 + 3 diagnosed in 2011 and treated with radiation therapy and hormonal therapy. Biochemical recurrence was diagnosed in 2014 with PSA of 1.36 ng/mL. PSA at the time the study was 20.3 ng/mL. Images were acquired after injection of 3.62 mCi of ^{68}Ga-RM2 and show focal uptake in right inguinal lymph nodes. Biopsy results indicated metastatic adenocarcinoma of prostate origin (*left panel*, maximum intensity projection; *top right panel*, axial T1 weighted image; *middle right panel*, axial PET image; *bottom right panel*, axial PET/MRI fused image).

excretion through the urinary bladder, highest radioactivity in the pancreas (in line with GRPR expression), and the production of three radioactive metabolites, which may alter distribution of the tracer. In terms of radiation dosimetry, ^{68}Ga-RM2 showed slightly higher radiation burden to other ^{68}Ga-labeled radiopharmaceuticals. The higher absorbed doses were detected in the urinary bladder wall (0.61 mSv/MBq) followed by the pancreas. In the same year, Kähkönen and colleagues[98] published the first human study with ^{68}Ga–RM2 PET/CT in 14 men with prostate cancer, 11 of whom were scheduled for radical prostatectomy (PSA levels ranging from 6.2 ng/mL to 45 ng/mL) and 3 had biochemical recurrence after surgery or hormonal therapy (PSA levels ranging from 0.36 ng/mL to 282 ng/mL). Quantitative analysis showed that average maximum standardized uptake value and mean standardized uptake value in pathologic lesions (6.6 $\pm$ 4.7 and 5.1 $\pm$ 3.7, respectively) were different from those of benign prostatic hypertrophy (2.4 $\pm$ 1.5 and 1.8 $\pm$ 1.2, respectively) and normal tissue of the peripheral zone (1.3 $\pm$ 1.0 and 1.0 $\pm$ 0.9, respectively); 2 patients underwent an ^{11}C-acetate PET/CT and 1 an ^{18}F-choline PET/CT. Results from the 2 studies were compared with those of ^{68}Ga–RM2 PET/CT. Using histology as gold standard, the investigators found a sensitivity of 88%, specificity of 81%, and accuracy of 83% for detection of primary prostate cancer and a sensitivity of 70% for the detection of metastatic lymph nodes. The comparison with ^{11}C-acetate and ^{18}F-choline showed concordance with the former, identifying local recurrence in the prostate bed and nodal relapse, and discordance with the latter, because of failure to detect multiple bone metastases in one patient.

The authors' group[100] recently published a pilot comparison of ^{68}Ga–RM2 PET/MR imaging with ^{68}Ga–PSMA-11 PET/CT in 7 patients with biochemically recurrent prostate cancer (PSA range 13.5 ng/mL $\pm$ 11.5 ng/mL) and noncontributory results on conventional imaging (bone scan, CT, and/or MR imaging). All patients underwent both ^{68}Ga–RM2 PET/MR imaging and ^{68}Ga–PSMA-11 PET/CT within a time period ranging from 13 days to 85 days. The study highlighted the known differences in biodistribution of the 2 PET radiopharmaceuticals, such as different excretion (both renal and hepatobiliary for PSMA-11 and mainly renal for RM2), which could have implications in the detection of pelvic and abdominal lesions. PSMA-11 clearance in the bowel made small retroperitoneal lymph nodes less conspicuous in 2 patients compared with RM2. The 2 radiopharmaceuticals showed similar but not identical uptake patterns of distribution in the suspected lesions, which may be due to the heterogeneous expression of PSMA and GRP, or to changes in expression of their receptors in the course of disease. In the authors' most recent experience with ^{68}Ga–RM2 PET/MR imaging, 30 patients were included with biochemical recurrence of prostate cancer and negative conventional imaging.[110]

^{68}Ga–RM2 PET identified recurrent disease in 20 of the 30 patients, whereas MR imaging found disease in 9 of the 30 patients.

FUTURE PERSPECTIVES

The research for a sensitive and specific PET radiopharmaceutical for prostate cancer imaging is still very active. All available tracers have drawbacks, such as difficulty of clearly differentiating malignant from benign prostate tissue, which limit their widespread clinical use. The discovery that GRPRs are highly expressed on prostate cancer cells, as opposed to normal prostate tissue and benign hypertrophy,[71] spurred great interest toward the development of bombesin/GRP analogs targeting the GRPR. An important aspect that needs to be taken into account is the presence of factors potentially altering expression of GRPRs on prostate cancer cells, such as the androgen regulation. A clear understanding of their correlation will help better define the role of bombesin analogs in imaging and therapy, because it may differ depending on stages of disease. More investigations are needed, therefore, in clarifying this aspect.

Several bombesin analogs have been developed to date for PET imaging of prostate cancer, and some have also been coupled to β-emitting radioisotopes for a theranostic approach to the disease. GRPR agonists were initially considered preferable to antagonists, due to their ability to be internalized in the cell. This characteristic was seen as a prerequisite for high in vivo uptake and led to the development of GRPR agonists for radiolabeling. As a result of the discovery that GRPR agonists have a mitogenic effect, and that antagonists have a higher tumor uptake and retention time in the cell, the latter category took priority in research.

^{68}Ga is one of the most interesting radioisotopes for PET imaging, due to several advantages, including on-demand production with low costs, convenient characteristics for PET imaging, and ease of the radiolabeling procedure. Furthermore, the combination chemistry of ^{68}Ga, which is similar to that of the β-emitting ^{177}Lu, makes it an ideal isotope for radiolabeling the same vector molecules for theranostic applications.[111] ^{68}Ga has been used for radiolabeling bombesin analogs in a large number of studies. Although several molecules targeting the GRPR have been developed, only a few of them have been translated into clinical settings. A few clinical studies have been conducted so far, and those available include small cohorts of patients. Further studies need to be carried out, either comparing different bombesin analogs, for identifying the most promising ones, or directly comparing them with other available prostate cancer imaging biomarkers. Because targeting the GRPR focuses on only 1 biological property of the malignant prostate cancer cell, perhaps a promising approach would be combining 2 different molecules targeting different antigens overexpressed on tumor cells using hybrid peptides.[112]

REFERENCES

1. Attard G, Parker C, Eeles RA, et al. Prostate cancer. Lancet 2016;387:70–82.
2. Siegel RL, Miller KD, Jemal A. Cancer statistics, 2016. CA Cancer J Clin 2016;66:7–30.
3. Surveillance, Epidemiology, and End Results (SEER) Program. SEER Stat Fact Sheets: Prostate. Available at: http://seer.cancer.gov/statfacts/ html/ prost.html. Accessed November 19, 2010.
4. Ward JF, Moul JW. Rising prostate-specific antigen after primary prostate cancer therapy. Nat Clin Pract Urol 2005;2:174–82.
5. Picchio M, Mapelli P, Panebianco V, et al. Imaging biomarkers in prostate cancer: role of PET/CT and MRI. Eur J Nucl Med Mol Imaging 2015;42:644–55.
6. Hayes JH, Barry MJ. Screening for prostate cancer with the prostate-specific antigen test: a review of current evidence. JAMA 2014;311:1143–9.
7. Draisma G, Etzioni R, Tsodikov A, et al. Lead time and overdiagnosis in prostate-specific antigen screening: importance of methods and context. J Natl Cancer Inst 2009;101:374–83.
8. Bill-Axelson A, Holmberg L, Ruutu M, et al. Radical prostatectomy versus watchful waiting in early prostate cancer. N Engl J Med 2011;364(18): 1708–17.
9. Wilt TJ, Brawer MK, Jones KM, et al. Radical prostatectomy versus observation for localized prostate cancer. N Engl J Med 2012;367(3):203–13.
10. Widmark A, Klepp O, Solberg A, et al. Endocrine treatment, with or without radiotherapy, in locally advanced prostate cancer (SPCG-7/SFUO-3): an open randomised phase III trial. Lancet (London, England) 2009;373(9660):301–8.
11. Warde P, Mason M, Ding K, et al. Combined androgen deprivation therapy and radiation therapy for locally advanced prostate cancer: a randomised, phase 3 trial. Lancet 2011;378(9809): 2104–11.
12. Horwitz EM, Bae K, Hanks GE, et al. Ten-year follow-up of radiation therapy oncology group protocol 92-02: a phase III trial of the duration of elective androgen deprivation in locally advanced prostate cancer. J Clin Oncol 2008; 26(15):2497–504.

13. Denham JW, Steigler A, Lamb DS, et al. Short-term neoadjuvant androgen deprivation and radiotherapy for locally advanced prostate cancer: 10-year data from the TROG 96.01 randomised trial. Lancet Oncol 2011;12(5):451–9.
14. Gillies RJ, Robey I, Gatenby RA. Causes and consequences of increased glucose metabolism of cancers. J Nucl Med 2008;49(Suppl 2):24S–42S.
15. Liu IJ, Zafar MB, Lai YH, et al. Fluorodeoxyglucose positron emission tomography studies in diagnosis and staging of clinically organ-confined prostate cancer. Urology 2001;57:108–11.
16. Salminen E, Hogg A, Binns D, et al. Investigations with FDG-PET scanning in prostate cancer show limited value for clinical practice. Acta Oncol 2002;41:425–9.
17. Oyama N, Akino H, Suzuki Y, et al. The increased accumulation of [18F]fluorodeoxyglucose in untreated prostate cancer. Jpn J Clin Oncol 1999; 29:623–9.
18. Jadvar H. Prostate cancer: PET with 18F-FDG, 18F- or 11C-acetate, and 18F- or 11C-choline. J Nucl Med 2011;52:81–9.
19. Fox JJ, Morris MJ, Larson SM, et al. Developing imaging strategies for castration resistant prostate cancer. Acta Oncol 2011;50(Suppl 1):39–48.
20. Morris MJ, Akhurst T, Osman I, et al. Fluorinated deoxyglucose positron emission tomography imaging in progressive metastatic prostate cancer. Urology 2002;59:913–8.
21. Oyama N, Akino H, Suzuki Y, et al. FDG PET for evaluating the change of glucose metabolism in prostate cancer after androgen ablation. Nucl Med Commun 2001;22:963–9.
22. Jadvar H, Desai B, Quinn D, et al. Treatment response assessment of metastatic prostate cancer with FDG PET/CT. J Nucl Med 2011;52(Suppl 1):1908.
23. Jadvar H, Gurbuz A, Li X, et al. Choline autoradiography of human prostate cancer xenograft: effect of castration. Mol Imaging 2008;7:147–52.
24. Breeuwsma AJ, Pruim J, Jongen MM, et al. In vivo uptake of [11C]choline does not correlate with cell proliferation in human prostate cancer. Eur J Nucl Med Mol Imaging 2005;32:668–73.
25. Schwarzenböck S, Souvatzoglou M, Krause BJ. Choline PET and PET/CT in primary diagnosis and staging of prostate cancer. Theranostics 2012;2(3):318–30.
26. Krause BJ, Souvatzoglou M, Tuncel M, et al. The detection rate of [11C]choline-PET/CT depends on the serum PSA-value in patients with biochemical recurrence of prostate cancer. Eur J Nucl Med Mol Imaging 2008;35:18–23.
27. Fuccio C, Castellucci P, Schiavina R, et al. Role of 11C-choline PET/CT in the re-staging of prostate cancer patients with biochemical relapse and negative results at bone scintigraphy. Eur J Radiol 2012;81:e893–6.
28. Segall GM. PET/CT with sodium 18F-fluoride for management of patients with prostate cancer. J Nucl Med 2014;55:531–3.
29. Poulsen MH, Petersen H, Hoilund-Carlsen PF, et al. Spine metastases in prostate cancer: comparison of technetium-99m-MDP whole-body bone scintigraphy, [(18) F]choline positron emission tomography(PET)/computed tomography (CT) and [(18) F]NaF PET/CT. BJU Int 2014;114:818–23.
30. Picchio M, Spinapolice EG, Fallanca F, et al. [11C] Choline PET/CT detection of bone metastases in patients with PSA progression after primary treatment for prostate cancer: comparison with bone scintigraphy. Eur J Nucl Med Mol Imaging 2012;39:13–26.
31. Yoshimoto M, Waki A, Yonekura Y, et al. Characterization of acetate metabolism in tumor cells in relation to cell proliferation: acetate metabolism in tumor cells. Nucl Med Biol 2001;28:117–22.
32. Song WS, Nielson BR. Normal organ standard uptake values in carbon-11 acetate PET imaging. Nucl Med Comm 2009;30(6):462–5.
33. Kato T, Tsukamoto E, Kuge Y, et al. Accumulation of [11C]acetate in normal prostate and benign prostatic hyperplasia: comparison with prostate cancer. Eur J Nucl Med Mol Imaging 2002;29:1492–5.
34. Kotzerke J, Volkmer BG, Neumaier B, et al. Carbon-11 acetate positron emission tomography can detect local recurrence of prostate cancer. Eur J Nucl Med Mol Imaging 2002;29:1380–4.
35. Oyama N, Miller TR, Dehdashti F, et al. 11C-acetate PET imaging of prostate cancer: detection of recurrent disease at PSA relapse. J Nucl Med 2003;44: 549–55.
36. Sandblom G, Sorensen J, Lundin N, et al. Positron emission tomography with 11C-acetate for tumor detection and localization in patients with prostate specific antigen relapse after radical prostatectomy. Urology 2006;67:996–1000.
37. Fricke E, Machtens S, Hofmann M, et al. Positron emission tomography with 11C-acetate and 18F-FDG in prostate cancer patients. Eur J Nucl Med Mol Imaging 2003;30:607–11.
38. Ross JS, Sheehan CE, Fisher HAG, et al. Correlation of primary tumor prostate-specific membrane antigen expression with disease recurrence in prostate cancer. Clin Cancer Res 2003;9:6357–62.
39. Horoszewicz JS, Kawinski E, Murphy GP. Monoclonal antibodies to a new antigenic marker in epithelial cells and serum of prostatic cancer patients. Anticancer Res 1987;7:927–36.
40. Lopes AD, Davis WL, Rosenstraus MJ, et al. Immunohistochemical and pharmacokinetic characterization of the site-specific immunoconjugate CYT-356 derived from antiprostate monoclonal antibody 7E11-C5. Cancer Res 1990;50:6423–9.

41. Israeli RS, Miller WH Jr, Su SL, et al. Sensitive nested reverse transcription polymerase chain reaction detection of circulating prostatic tumor cells: comparison of prostate-specific membrane antigen and prostate-specific antigen-based assays. Cancer Res 1994;54:6306–10.
42. Silver DA, Pellicer I, Fair WR, et al. Prostate specific membrane antigen expression in normal and malignant human tissues. Clin Cancer Res 1997;3: 81–5.
43. Troyer JK, Beckett ML, Wright GL Jr. Detection and characterization of the prostate-specific membrane antigen (PSMA) in tissue extracts and body fluids. Int J Cancer 1995;62:552–8.
44. Afshar-Oromieh A, Zechmann CM, Malcher A, et al. Comparison of PET imaging with a (68)Ga-labelled PSMA ligand and (18)F-choline-based PET/CT for the diagnosis of recurrent prostate cancer. Eur J Nucl Med Mol Imaging 2014;41(1):11–20.
45. Eiber M, Weirich G, Holzapfel K, et al. Simultaneous Ga-PSMA HBED-CC PET/MRI improves the localization of primary prostate cancer. Eur Urol 2016;70(5):829–36.
46. Maurer T, Gschwend JE, Rauscher I, et al. Diagnostic efficacy of gallium-PSMA positron emission tomography compared to conventional imaging in lymph node staging of 130 consecutive patients with intermediate to high risk prostate cancer. J Urol 2016;195(5):1436–43.
47. Eiber M, Maurer T, Souvatzoglou M, et al. Evaluation of hybrid (6)(8)Ga-PSMA ligand PET/CT in 248 patients with biochemical recurrence after radical prostatectomy. J Nucl Med 2015;56(5): 668–74.
48. Afshar-Oromieh A, Avtzi E, Giesel FL, et al. The diagnostic value of PET/CT imaging with the (68) Ga-labelled PSMA ligand HBED-CC in the diagnosis of recurrent prostate cancer. Eur J Nucl Med Mol Imaging 2015;42(2):197–209.
49. Roethke MC, Kuru TH, Afshar-Oromieh A, et al. Hybrid positron emission tomography-magnetic resonance imaging with gallium 68 prostate-specific membrane antigen tracer: a next step for imaging of recurrent prostate cancer-preliminary results. Eur Urol 2013;64(5):862–4.
50. Maurer T, Eiber M, Schwaiger M, et al. Current use of PSMA–PET in prostate cancer management. Nat Rev Urol 2016;13:226–35.
51. Eiber M, Pyka T, Okamoto S, et al. 68 Gallium-HBED-CC-PSMA PET compared to conventional bone scintigraphy for evaluation of bone metastases in prostate cancer patients. Eur Urol Supplements 2016;15(3).
52. Pyka T, Okamoto S, Dahlbender M, et al. Comparison of bone scintigraphy and 68Ga-PSMA PET for skeletal staging in prostate cancer. Eur J Nucl Med Mol Imaging 2016;43(12):2114–21.
53. Kulkarni H, Singh A, Niepsch K, et al. PSMA radioligand therapy (PRLT) of metastatic castration-resistant prostate cancer: first results using the PSMA Inhibitor 617. J Nucl Med 2016;57:139.
54. Rahbar K, Bode A, Weckesser M, et al. Radioligand therapy with Lu-177-PSMA-617 may improve survival in patients with metastatic prostate Cancer. J Nucl Med 2016;57:142.
55. Rahbar K, Schmidt M, Heinzel A, et al. Response and tolerability after a single dose of Lu-177-PSMA-617 in patients with metastatic castration resistant prostate cancer: a multicenter Study. J Nucl Med 2016;57:140.
56. Kiess A, Minn IL, Vaidyanathan G, et al. [211At]YC-I-27 for PSMA-targeted alpha-particle radiopharmaceutical therapy. J Nucl Med 2016;57:143.
57. Chatalic K, Nonnekens J, Bruchertseifer F, et al. 213Bi-labeled PSMA-targeting agents for alpha radionuclide therapy of prostate cancer. J Nucl Med 2016;57:137.
58. Okudaira H, Oka S, Ono M, et al. Accumulation of trans-1-amino-3-[(18)F]fluorocyclobutanecarboxylic acid in prostate cancer due to androgen-induced expression of amino acid transporters. Mol Imaging Biol 2014;16(6):756–64.
59. Schuster DM, Votaw JR, Nieh PT, et al. Initial experience with the radiotracer anti-1-amino-3-18F-fluorocyclobutane-1-carboxylic acid with PET/CT in prostate carcinoma. J Nucl Med 2007;48(1):56–63.
60. Sörensen J, Owenius R, Lax M, et al. Regional distribution and kinetics of [18F]fluciclovine (anti-[18F]FACBC), a tracer of amino acid transport, in subjects with primary prostate cancer. Eur J Nucl Med Mol Imaging 2013;40(3):394–402.
61. Turkbey B, Mena E, Shih J, et al. Localized prostate cancer detection with 18F FACBC PET/CT: comparison with MR imaging and histopathologic analysis. Radiology 2014;270(3):849–56.
62. Nanni C, Schiavina R, Boschi S, et al. Comparison of 18F-FACBC and 11C-choline PET/CT in patients with radically treated prostate cancer and biochemical relapse: preliminary results. Eur J Nucl Med Mol Imaging 2013;40(Suppl 1):11–7.
63. Schuster DM, Savir-Baruch D, Nieh P, et al. Detection of recurrent prostate carcinoma with anti-3-18F-fluorocyclobutane-1-carboxylic acid PET/CT and 111In-capromab pendetide SPECT/CT. Radiology 2011;259:852–61.
64. Erspamer V, Erpamer GF, Inselvini M. Some pharmacological actions of alytesin and bombesin. J Pharm Pharmacol 1970;22(11):875–6.
65. Bologna M, Festuccia C, Muzi P, et al. Bombesin stimulates growth of human prostatic cancer cells in vitro. Cancer 1989;63(9):1714–20.
66. Erspamer V. Discovery, isolation, and characterization of bombesin-like peptides. Ann N Y Acad Sci 1988;547:3–9.

67. Brown M, Marki W, Rivier J. Is gastrin releasing peptide mammalian bombesin? Life Sci 1980; 27(2):125–8.
68. McDonald TJ, Jornvall H, Nilsson G, et al. Characterization of a gastrin releasing peptide from porcine non-antral gastric tissue. Biochem Biophys Res Commun 1979;90(1):227–33.
69. McDonald TJ, Nilsson G, Vagne M, et al. A gastrin releasing peptide from the porcine nonantral gastric tissue. Gut 1978;19(9):767–74.
70. Jensen RT, Battey JF, Spindel ER, et al. International Union of Pharmacology. LXVIII. Mammalian bombesin receptors: nomenclature, distribution, pharmacology, signaling, and functions in normal and disease states. Pharmacol Rev 2008;60(1): 1–42.
71. Ohki-Hamazaki H, Iwabuchi M, Maekawa F. Development and function of bombesin-like peptides and their receptors. Int J Dev Biol 2005;49(2–3): 293–300.
72. Schroeder RP, van Weerden WM, Krenning EP, et al. Gastrin-releasing peptide receptor-based targeting using bombesin analogues is superior to metabolism-based targeting using choline for in vivo imaging of human prostate cancer xenografts. Eur J Nucl Med Mol Imaging 2011;38(7): 1257–66.
73. Markwalder R, Reubi JC. Gastrin-releasing peptide receptors in the human prostate: relation to neoplastic transformation. Cancer Res 1999; 59(5):1152–9.
74. Gugger M, Reubi JC. Gastrin-releasing peptide receptors in non-neoplastic and neoplastic human breast. Am J Pathol 1999;155(6):2067–76.
75. Moody TW, Zia F, Venugopal R, et al. GRP receptors are present in non small cell lung cancer cells. J Cell Biochem Suppl 1996;24:247–56.
76. Sun B, Halmos G, Schally AV, et al. Presence of receptors for bombesin/gastrin-releasing peptide and mRNA for three receptor subtypes in human prostate cancers. Prostate 2000;42(4):295–303.
77. Pansky A, De Weerth A, Fasler-Kan E, et al. Gastrin releasing peptide-preferring bombesin receptors mediate growth of human renal cell carcinoma. J Am Soc Nephrol 2000;11(8):1409–18.
78. Reubi JC, Wenger S, Schmuckli-Maurer J, et al. Bombesin receptor subtypes in human cancers: detection with the universal radioligand (125)I-[D-TYR(6), beta-ALA(11), PHE(13), NLE(14)] bombesin(6-14). Clin Cancer Res 2002;8(4):1139–46.
79. Levine L, Lucci JA 3rd, Pazdrak B, et al. Bombesin stimulates nuclear factor kappa B activation and expression of proangiogenic factors in prostate cancer cells. Cancer Res 2003;63(13):3495–502.
80. Stangelberger A, Schally AV, Djavan B. New treatment approaches for prostate cancer based on peptide analogues. Eur Urol 2008;53(5):890–900.
81. Maecke HR, Hofmann M, Haberkorn U. (68)Ga-labeled peptides in tumor imaging. J Nucl Med 2005;46(Suppl 1):172s–8s.
82. Gleason GI. A positron cow. Int J Appl Radiat Isotopes 1960;8:90–4.
83. Yano Y, Anger HO. A gallium-68 positron cow for medical use. J Nucl Med 1964;5:484–7.
84. Greene WT, Tucker WD. An improved gallium-68 cow. Int J Appl Radiat Isotopes 1961;12:62–3.
85. Chakravarty R, Chakraborty S, Ram R, et al. Detailed evaluation of different (68)Ge/(68)Ga generators: an attempt toward achieving efficient (68) Ga radiopharmacy. J Labeled Compd Radiopharm 2016;59(3):87–94.
86. Asti M, Iori M, Capponi PC, et al. Influence of different chelators on the radiochemical properties of a 68-Gallium labelled bombesin analogue. Nucl Med Biol 2014;41(1):24–35.
87. Baum R, Parsad V, Mutloka N, et al. Molecular imaging of bombesin receptors in various tumors by Ga-68 AMBA PET/CT: first results. J Nucl Med 2007;48(Suppl 2):79. Available at: http://jnm.snmjournals.org/content/48/supplement_2/79P.2.
88. Lantry LE, Cappelletti E, Maddalena ME, et al. ^{177}Lu-AMBA: synthesis and characterization of a selective ^{177}Lu-labeled GRP-R agonist for systemic radiotherapy of prostate cancer. J Nucl Med 2006; 47:1144–52.
89. Chen J, Linder KE, Cagnolini A, et al. Synthesis, stabilization and formulation of [^{177}Lu]Lu-AMBA, a systemic radiotherapeutic agent for gastrin releasing peptide receptor positive tumors. Appl Radiat Isot 2008;66:497–505.
90. Maddalena ME, Fox J, Chen J, et al. 177Lu-AMBA biodistribution, radiotherapeutic efficacy, imaging, and autoradiography in prostate cancer models with low GRP-R expression. J Nucl Med 2009; 50(12):2014–7.
91. Ginj M, Zhang H, Waser B, et al. Radiolabeled somatostatin receptor antagonists are preferable to agonists for in vivo peptide receptor targeting of tumors. Proc Natl Acad Sci U S A 2006;103: 16436–41.
92. Llinares M, Devin C, Chaloin O, et al. Syntheses and biological activities of potent bombesin receptor antagonists. J Pept Res 1999;53:275–83.
93. Azay J, Nagain C, Llinares M, et al. Comparative study of in vitro and in vivo activities of bombesin pseudopeptide analogs modified on the C-terminal dipeptide fragment. Peptides 1998;19(1):57–63.
94. Tokita K, Katsuno T, Hocart SJ, et al. Molecular basis for selectivity of high affinity peptide antagonists for the gastrin-releasing peptide receptor. J Biol Chem 2001;276(39):36652–63.
95. Azay J, Gagne D, Devin C, et al. JMV641: a potent bombesin receptor antagonist that inhibits Swiss 3T3 cell proliferation. Regul Pept 1996;65(1):91–7.

96. Mansi R, Wang X, Forrer F, et al. Evaluation of a 1,4,7,10- tetraazacyclododecane-1,4,7,10-tetraacetic acid-conjugated bombesin-based radioantagonist for the labeling with single-photon emission computed tomography, positron emission tomography, and therapeutic radionuclides. Clin Cancer Res 2009;15(16): 5240–9.
97. Mansi R, Wang X, Forrer F, et al. Development of a potent DOTA-conjugated bombesin antagonist for targeting GRPr-positive tumours. Eur J Nucl Med Mol Imaging 2011;38(1):97–107.
98. Kähkönen E, Jambor I, Kemppainen J, et al. In vivo imaging of prostate cancer using [68Ga]-labeled bombesin analog BAY86-7548. Clin Cancer Res 2013;19:5434–43.
99. Roivainen A, Kähkönen E, Luoto P, et al. Plasma pharmacokinetics, whole-body distribution, metabolism, and radiation dosimetry of 68Ga bombesin antagonist BAY 86-7548 in healthy men. J Nucl Med 2013;54(6):867–72.
100. Minamimoto R, Hancock S, Schneider B, et al. Pilot comparison of ^{68}Ga-RM2 PET and ^{68}Ga-PSMA-11 PET in patients with biochemically recurrent prostate Cancer. J Nucl Med 2016;57:557–62.
101. Varasteh Z, Velikyan I, Lindeberg G, et al. Synthesis and characterization of a high-affinity NOTA-conjugated bombesin antagonist for GRPR-targeted tumor imaging. Bioconjug Chem 2013;24:1144–53.
102. Gourni E, Mansi R, Jamous M, et al. N-terminal modifications improve the receptor affinity and pharmacokinetics of radiolabeled peptidic gastrin-releasing peptide receptor antagonists: examples of 68Ga- and 64Cu-labeled peptides for PET imaging. J Nucl Med 2014;55(10):1719–25.
103. Sun Y, Ma X, Zhang Z, et al. Preclinical study on GRPR-targeted ^{68}Ga-probes for PET imaging of prostate cancer. Bioconjug Chem 2016;27(8): 1857–64.
104. Maina T, Bergsma H, Kulkarni HR, et al. Preclinical and first clinical experience with the gastrin-releasing peptide receptor-antagonist [(68)Ga] SB3 and PET/CT. Eur J Nucl Med Mol Imaging 2016;43(5):964–73.
105. Pan D, Xu XP, Yang RH, et al. A new (68)Ga-labeled BBN peptide with a hydrophilic linker for GRPR-targeted tumor imaging. Amino Acids 2014;46(6):1481–9.
106. Sun Y, Hong X, Cheng Z. Development a clinical translatable 68-Ga-labeled and GRPR-targeted probe for PET imaging of prostate cancer [abstract]. J Nucl Med 2016;57(Suppl 2):1194.
107. Dalm S, Bakker I, de Blois, et al. 68Ga/177Lu-Neo-BOMB1, a novel radiolabeled GRPR antagonist for theranostic use in oncology. J Nucl Med 2016; 57(Suppl 2):331.
108. Hofmann M, Machtens S, Stief C, et al. Feasibility of Ga-68-DOTABOM PET in prostate carcinoma patients [abstract]. J Nucl Med 2004;45:449.
109. Nock BA, Kaloudi A, Lymperis E, et al. Theranostic perspectives in prostate cancer with the GRPR-antagonist NeoBOMB1 – preclinical and first clinical results [abstract]. J Nucl Med 2016. [Epub ahead of print].
110. Iagaru A, Minamimoto R, Loening A, et al. Biochemically recurrent prostate cancer: 68Ga-RM2 (formerly known as 68Ga-Bombesin or BAY86-7548) PET/MRI is superior to conventional imaging [abstract]. J Nucl Med 2016;57(Suppl 2):466.
111. Velikyan I. Prospective of 68Ga-radiopharmaceutical development. Theranostics 2014;4(1):47–80.
112. Zhang J, Niu G, Lang L, et al. Clinical translation of a dual integrin αvβ3 and GRPR targeting PET radiotracer 68Ga-NOTA-BBN-RGD [abstract]. J Nucl Med 2016. [Epub ahead of print].

Imaging of Prostate Cancer Using ^{18}F-Choline PET/Computed Tomography

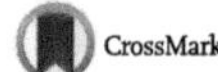

Marina Hodolič, MD, PhD[a,b,*]

KEYWORDS

• Prostate cancer • Choline • ^{18}F-choline • FCH (fluorocholine) • PET/CT

KEY POINTS

- ^{18}F-fluorocholine (FCH) PET/computed tomography (CT) may be considered a valuable imaging modality in patients with prostate cancer disease.
- Its main role is in restaging of patients with biochemical recurrence of prostate cancer disease after radical prostatectomy or external beam radiotherapy.
- ^{18}F-FCH PET/CT is strengthening its position in the initial staging, biopsy target definition, and radiotherapy planning, as well as therapy monitoring of prostate cancer disease.
- Gleason score and prostate-specific antigen value, doubling time, and velocity can influence positivity of 18F-FCH PET/CT.

In 2012, the *World Cancer Statistics* reported that lung, prostate, and colorectal cancers contributed to 42% of all cancers in men, excluding nonmelanoma skin cancer.[1] Prostate cancer is the second most frequent cancer and the sixth leading cause of cancer death in men worldwide. Despite improved methods of early diagnosis, evaluation, and management of patients with prostate cancer, in the United States approximately 1 in 10 men will ultimately die of prostate cancer.

Initiatives for screening and availability of new treatment modalities have a major impact on disease epidemiology. Approximately 68% of patients with prostate cancer are from more developed countries. Prostate cancer tends to develop in men older than age 50 years and it is diagnosed in 80% of men by the age of 80 years. It is usually slow growing and it is frequently asymptomatic. As a consequence, some men affected with this malignancy receive no diagnosis or therapy and they usually die of other unrelated causes. In the development of prostate cancer, many factors have been implicated but yet there is no established relationship between any environmental factor and the incidence or aggressive nature of prostate cancer.

CLINICAL MANAGEMENT OF PATIENTS WITH PROSTATE CANCER

In most cases, in the early stages, prostate cancer is harmless and seems to be symptom free. For this reason, sensitive diagnostic procedures are crucial for appropriate management and a good survival rate.

Prostate-specific antigen (PSA), a serum marker, can be an early clue to the presence of prostate cancer. Although a nonspecific biomarker, an elevated PSA level should lead to other diagnostic procedures. Using PSA alone, a 70% to 80% specificity and a 70% sensitivity is mediocre.[2–4] However, PSA level measurement and digital rectal examination followed by endorectal ultrasound (US) and biopsy are still basic procedures performed in patients with suspicion of prostate cancer. Ultrasound, computed tomography (CT) scan, and MR

Disclosure Statement: The author has nothing to disclose.

[a] Nuclear Medicine Research Department, Iason, Graz, Austria; [b] Department of Nuclear Medicine, Palacký University Olomouc, Olomouc, Czech Republic
* Poljanska cesta 19, Ljubljana 1000, Slovenia.
E-mail address: marina.hodolic@gmail.com

PET Clin 12 (2017) 173–184
http://dx.doi.org/10.1016/j.cpet.2016.11.004

imaging have shown their importance in the detection of primary disease but still remain weak in early detection of affected lymph nodes and distal metastases.[5] Identification of lymph node involvement by either CT or MR imaging is based primarily on size and shape criteria. Also, these modalities cannot determine the degree of aggressiveness of the tumor, a feature that is important to guide therapy (to avoid underestimating or overestimating therapeutic options). In accordance with European[6,7] and American guidelines,[8] to assess the extent of disease in patients with prostate cancer, nuclear medicine has traditionally been limited to bone scintigraphy (BS) with Tc-99m methylene diphosphonate or Tc-99m 3,3-diphosphono-1,2-propanodicarboxylicacid. Their sensitivity and specificity remains low. Also, patients with low-risk prostate cancer are unlikely to have metastatic bone involvement. Some studies support the statement that BS is sensitive at PSA levels greater than 20 ng/mL.[9] This conventional nuclear medicine modality is mainly reserved for patients with high-risk prostate cancer, bone pain, elevated serum alkaline phosphatase levels, or equivocal bone lesions on other imaging modalities.[10] Therefore, the routine use of BS for primary staging in all patients with newly diagnosed prostate cancer is questionable. Regardless of whether it is positive or negative, BS does not exclude soft tissue involvement.

Currently, more than 95% of PET studies worldwide are performed using ^{18}F-fluorocholine (FDG). The role of ^{18}F-FDG PET/CT in patients with prostate cancer is still reserved for patients who are at high risk for having poorly differentiated prostate cancer (based on a high Gleason score [GS] of biopsied prostate tissue), high PSA values, or even in the presence of castrate-resistant lesions. Because ^{18}F-FDG uptake correlates with tumor aggressiveness, identification of metastatic prostate cancer disease with an ^{18}F-FDG PET/CT scan indicates a poor prognosis for the patient. Nuclear medicine physicians should be alert to the incidental finding of focal ^{18}F-FDG uptake in the prostate because it may represent prostate malignancy.

Despite widespread use of ^{18}F-FDG, the need for a more sensitive and specific tracer to increase overall diagnostic accuracy is permanently present. For this reason, application of radiotracers other than ^{18}F-FDG in patients with prostate cancer is crucial.

CHOLINE, ^{11}C-CHOLINE, AND ^{18}F-CHOLINE

Choline, a quaternary ammonium cation, is an essential nutrient for humans and is mostly derived from the diet.[11,12] Radiolabeled choline is among the most commonly applied PET tracers for prostate cancer imaging in Europe. Choline is a substrate for the synthesis of phosphatidylcholine, a major phospholipid in the cell membrane. Radiolabeled choline is incorporated into tumor cells by active transport, phosphorylated in the cells, and integrated into phospholipids. In this way, uptake of radiolabeled choline reflects proliferative activity of membrane lipid synthesis. In 1997, choline was labeled with ^{11}C, short-lived isotope (half-life 20 minutes). In the early 2000s, DeGrado and colleagues[13] took advantage of longer-lived radionuclide ^{18}F (half-life 110 minutes) and synthesized no carrier-added choline analogue, [18F]-fluoromethyl-dimethyl-2-hydroxyethylammonium (FCH). Hara[14] synthetized 2-[18F]-fluoroethyldimethyl-2-hydroxyethylammonium (FEC). Both compounds showed the similar properties of rapid uptake in prostate cancer tissue and rapid blood clearance, with minor differences, such as FEC showing later peak uptake in the prostate.

In comparison with ^{11}C-choline, the longer half-life of ^{18}F allows ^{18}F-choline analogues to be distributed to centers lacking an onsite cyclotron. Additionally, shorter positron range of ^{18}F provides better spatial resolution and better imaging quality. In comparison with ^{11}C-choline, the weak point of ^{18}F-choline analogues is that they are eliminated via the kidneys so urinary activity can obscure, or they can be mistaken for malignant processes in the pelvis. This effect can be minimized with early acquisition before tracer appearance in the bladder and delayed imaging after voiding, as well as use of diuretics.

RADIATION DOSIMETRY OF ^{18}F-FLUOROCHOLINE: TOXICITY STUDIES

Based on the biokinetic compartmental model in patients with prostate cancer, dosimetry of ^{18}F-FCH has been calculated. The distribution of radioactivity varies in various organs; kidneys and liver are critical organs. The highest radioactivity has been found in the kidneys (reference patient, 0.079 mGy/MBq; individual values, 0.033–0.105 mGy/MBq) and liver (reference patient, 0.062 mGy/MBq; individual values, 0.036–0.082 mGy/MBq).[15] The urinary bladder wall of the reference patient received a dose between 0.017 and 0.030 mGy/MBq, depending on frequency of voiding. Radiation dosimetry limits administrations levels of ^{18}F-FCH to 4.07 MBq/kg (0.110 μCi/kg) in human research studies. The effective whole-body dose equivalent from administration of 4.07 MBq/kg is approximately 0.01 Sv.[16] Prostate cancer tissue uptake is rapid and already significant after 1.5 minutes. Optimal tumor-to-background contrast is reached within

5 to 7 minutes after injection of tracer. This allows early acquisition and provides scans of good diagnostic quality.

In acute toxicity studies, neither death nor behavioral or movement abnormalities were noted for up to 48 hours after administration of 1 mg/kg of body weight of nonradioactive [^{19}F]FCH into mice. Based on these findings, it has been estimated that normal dose of ^{18}F-FCH in the radiotracer preparation would be a factor of 300,000 times lower than the dose given in toxicity study of DeGrado and colleagues.[16]

PATIENT PREPARATION AND ^{18}F-FLUOROCHOLINE PET/COMPUTED TOMOGRAPHY SCAN ACQUISITION PROTOCOLS

Before ^{18}F-FCH PET/CT scanning, patients should be well hydrated (approximately 1 L of liquid). To minimize physiologic distribution of the tracer in the in the bowel, fasting is recommended for 6 to 10 hours before acquisition. The influence of androgen deprivation therapy (ADT) on choline uptake in patients with prostate cancer disease has not yet been clarified (see later discussion). Most European nuclear medicine centers recommend intravenous administrations of 2.5 to 4 MBq/kg of ^{18}F-FCH. At present, there is no standardized ^{18}F-FCH PET/CT scan acquisition protocol; however, many protocols incorporate late with early imaging (0–15 minutes after tracer injection) to avoid interference visualization of the pelvic disease with interference from physiologic filling of urinary activity in the bladder. Late acquisition is usually performed 45 to 60 minutes after tracer injection. Late acquisition allows better sensitivity for distal disease.[17–19] Early and late PET imaging, as well as coregistered low-dose CT scan data, are sufficient for good scan interpretation.

PHYSIOLOGIC DISTRIBUTION OF ^{18}F-FLUOROCHOLINE

Physiologic ^{18}F-FCH uptake (**Fig. 1**) is noted in the salivary glands, liver, pancreas, renal parenchyma, and urinary bladder. Faint uptake is seen in the spleen, bone marrow, and muscles. Bowel activity is variable and depends on duration of fasting before acquisition. There is no physiologic uptake of ^{18}F-FCH in the brain.

PROBLEMS AND PITFALLS IN THE INTERPRETATION OF ^{18}F-FLUOROCHOLINE PET/COMPUTED TOMOGRAPHY SCANS

In patients with prostate cancer disease, results of an ^{18}F-FCH PET/CT scan can be either false-negative (mainly in lesions less than 5 mm or minimally involved lymph nodes) or false-positive (reactive lymph nodes or benign prostatic lesions). Additionally, to avoid nonspecific ^{18}F-FCH uptake, correct timing for an ^{18}F-FCH PET/CT scan in patients who have undergone surgery, radiotherapy, or chemotherapy is required.

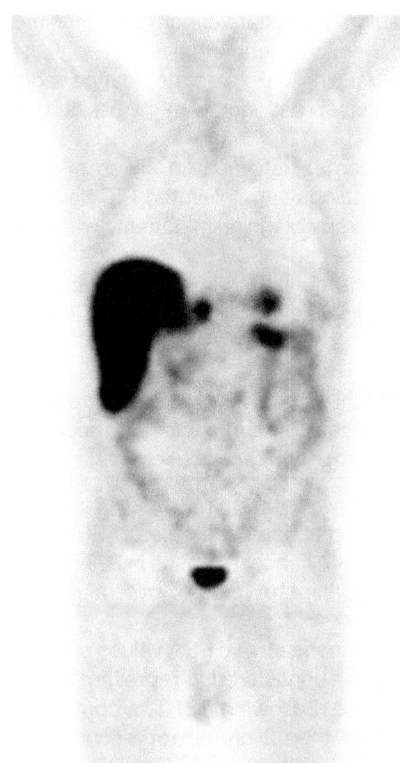

Fig. 1. ^{18}F-FCH PET/CT scan showing physiologic distribution of ^{18}F-FCH in healthy men.

CLINICAL INDICATION FOR ^{18}F-FLUOROCHOLINE PET/COMPUTED TOMOGRAPHY SCANS IN PATIENTS WITH PROSTATE CANCER

Patients' referral criteria for an ^{18}F-FCH PET/CT scan still have to be defined. However, there is no threshold for serum PSA level (nanograms per milliliter) and, with an ^{18}F-FCH PET/CT scan, it should not be used. Also, the importance of the GS, the influence of hormonal treatment (antiandrogen therapy), PSA velocity (PSAve), and PSA doubling time (PSAdt) should be clarified.

Despite a lack of precise guidelines about when to use an ^{18}F-FCH PET/CT scan in patients with prostate cancer disease, the most important clinical indications can be roughly divided into

1. Restaging of prostate cancer disease (in cases of biochemical recurrence)
2. Initial staging of prostate cancer disease (in cases of patients with high-risk prostate cancer)
3. Biopsy target definition (in cases of repeated negative biopsy and elevated PSA level)
4. Radiotherapy planning in patients with prostate cancer disease
5. Treatment monitoring in patients with prostate cancer disease.

^{18}F-Fluorocholine PET/Computed Tomography Scans in Restaging of Prostate Cancer Disease (Cases of Biochemical Recurrence)

Despite highly successful radical prostatectomy (RP) and external beam radiotherapy (EBRT) treatments, prostate cancer relapses in 20% up to 40% of patients within 10 years of potentially curative local therapy.[20,21]

After RP, 2 consecutive PSA values of 0.2 ng/mL and above are considered to represent recurrence of the disease. Following EBRT, a confirmed PSA value greater than 2 ng/mL represents recurrent prostate cancer disease.[22,23] The PSA level measurement, as well as PSA kinetics after RP or EBRT, is routinely performed for detecting prostate cancer recurrence (ie, biochemical recurrence), although it cannot distinguish between local, regional, or distant recurrence. A recent article on 187 subjects[24] showed that endorectal-coil MR imaging should be considered as the first imaging evaluation for biochemical recurrence for identifying patients suitable for localized salvage therapy. Endorectal-coil MR imaging showed a high level of sensitivity in identifying local recurrence of prostate cancer following RP, even at low PSA levels. For patients with a PSA less than 0.4 ng/mL the sensitivity of endorectal-coil MR imaging was 86%.[24]

Currently, there are no guidelines regarding nuclear medicine imaging procedures in patients with biochemical relapse of prostate cancer. However, in Europe many hospitals successfully applied the ^{18}F-FCH PET/CT scan as a first-line imaging modality in patients with biochemical relapse, of prostate cancer (**Fig. 2**). Unfortunately, the ^{18}F-FCH PET/CT scan has low sensitivity at low PSA levels.[25–28] In patients with a PSA less than 2 ng/mL, the detection rate is only 30% to 40%.[27] Some investigators proved that an ^{18}F-FCH PET/CT scan is a sensitive modality to detect recurrent prostate cancer disease if the PSA is higher than 2 ng/mL.[29,30] A study on 1000 subjects[31] showed that an ^{18}F-FCH PET/CT scan detection rate is not linked just to PSA serum level but also to the GS. For suspected recurrence of prostate cancer, a high GS at diagnosis can be associated with positive ^{18}F-FCH PET/CT scan results, regardless of the serum PSA level at the time of imaging. Therefore, the GS is an independent predictive factor for a positive ^{18}F-FCH PET/CT scan, even at low PSA levels (<1 ng/mL; detection rate: 47%).[31] Positivity of an ^{18}F-FCH PET/CT scan is also influenced by PSAve (the time it takes for PSA to rise to a certain level) and PSAdt (the time it takes for PSA levels to double). Schillaci and colleagues[32] recommended an ^{18}F-FCH PET/CT scan in patients with a PSA greater than 2 ng/mL, a PSAdt up to 6 months, and a PSAve greater than 2 ng/mL per year. The detection rate is higher in cases of high PSAve (>5 ng/ml/y) and short PSAdt (<2 or 3 months). PSAdt is also an independent predictor of positivity of an ^{18}F-FCH PET/CT scan in patients with normal PSA level.[33]

In conclusion, in patients with recurrent prostate cancer disease, the overall sensitivity of an ^{18}F-FCH PET/CT scan seems to be higher among patients with a higher PSA, a higher initial GS, and a shorter PSAdt.

^{18}F-Fluorocholine PET/Computed Tomography Scan in the Initial Staging of Prostate Cancer Disease (Cases of Patients with High-Risk Prostate Cancer)

Approximately 1.5% of patients who are diagnosed with prostate cancer have clinically evident

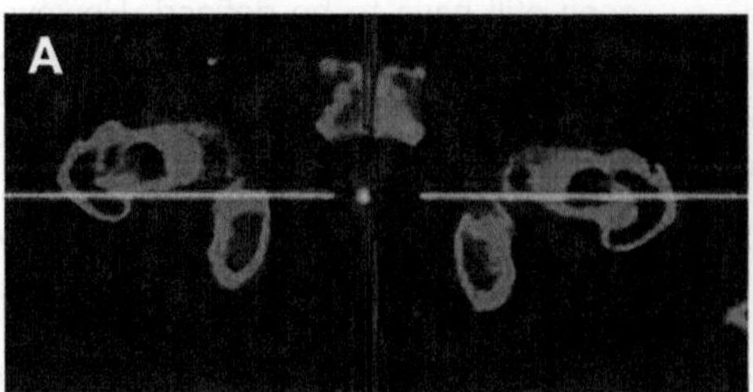

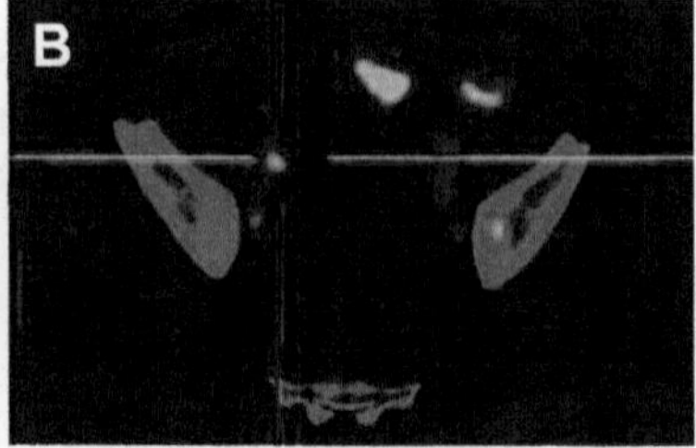

Fig. 2. (*A*) ^{18}F-FCH PET/CT scan showing focal tracer uptake in the prostatic bed (patient after RP; PSA = 0.8 ng/mL). (*B*) ^{18}F-FCH PET/CT scan showing increased tracer uptake in the right iliac lymph nodes (patient after RP; PSA = 1.5 ng/mL).

metastatic disease.[34] The pelvic and retroperitoneal lymph nodes, prostatic bed, and skeleton are the most frequently affected sites of metastatic spread, relating to 66%, 34%, and 29% of patients, respectively.[35] The demonstration that the disease is localized to the prostate gland or that it also has extraglandular spread is of key importance when defining the therapeutic approach. PSA is able to determine presence of the disease but not the disease extension. Therefore, imaging modalities play a main role in the initial staging of patients with prostate cancer. Their optimal use is still under debate because their diagnostic value (ie, sensitivity and specificity) is not agreed on.[36,37] The spread within the pelvis is most often evaluated by CT scan or MR imaging. However, meta-analysis from Hovels and colleagues[38] showed that the pooled sensitivity of CT scans in predicting lymph-node metastases is only 42%. On the other hand, MR imaging can detect extracapsular prostatic extension, seminal vesicle invasion, and the presence of enlarged locoregional lymph nodes, and can quantify the spectrum of cancer metabolites using spectroscopic techniques. Endorectal MR imaging allows imaging of spread of the disease to the prostatic capsule and seminal vesicles.

Despite different opinions in numerous studies, the ^{18}F-FCH PET/CT scan seems to have a role in the initial staging in patients with biopsy-proven intermediate to high-risk prostate cancer. Its unique whole-body imaging modality shows the extent of prostate cancer disease in the entire body, both in soft tissue and the skeleton. A retrospective study from Evangelista and colleagues[39] showed higher sensitivity in detection of bone metastases and lymph nodes disease involvement with ^{18}F-FCH PET/CT scans in subjects with intermediate to high-risk prostate cancer. In comparison with a dedicated CT scan, an ^{18}F-FCH PET/CT scan showed a higher sensitivity and a similar specificity: 46.2% versus 69.2% and 92.3% versus 92.3%, respectively, in detecting lymph node involvement. Moreover, the sensitivity and specificity of ^{18}F-FCH PET/CT scans were higher than those of bone scan: 100% versus 90% and 86.4% versus 77.2%, respectively. The overall accuracy of ^{18}F-FCH PET/CT scans for lymph-node involvement was 83.3%. In contrast to CT scan and BS, ^{18}F-FCH PET/CT scans changed the staging of the prostate cancer disease in 33.3% patients. In cases of occult lymph node metastases, the study of Hacker and colleagues[40] showed that an ^{18}F-FCH PET/CT scan is not a useful tool in searching for occult lymph node metastases in clinically confirmed prostate cancer (a sensitivity of only 10% and a specificity of 80% was observed). In this study, a sentinel node-guided pelvic lymph node dissection allowed the detection of even small lymph node metastases. In a large study involving 912 lymph node samples in 130 subjects with intermediate or high-risk prostate cancer, better sensitivity to detect lymph node involvement using an ^{18}F-FCH PET/CT scan was found in the lymph nodes 0.5 cm or larger in diameter: sensitivity, specificity, and positive and negative predictive value was: 66%, 96%, 82%, and 92%, respectively. An ^{18}F-FCH PET/CT scan led to a change in therapy in 15% of all subjects and 20% of high-risk subjects.[18] The same group of investigators assessing bone metastases with ^{18}F-FCH PET/CT scans and diagnostic CT scans alone showed that 24% of bone lesions detectable on an ^{18}F-FCH PET/CT scan had no detectable morphologic changes on CT scan, probably due to bone marrow metastases. In this study, the sensitivity, specificity, and accuracy of ^{18}F-FCH PET/CT scans in detecting bone metastases from prostate cancer was 79%, 97%, and 84%, respectively.[41] Finally, based on the published data, the change in management by the inclusion of ^{18}F-FCH PET/CT scan for the initial staging of patients with prostate cancer ranged between 5%[42] and 36%.[43]

Therefore, ^{18}F-FCH PET/CT scans at initial staging can help to determine appropriate method of treatment (RP, EBRT, antiandrogen treatment, salvage surgery, chemotherapy, or a combination of these) and, despite different opinions in various studies, it seems to have a role in the initial staging, especially in patients with biopsy-proven high-risk prostate cancer (**Fig. 3**).

^{18}F-Fluorocholine PET/Computed Tomography Scan in Biopsy Target Definition (Cases of Repeated Negative Biopsy and Elevated Prostate-Specific Antigen Level)

Twenty percent of patients with prostate cancer who undergo fine-needle biopsy will have false-negative biopsy result.[44] Several studies have shown that a significant number of patients with an initial negative prostate needle biopsy and persistently elevated serum PSA levels will have prostatic malignancy found on subsequent biopsy.[45,46] The operator's ability in guiding the biopsy needle is of great importance. Because of a possible source of error, different morphologic imaging modalities have been implemented in localization of prostate cancer; for example, US (transrectal, color-flow Doppler, power Doppler) and multiparametric MR Imaging.

None of them totally solved the problem of precise localization of malignant process in the prostate. PET/CT scan modality with choline analogues can be potentially helpful for localization of

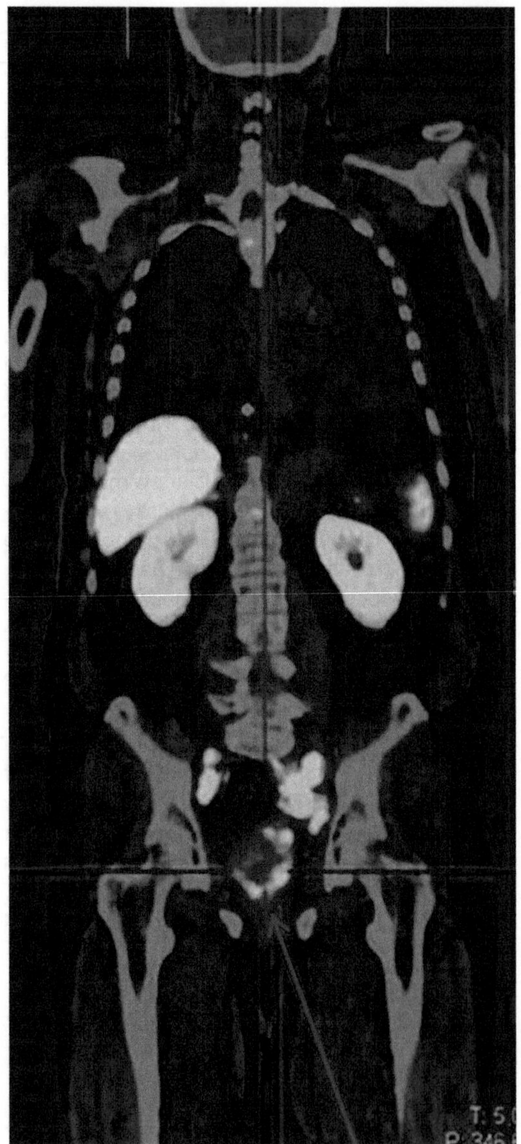

Fig. 3. ^{18}F-FCH PET/CT scan showing increased tracer uptake in multiple enlarged iliac lymph nodes bilaterally (patient at initial staging; PSA = 22 ng/mL; GS = 9).

malignant process in the prostate, especially when morphologic diagnostic methods are inconclusive. A study of 20 subjects with elevated PSA level and negative biopsy showed that an ^{18}F-FCH PET/CT scan was able to identify the malignant zone in the prostate in only 25%.[47] In Igerc and colleagues[47] study, neither semiquantitative analysis (SUVmax) nor dual-phase protocol (early acquisition 3–5 minutes and late acquisition 30 minutes after tracer injection) was helpful. Image analysis was performed visually and described focal, multifocal, or inhomogeneous tracer uptake. In the group of subjects who had a focal tracer uptake, ^{18}F-FCH PET/CT scans had a sensitivity of 100%, a specificity of 46.7%, and a positive predictive value of 38.5% for the detection of prostate cancer; however, this was validated by biopsy and not histology.[47] Another study dealing with this topic[48] found that imaging delayed 1 hour leads to an improvement of malignant to benign contrast ratio of uptake in the prostate. The investigators reported decreasing SUVmax over 1 hour in benign zones and either stable or increasing SUVmax in malignant zones. Dual time point imaging in this setting requires further investigation and evaluation.

In 80% of cases, prostate cancer is located in the peripheral zone of the prostate. In the additional 20% of cases, prostate cancer is developed anterior to the urethra.[49] This area is difficult to assess using ^{18}F-FCH because of urinary excretion of the tracer. Also, ^{18}F-FCH uptake seems to be present in benign changes (prostatitis and prostatic hypertrophy), as well as in prostate cancer. Therefore, because the tracer is not specific, ^{18}F-FCH PET/CT scans cannot be generally recommended as the primary procedure for the localization of prostate cancer.

In conclusion, currently, the routine use of ^{18}F-FCH PET/CT scans cannot be recommended as a first-line screening procedure for primary prostate cancer. A potential application of ^{18}F-FCH PET/CT scans may be to increase the detection rate of clinically suspected prostate cancer with multiple negative prostate biopsies (**Fig. 4**). New procedures such as ^{18}F-FCH MR imaging/PET are being evaluated in imaging of primary prostate cancer.[50]

^{18}F-Fluorocholine PET/Computed Tomography Scan in Radiotherapy Planning in Patients with Prostate Cancer Disease

For many years, MR imaging, as well as magnetic resonance spectroscopy, have been proposed as first-line modalities in precise definition of intraprostatic lesions.[51,52] Precise detection of the site of prostate cancer process is crucial for a good radiotherapy treatment outcome. Additionally, organs at risk, such as the rectum and bladder, need to be protected. In their review article, Schwarzenböck and colleagues[53] presented most common indication for radiotherapy use in patients with prostate cancer: (1) irradiation of the former prostate bed with enlargement of the irradiation field to the pelvic lymphatics to include all pelvic lymph nodes with or without a boost to PET-positive lymph nodes, (2) irradiation of the former prostate bed and PET-positive lymph nodes and the corresponding lymphatic drainage vessels, and (3) irradiation of the former prostate bed and irradiation of PET-positive lymph nodes only (without irradiation of any

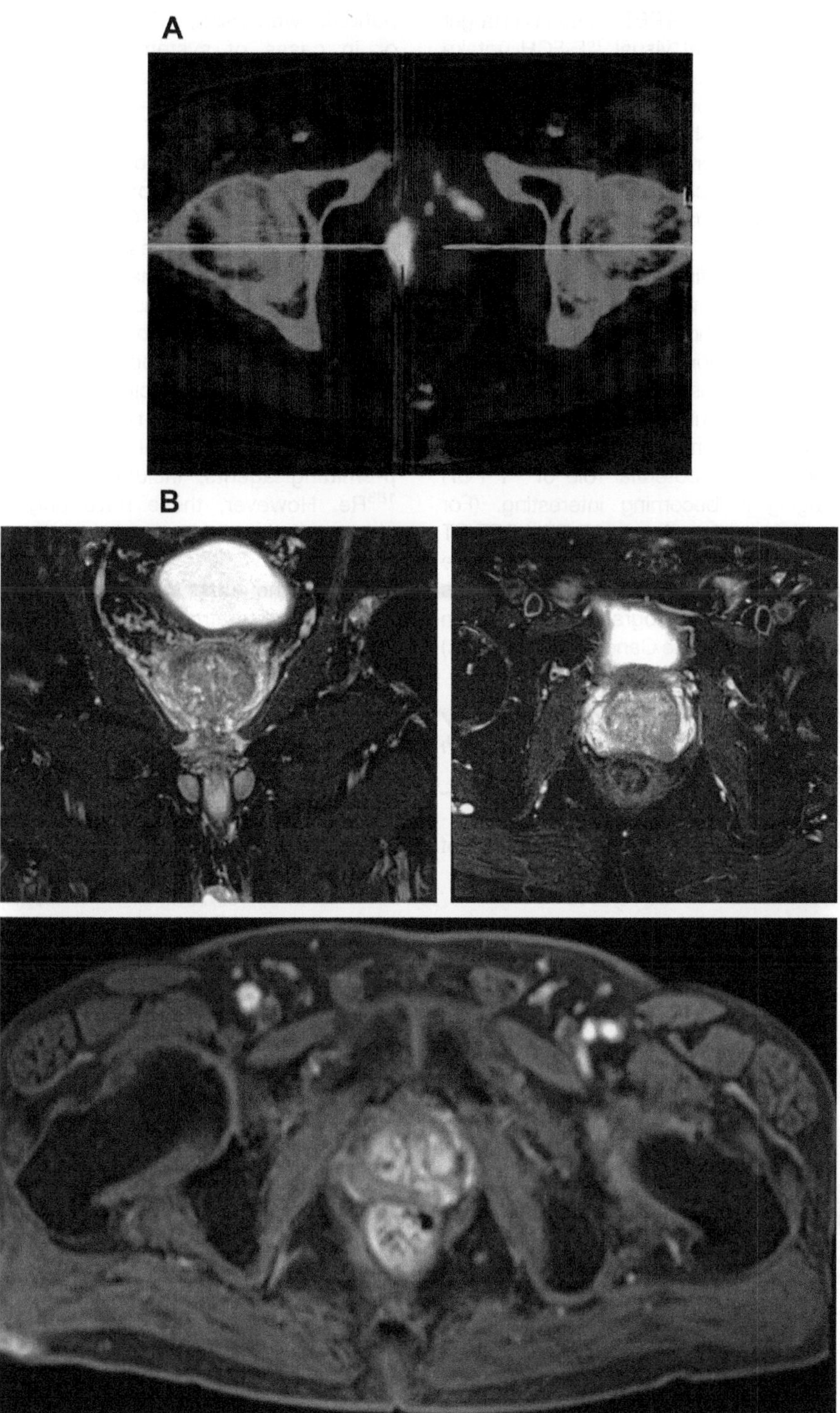

Fig. 4. (*A*) ^{18}F-FCH PET/CT scan showing increased tracer uptake in the right lobe of prostate (patient with PSA = 10.2 ng/mL) and after negative biopsy and negative MR imaging scan (*B*).

lymphatic drainage vessels).[53] According to the available scientific sources, neither ^{11}C-choline nor ^{18}F-FCH PET/CT scan is strongly recommended for target volume definition for primary or recurrent prostate cancer. However, several articles are showing promising results for choline PET/CT scan as an image-guide tool for the irradiation of prostate cancer relapse.[54–60]

The weak point of ^{18}F-FCH PET/CT scans in target volume delineation is that visual ^{18}F-FCH uptake does not totally correlate with malignant process, inflammation can be still present. The study of Bundschuh and colleagues[61] showed that the choline uptake pattern corresponded to the histologic localization of prostate cancer in fewer than 50% of lesions and that SUVmax thresholding with standard algorithms did not lead to satisfying results with respect to defining tumor tissue in the prostate. However, prospective, comparative studies with histopathological specimens are required to validate various approaches in the use of ^{18}F-FCH PET/CT scans in target volume delineation of primary and recurrent prostate cancer, as well as in the identification of prostate cancer lymph node involvement. The potential role of ^{18}F-FCH PET/MR imaging is becoming interesting. (For more detailed information about 18F-FCH PET/CT in radiotherapy planning in patients with prostate cancer disease, please see Kalevi J.A. Kairemo's article, "PET/Computed Tomography for Radiation Therapy Planning of Prostate Cancer," in this issue.)

^{18}F-Fluorocholine PET/Computed Tomography Scan in Treatment Monitoring in Patients with Prostate Cancer Disease

Over the past decades, different therapeutic options have been included in the management of patients with rising PSA after primary therapy or in cases of systemic spread of prostate cancer disease. For this purpose, ADT is used with luteinizing hormone-releasing hormone agonists and antagonists, as well as androgen receptor blockers. Androgens stimulate growth, function, and proliferation in normal and malignant prostate cells. On the other hand, deprivation of androgens induces prostate cell apoptosis.[62] Despite treatment with ADT, most men will progress to castrate-resistant prostate cancer. This group of patients undergoes chemotherapy with docetaxel or cabazitaxel (**Fig. 5**). As therapy, nuclear medicine proposes treatment of skeletal metastases with an α-emitting radiopharmaceutical ^{223}Ra, as well as some β-emitting agents, including ^{82}Sr, ^{153}Sa, and ^{188}Re. However, these have only a palliative characteristics, with no impact on patient survival.

PSA is the most commonly used marker for evaluation of treatment response in patients with progressive prostate cancer disease. PSA alone is not sufficiently reliable for monitoring disease activity in patients with castrate-resistant prostate cancer because visceral metastases may develop in men even without an increase in PSA level.[63] Is there a role for nuclear medicine in evaluation of therapeutic response of ADT or chemotherapy in patients with rising PSA after primary therapy or

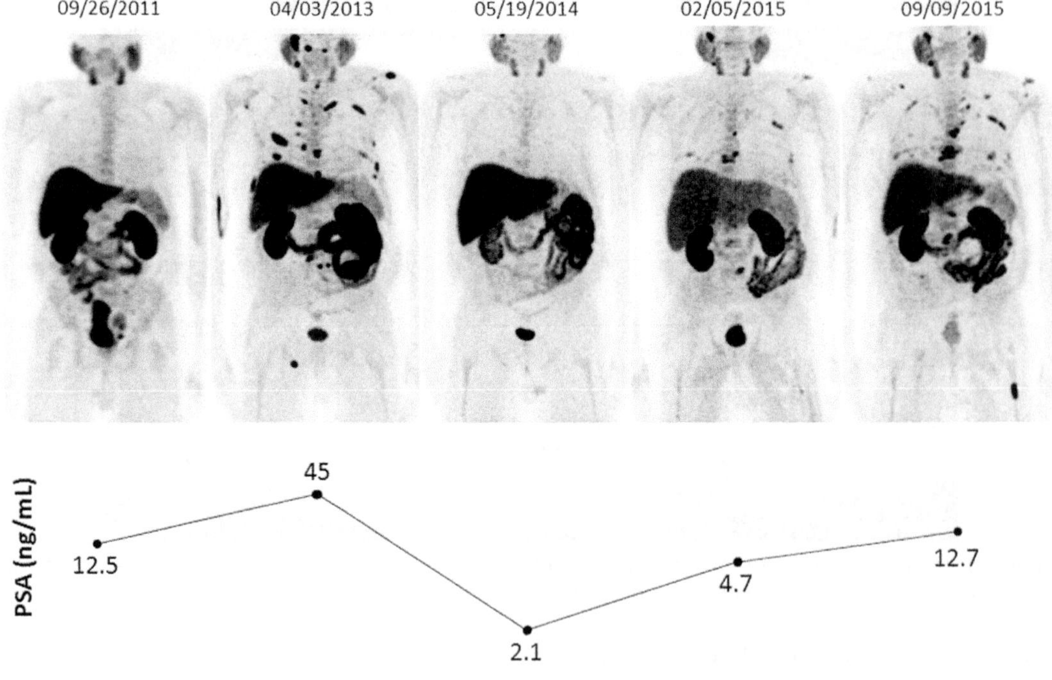

Fig. 5. ^{18}F-FCH PET/CT scan showing treatment monitoring in patient with prostate cancer disease.

with disseminated prostate cancer disease? In the guidelines from the European Association of Urology, 2014, there is no precise indication for choline PET/CT scans in patients with castrate-resistant prostate cancer.[7] In 2015, the Prostate Cancer Clinical Trials Working Group 2 recommended a combination of BS, CT scan, PSA measurements, and clinical findings in patients with metastatic castrate-resistant prostate cancer.[64] For this group of patients, the guidelines presented MR imaging and PET as useful techniques. The St. Gallen's Consensus Conference recommended BS and CT scan as baseline investigations. PSA should be considered for monitoring treatment response in conjunction with alkaline phosphatase and lactate dehydrogenase.[65]

Up to 45% of the patients going for choline PET/CT scans are undergoing ADT at the time of the examination. In this regard, there is a question whether ADT influences the choline uptake and, therefore, whether ADT should be withdrawn before PET. Some studies support the theory that there is no influence of ADT on the detection rate of ^{18}F-FCH PET/CT scans; therefore, it is not necessary to withdraw ADT before performing ^{18}FCH PET/CT scan.[62,66–68]

On the other hand, some investigators postulate an inhibitory effect of ADT on choline uptake and thus recommend that the choline PET scan should be performed either before starting ADT or the treatment should be interrupted for a certain amount of time before the scan.[69,70] It remains unclear if differences in choline uptake can be contributed to an effect caused by the therapeutic effect of ADT; for example, the reduced tumor volume or changes in metabolism.[71]

Patients who do not respond to ADT and who present with PSA elevation despite the ongoing ADT are the main candidates for choline PET.[62] In their study, McCarthy and colleagues[72] showed better sensitivity of an ^{18}F-FCH PET/CT scan in comparison with conventional imaging modalities (CT scan and BS) in follow-up of patients with castration-resistant prostate carcinoma. The ^{18}F-FCH PET/CT scan showed good initial concordance (81%) with BS and CT scan in the detection of active metastatic prostate carcinoma. Follow-up of the cases in which ^{18}F-FCH was initially discordant, with subsequent BS or CT scan, shows that ^{18}F-FCH is accurate in determining the presence or absence of prostate metastasis in 79% of lesions. Another group of investigators showed that the combination of decrease in PSA level and an ^{18}F-FCH PET/CT scan can be an early predictor of outcome in patients with castrate-resistant prostate cancer treated with enzalutamide.[73]

It seems that a role is still being sought for ^{18}F-FCH PET/CT scans in the therapy monitoring of patients with rising PSA after primary therapy or in cases of systemic spread of prostate cancer disease. Nevertheless, it seems that ^{18}F-FCH PET/CT scans have a role in a selected group of patients.

SUMMARY

In conclusion, an ^{18}F-FCH PET/CT scan may be considered a valuable imaging modality in patients with prostate cancer disease. Probably, its main role is in restaging of patients with biochemical recurrence of prostate cancer disease after RP or EBRT. At the same time, the ^{18}F-FCH PET/CT scan is strengthening its position in the initial staging, biopsy target definition, and radiotherapy planning, as well as therapy monitoring of prostate cancer disease. PSA value, PSAdt, and PSAve, as well as GS, can influence the positivity of ^{18}F-FCH PET/CT scans. The influence of ADT on choline uptake in patients with prostate cancer disease has not yet been precisely clarified.

Last but not least, collaboration between nuclear medicine physicians, radiologists, urologists, oncologists, and radiotherapists is crucial to the intention to help patients with prostate cancer disease.

ACKNOWLEDGMENTS

The author would like to thank Jure Fettich, MD, PhD, for his invaluable suggestions and support during writing this article; Laura Evangelista MD, PhD, for providing ^{18}F-FCH PET/CT scan examples for this article; Christoph Artner for supporting my ideas in work with ^{18}F-FCH.

REFERENCES

1. Available at: http://www.wcrf.org/int/cancer-facts-figures/worldwide-data.
2. Catalona WJ, Smith DS, Ratliff TL, et al. Measurement of prostate-specific antigen in serum as a screening test for prostate cancer. N Engl J Med 1991;324(17):1156–61.
3. Brawer MK, Chetner MP, Beatie J, et al. Screening for prostatic carcinoma with prostate specific antigen. J Urol 1992;147:841–5.
4. Roscigno M, Scattoni V, Bertini R, et al. Diagnosis of prostate cancer. State of the art. Minerva Urol Nefrol 2004;56:123–45.
5. Beauregard JM, Williams SG, Degrado TR, et al. Pilot comparison of F-fluorocholine and F-fluorodeoxyglucose PET/CT with conventional imaging in prostate cancer. J Med Imaging Radiat Oncol 2010;54:325–32.

6. Heidenreich A, Bastian PJ, Bellmunt J, et al, European Association of Urology. EAU guidelines on prostate cancer. Part 1: screening, diagnosis, and local treatment with curative intent—update 2013. Eur Urol 2014;65:124–37.
7. Heidenreich A, Bastian PJ, Bellmunt J, et al. EAU guidelines on prostate cancer. Part II: treatment of advanced, relapsing, and castration-resistant prostate cancer. Eur Urol 2014;65:467–79.
8. Mohler JL, Kantoff PW, Armstrong AJ, et al. Prostate cancer, version 2. 2014. J Natl Compr Canc Netw 2014;12:686–718.
9. Bott SR. Management of recurrent disease after radical prostatectomy. Prostate Cancer Prostatic Dis 2004;7(3):211–6.
10. Even-Sapir E, Metser U, Mishani E, et al. The detection of bone metastases in patients with high-risk prostate cancer: 99mTc-MDP (Planar) bone scintigraphy, single- and (multi-field-of-view) SPECT, 18F-fluoride PET and 18F-fluoride PET/CT. J Nucl Med 2006;47(2):287–97.
11. Bathen TF, Sitter B, Sjøbakk TE, et al. Magnetic resonance metabolomics of intact tissue: a biotechnological tool in cancer diagnostics and treatment evaluation. Cancer Res 2010;70:6692–6.
12. Li Z, Vance DE. Phosphatidylcholine and choline homeostasis. J Lipid Res 2008;49(6):1187–94.
13. DeGrado TR, Coleman RE, Wang S, et al. Synthesis and evaluation of 18F-labeled choline as an oncologic tracer for positron emission tomography: initial findings in prostate cancer. Cancer Res 2001;61(1):110–7.
14. Hara T. 18F-fluorocholine: a new oncologic PET tracer. J Nucl Med 2001;42(12):1815–7.
15. Giussani A, Janzen T, Uusijärvi-Lizana H, et al. A compartmental model for biokinetics and dosimetry of ^{18}F-choline in prostate cancer patients. J Nucl Med 2012;53:985–93.
16. DeGrado T, Reiman R, Price D, et al. Pharmacokinetics and radiation dosimetry of ^{18}F-fluorocholine. J Nucl Med 2002;43:92–6.
17. DeGrado T, Kwee S, Coel M, et al. Impact of urinary excretion of (18)F-labeled choline analogs. J Nucl Med 2007;48:1225.
18. Beheshti M, Imamovic L, Broinger G, et al. 18F choline PET/CT in the preoperative staging of prostate cancer in patients with intermediate or high risk of extracapsular disease: a prospective study of 130 patients. Radiology 2010;254:925–33.
19. Steiner C, Vees H, Zaidi H, et al. Three-phase 18F-fluorocholine PET/CT in the evaluation of prostate cancer recurrence. Nuklearmedizin 2009;48:1–9.
20. Han M, Partin AW, Pound CR, et al. Long-term biochemical disease-free and cancer-specific survival following anatomic radical retropubic prostatectomy: the 15-year Johns Hopkins experience. Urol Clin North Am 2001;28:555–65.
21. Ward JF, Moul JW. Rising prostate-specific antigen after primary prostate cancer therapy. Nat Clin Pract Urol 2005;2:174–82.
22. Stephenson AJ, Kattan MW, Eastham JA, et al. Defining biochemical recurrence of prostate cancer after radical prostatectomy: a proposal for a standardized definition. J Clin Oncol 2006;24(24):3973–8.
23. Roach M, Hanks G, Thames H, et al. Defining biochemical failure following radiotherapy with or without hormonal therapy in men with clinically localized prostate cancer: recommendations of the RTOG-ASTRO Phoenix Consensus Conference. Int J Radiat Oncol Biol Phys 2006;65:965–74.
24. Linder BJ, Kawashima A, Woodrum DA, et al. Early localization of recurrent prostate cancer after prostatectomy by endorectal coil magnetic resonance imaging. Can J Urol 2014;21(3):7283–9.
25. Cimitan M, Bortolus R, Morassut S, et al. 18F-fluorocholine PET/CT imaging for the detection of recurrent prostate cancer at PSA relapse: experience in 100 consecutive patients. Eur J Nucl Med Mol Imaging 2006;33:1387–98.
26. Vees H, Buchegger F, Albrecht S, et al. 18F-Choline and/or 11C-acetate positron emission tomography: detection of residual or progressive subclinical disease at very low prostate-specific antigen values (<1 ng/ml) after radical prostatectomy. BJU Int 2007;99:1415–20.
27. Heinisch M, Dirisamer A, Loidl W, et al. Positron emission tomography/computed tomography with F-18-fluorocholine for restaging of prostate cancer patients: meaningful at PSA < 5 ng/ml? Mol Imaging Biol 2006;8:43–8.
28. Pelosi E, Arena V, Skanjeti A, et al. Role of whole-body 18F-choline PET/CT in disease detection in patients with biochemical relapse after radical treatment for prostate cancer. Radiol Med 2008;113:895–904.
29. Heidenreich A, Bellmunt J, Bolla M, et al. EAU guidelines on prostate cancer. Part I: screening, diagnosis, and treatment of clinically localised disease. Actas Urol Esp 2011;35:501–14.
30. Husarik D, Miralbell R, Dubs M, et al. Evaluation of [(18)F]-choline PET/CT for staging and restaging of prostate cancer. Eur J Nucl Med Mol Imaging 2008;35:253–63.
31. Cimitan M, Evangelista L, Hodolič M, et al. Gleason score at diagnosis predicts the rate of detection of 18F-choline PET/CT performed when biochemical evidence indicates recurrence of prostate cancer: experience with 1,000 patients. J Nucl Med 2015;56(2):209–15.
32. Schillaci O, Calabria F, Tavolozza M, et al. Influence of PSA, PSA velocity and PSA doubling time on contrast-enhanced 18F-choline PET/CT detection rate in patients with rising PSA after radical prostatectomy. Eur J Nucl Med Mol Imaging 2012;39(4):589–96.

33. Hodolič M, Maffione AM, Fettich J, et al. Metastatic prostate cancer proven by 18F-FCH PET/CT staging scan in patient with normal PSA but high PSA doubling time. Clin Nucl Med 2013;38: 739–40.
34. Ryan CJ, Elkin EP, Small EJ, et al. Reduced incidence of bony metastasis at initial prostate cancer diagnosis: data from CaPSURE. Urol Oncol 2006; 24:396–402.
35. Giovacchini G, Picchio M, Coradeschi E, et al. Predictive factors of (11C)choline PET/CT in patients with biochemical failure after radical prostatectomy. Eur J Nucl Med Mol Imaging 2010;37:301–9.
36. Abuzallouf S, Dayes I, Lukka H. Baseline staging of newly diagnosed prostate cancer: a summary of the literature. J Urol 2004;171:2122–7.
37. Hricak H, Choyke P, Eberhardt SC, et al. Imaging prostate cancer: a multidisciplinary perspective. Radiology 2007;243:28–53.
38. Hovels AM, Heesakkers RA, Adang EM, et al. The diagnostic accuracy of CT and MRI in the staging of pelvic lymph nodes in patients with prostate cancer: a meta-analysis. Clin Radiol 2008;63:387–95.
39. Evangelista L, Cimitan M, Zattoni F, et al. Comparison between conventional imaging (abdominal-pelvic computed tomography and bone scan) and [(18)F] choline positron emission tomography/computed tomography imaging for the initial staging of patients with intermediate- to high-risk prostate cancer: a retrospective analysis. Scand J Urol 2015;49(5): 345–53.
40. Hacker A, Jeschke S, Leeb K, et al. Detection of pelvic lymph node metastases in patients with clinically localized prostate cancer: comparison of [18F]fluoro choline positron emission tomography-computerized tomography and laparoscopic radioisotope guided sentinel lymph node dissection. J Urol 2006;176: 2014–9.
41. Beheshti M, Vali R, Waldenberger P, et al. The use of F-18 choline PET in the assessment of bone metastases in prostate cancer: correlation with morphological changes on CT. Mol Imaging Biol 2010;12: 98–107.
42. Beheshti M, Vali R, Waldebìnberger P, et al. Detection of bone metastases in patients with prostate cancer by 18F fluorocholine and 18F fluoride PET-CT: a comparative study. Eur J Nucl Med Mol Imaging 2008;35:1766–74.
43. Evangelista L, Zattoni F, Guttilla A, et al. High risk and very high risk prostate cancer and the role of choline PET/CT at initial staging. EANM Congress 2013;40:P271.
44. Rabbani F, Stroumbakis N, Kava BR, et al. Incidence and clinical significance of false-negative sextant prostate biopsies. J Urol 1998;159:1247–50.
45. Ellis WJ, Brawer MK. Repeat prostate needle biopsy: who needs it? J Urol 1995;153(5):1496–8.
46. Fleshner NE, O'Sullivan M, Fair WR. Prevalence and predictors of a positive repeat transrectal ultrasound guided needle biopsy of the prostate. J Urol 1997; 158(2):505–8 [discussion: 508–9].
47. Igerc I, Kohlfürst S, Gallowitsch HJ, et al. The value of 18F-Choline PET/CT in patients with elevated PSA-level and negative prostate needle biopsy for localisation of prostate cancer. Eur J Nucl Med Mol Imaging 2008;35:976–83.
48. Kwee SA, DeGrado T. Prostate biopsy guided by 18F-fluorocholine PET in men with persistently elevated PSA levels. Eur J Nucl Med Mol Imaging 2008;35:1567–9.
49. Volkin D, Turkbey B, Hoang AH, et al. Multiparametric magnetic resonance imaging (MRI) and subsequent MRI/ultrasonography fusion-guided biopsy increase the detection of anteriorly located prostate cancers. BJU Int 2014;114:E43–9.
50. Piert M, Montgomery J, Kunju LP, et al. 18F-Choline PET/MRI: the additional value of PET for MRI-guided transrectal prostate biopsies. J Nucl Med 2016; 57(7):1065–70.
51. Fonteyne V, Villeirs G, Speleers B, et al. Intensity-modulated radiotherapy as primary therapy for prostate cancer: report on acute toxicity after dose escalation with simultaneous integrated boost to intraprostatic lesion. Int J Radiat Oncol Biol Phys 2008;72(3):799–807.
52. Van Lin EN, Futterer JJ, Heijmink SW, et al. IMRT boost dose planning on dominant intraprostatic lesions: gold marker-based three-dimensional fusion of CT with dynamic contrast-enhanced and 1H-spectroscopic MRI. Int J Radiat Oncol Biol Phys 2006; 65(1):291–303.
53. Schwarzenböck SM, Kurth J, Gocke Ch, et al. Role of choline PET/CT in guiding target volume delineation for irradiation of prostate cancer. Eur J Nucl Med Mol Imaging 2013;40(Suppl 1):S28–35.
54. Picchio M, Giovannini E, Crivellaro C, et al. Clinical evidence on PET/CT for radiation therapy planning in prostate cancer. Radiother Oncol 2010;96(3):347–50.
55. Pinkawa M, Holy R, Piroth MD, et al. Intensity-modulated radiotherapy for prostate cancer implementing molecular imaging with 18F-choline PET-CT to define a simultaneous integrated boost. Strahlenther Onkol 2010;186(11):600–6.
56. Ciernik IF, Brown DW, Schmid D, et al. 3D-segmentation of the 18F-choline PET signal for target volume definition in radiation therapy of the prostate. Technol Cancer Res Treat 2007;6(1):23–30.
57. Niyazi M, Bartenstein P, Belka C, et al. Choline PET based dose-painting in prostate cancer–modelling of dose effects. Radiat Oncol 2010;5:23.
58. Rischke HC, Knippen S, Kirste S, et al. Treatment of recurrent prostate cancer following radical prostatectomy: the radiation-oncologists point of view. Q J Nucl Med Mol Imaging 2012;56(5):409–20.

59. Würschmidt F, Petersen C, Wahl A, et al. [18F]fluoroethylcholine-PET/CT imaging for radiation treatment planning of recurrent and primary prostate cancer with dose escalation to PET/CT-positive lymph nodes. Radiat Oncol 2011;6:44.
60. Wang H, Vees H, Miralbell R, et al. 18F-fluorocholine PET-guided target volume delineation techniques for partial prostate re-irradiation in local recurrent prostate cancer. Radiother Oncol 2009;93(2):220–5.
61. Bundschuh RA, Wendl CM, Weirich G, et al. Tumour volume delineation in prostate cancer assessed by [11C]choline PET/CT: validation with surgical specimens. Eur J Nucl Med Mol Imaging 2013; 40(6):824–31.
62. Chondrogiannis S, Marzola MC, Ferretti A, et al. Is the detection rate of 18F-choline PET/CT influenced by androgen-deprivation therapy? Eur J Nucl Med Mol Imaging 2014;41(7):1293–300.
63. Pezaro CJ, Omlin A, Lorente D, et al. Visceral disease in castration-resistant prostate cancer. Eur Urol 2014;65:270–3.
64. NCCN. NCCN clinical practice guidelines in oncology. Prostate cancer. 2015. Available at: http://www.nccn.org/professionals/physician_gls/f_guidelines.asp. Accessed July 21, 2015.
65. Gillessen S, Omlin A, Attard G, et al. Management of patients with advanced prostate cancer: recommendations of the St Gallen Advanced Prostate Cancer Consensus Conference (APCCC) 2015. Ann Oncol 2015;26:1589–604.
66. Beheshti M, Haim S, Zakavi R, et al. Impact of 18F-choline PET/CT in prostate cancer patients with biochemical recurrence: influence of androgen deprivation therapy and correlation with PSA kinetics. J Nucl Med 2013;54(6):833–40.
67. Price DT, Coleman E, Liao RP, et al. Comparison of [18F]fluorocholine and [18F]fluorodeoxyglucose for positron emission tomography of androgen dependent and androgen independent prostate cancer. J Urol 2002;168:273–80.
68. Henninger B, Vesco P, Putzer D, et al. [18F]choline positron emission tomography in prostate cancer patients with biochemical recurrence after radical prostatectomy: influence of antiandrogen therapy–a preliminary study. Nucl Med Commun 2012;33:889–94.
69. Giovacchini G, Picchio M, Coradeschi E, et al. [(11)C]Choline uptake with PET/CT for the initial diagnosis of prostate cancer: relation to PSA levels, tumour stage and anti-androgenic therapy. Eur J Nucl Med Mol Imaging 2008;35:1065–73.
70. Fuccio C, Schiavina R, Castellucci P, et al. Androgen deprivation therapy influences the uptake of 11C-choline in patients with recurrent prostate cancer: the preliminary results of a sequential PET/CT study. Eur J Nucl Med Mol Imaging 2011;38:1985–9.
71. Dost RJ, Glaudemans AW, Breeuwsma AJ, et al. Influence of androgen deprivation therapy on choline PET/CT in recurrent prostate cancer. Eur J Nucl Med Mol Imaging 2013;40(Suppl 1):S41–7.
72. McCarthy M, Siew T, Campbell A, et al. (18)F-Fluoromethylcholine (FCH) PET imaging in patients with castration-resistant prostate cancer: prospective comparison with standard imaging. Eur J Nucl Med Mol Imag 2011;38:14–22.
73. De Giorgi U, Caroli P, Scarpi E, et al. (18)F-Fluorocholine PET/CT for early response assessment in patients with metastatic castration-resistant prostate cancer treated with enzalutamide. Eur J Nucl Med Mol Imaging 2015;42(8):1276–83.

Clinical Applications of Molecular Imaging in the Management of Prostate Cancer

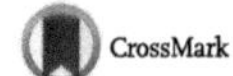

Michael A. Gorin, MD[a,*], Steven P. Rowe, MD, PhD[b], Samuel R. Denmeade, MD[c]

KEYWORDS

• Molecular imaging • Prostate cancer • PET • Cancer staging

KEY POINTS

- Prostate cancer is a common malignancy with a number of varied clinical states for which there are a multitude of treatment options.
- In selecting an ideal mode of treatment for a given patient, it is critical to accurately determine the locations and extent of their disease.
- Molecular imaging offers the promise of improved sensitivity over conventional imaging modalities for detecting sites of prostate cancer.
- Molecular imaging also offers the potential to determine additional information about a patient's prostate cancer such as Gleason score or the abundance of a molecular therapeutic target.

INTRODUCTION

Prostate cancer is the most common noncutaneous malignancy in men, accounting for 1 in 10 of all cancer diagnoses.[1] Worldwide, approximately 1.1 million cases are diagnosed annually.[2] Because of the widespread use of prostate-specific antigen (PSA) screening, nearly 80% of patients will be found to have clinically localized disease at the time of initial presentation.[3] Despite local treatment with either radiation therapy or radical prostatectomy, 20% to 30% of men with prostate cancer will recur biochemically within 10 years.[4–7] For patients with recurrent disease, treatment options include salvage local therapy and systemic treatment with androgen deprivation.[8,9] Fortunately, because of the slow natural history of prostate cancer, only half of all men who recur biochemically will progress to overt metastatic disease.[4–7] A proportion of these patients, however, will develop castration resistance and require secondary treatment with a novel antiandrogen or cytotoxic chemotherapy.[10–12]

Given the wide range of disease states and available treatment options for men with prostate cancer, there is a need for improved imaging techniques capable of accurately and precisely defining a patient's extent of disease. Molecular imaging with PET offers this promise. In oncology, molecular imaging is most commonly performed with 2-deoxy-2-[^{18}F]-fluoro-D-glucose PET. When performed in combination with x-ray computed

Dr M.A. Gorin has served a consultant to Progenics Pharmaceuticals.

[a] Department of Urology, Johns Hopkins University School of Medicine, 600 North Wolfe Street, Marburg 118, Baltimore, MD 21287, USA; [b] The Russell H. Morgan Department of Radiology and Radiological Science, Johns Hopkins University School of Medicine, Baltimore, MD 21287, USA; [c] The Sidney Kimmel Comprehensive Cancer Center, Johns Hopkins University School of Medicine, Baltimore, MD 21287, USA

* Corresponding author.

E-mail address: mgorin1@jhmi.edu

PET Clin 12 (2017) 185–192

http://dx.doi.org/10.1016/j.cpet.2016.11.001

1556-8598/17/

tomography (CT), this imaging test allows for the highly sensitive localization of rapidly dividing cells undergoing glycolysis.[13] This test, however, has offered little in the way of clinical utility for imaging prostate cancer. This lack of utility has been attributed to several factors, including the slow-growing nature of prostate cancer and its relatively low level of glycolytic activity in the castrate-sensitive state.[14,15] As a result, the field has witnessed a flurry of activity in the development of novel PET radiotracers for prostate cancer imaging. These radiotracers include agents targeting fatty-acid synthesis (eg, ^{11}C-choline, ^{18}F-choline, and ^{11}C-acetate), amino acid transport (eg, ^{18}F-FACBC), and the transmembrane protein prostate-specific membrane antigen (PSMA; eg, ^{68}Ga-PSMA-11 and ^{18}F-DCFPyL). This article reviews the current uses of imaging in the management of men with prostate cancer and outlines potential ways in which molecular imaging can be used to improve patient outcomes.

INITIAL PROSTATE CANCER STAGING WITH CONVENTIONAL IMAGING

According to current guidelines from the National Comprehensive Cancer Network,[16] the decision to perform staging imaging of patients with newly diagnosed prostate cancer should be based on a combination of digital rectal examination findings (ie, clinical T stage), serum PSA level, and biopsy Gleason sum. Per these guidelines, staging with cross-sectional imaging, including CT or MR imaging, is only recommended for patients with clinical T3 or T4 disease or those with clinical T1 or T2 disease who have a ≥10% risk of lymph node involvement. Most commonly, the Partin tables[17] or Briganti nomogram[18] are used to estimate this risk. Additionally, assessment for bone metastases using technetium-99m (^{99m}Tc)-methylene diphosphonate bone scan is recommended for patients with any of the following: bone pain, Gleason ≥8 cancer on biopsy, clinical T1 disease with a PSA ≥20 ng/mL, clinical T2 disease with a PSA ≥10 ng/mL, or clinical T3 to T4 disease. The goal of this and similar staging guidelines is to prevent the indiscriminate and costly use of imaging in patients who are at low risk of harboring metastases. In fact, the appropriate use of staging imaging in men with prostate cancer is among the items highlighted by the American Board of Internal Medicine's Choosing Wisely Campaign.[19]

Following a complete staging evaluation, patients found to have clinically localized prostate cancer should be further substratified based on their risk of progression to systemic disease. The most current version of the National Comprehensive Cancer Network guidelines[16] includes 5 risk categories: very low risk, low risk, intermediate risk, high risk, and very high risk (defined in **Table 1**). In general terms, patients with clinically localized intermediate or higher-risk prostate cancer should be offered treatment with either radiation therapy (external beam or brachytherapy with or without androgen deprivation depending on the risk category) or surgery with radical prostatectomy. Patients in the very low and low-risk groups may also be offered these treatment options; however, given the indolent nature of their disease, these men should also be presented with the option of active surveillance with selective delayed intervention. In fact, because of the significant morbidity associated with treatment (ie, urinary incontinence and erectile dysfunction), active surveillance has in recent years emerged as the de facto standard of care in this patient population. This trend has followed the publication of several reports that have shown the safety of active surveillance in appropriately selected men with low-risk prostate cancer.[20–26]

Table 1
Risk categories of localized prostate cancer as defined by the National Comprehensive Cancer Network (Version 3.2016)

Risk Category	Clinical T Stage	Gleason Score	PSA (ng/mL)
Very low[a]	T1c	≤6 (Fewer than 3 cores each with ≤50% cancer)	<10 (PSA density <0.15 ng/mL/g)
Low[b]	T1-T2a	≤6	<10
Intermediate[b]	T2b–T2c	7	10–20
High[b]	T3a	8–10	>20
Very high[b]	T3b–T4	Primary pattern 5 or >4 cores with Gleason score 8–10	—

[a] Patients must meet all criteria to be included in the very low risk group.
[b] Patients meeting any of the listed criteria are included in the risk group.

MOLECULAR IMAGING OF PATIENTS WITH CLINICALLY LOCALIZED DISEASE

In considering the role of molecular imaging the management of men with clinically localized prostate cancer, there are 3 main areas in which such imaging may be of relative value.

Pretreatment Staging

One potential use of molecular imaging is in the pretreatment staging of men with clinically localized prostate cancer who are at risk of harboring occult metastatic disease. The need for improved staging methods is perhaps best exemplified by surgical series data demonstrating that up to 20% of patients with high-risk prostate cancer will harbor occult lymph node metastases.[17,18] Molecular imaging has already shown promise for this application. Notably, recent experience with PSMA-targeted PET/CT has found an average sensitivity in the range of 60% for detecting clinically occult disease-involved lymph nodes at the time of radical prostatectomy.[27–30] The preoperative detection of these nodes is of prognostic relevance and can aid in counseling patients regarding the likelihood of requiring additional therapy after surgery. Additionally, molecular imaging may allow for the pretreatment identification of patients for whom surgery would likely prove futile (eg, those with bone metastases or large-volume nodal disease). The use of molecular imaging as a marker for identifying patients who are at risk of failure from local therapy was nicely illustrated in a report by Haseebuddin and colleagues.[31] In this study, the authors found that the preoperative detection of positive lymph nodes with ^{11}C-acetate PET/CT was associated with a more than 3-fold hazard of treatment failure independent of both preoperative and postoperative clinicopathologic variables.

Selection of Patients for Active Surveillance

A second area in which molecular imaging may have utility is in the selection of candidates for active surveillance. Currently, patients are selected for this approach based entirely on clinicopathologic parameters. At our institution, for example, we used the Epstein criteria for this purpose.[32,33] These criteria mandate that appropriate active surveillance candidates have Gleason 6 disease in less than 3 cores with $\leq$50% cancer in each core, a PSA less than 10 ng/mL, a PSA density less than 0.15 ng/mL/g, and a clinical examination of T1c. With use of these criteria, only 0.6% of active surveillance enrollees have developed metastatic disease at 10 years of follow-up.[24] At other institutions, this rate has been reported as high as 2% to 3% when patients with pattern 4 cancer are allowed to proceed with active surveillance.[23] These data underscore the importance of accurately determining Gleason score when selecting candidates for this observational approach. There are, however, concerns regarding the undergrading of prostate cancer using standardly performed ultrasound-guided template biopsy.[34,35] This has led many in the field to also rely on multiparametric MR imaging in the evaluation potential active surveillance candidates.[36–38] In studies in which whole-mount sections of the prostate are used as a reference standard, multiparametric MR imaging has a sensitivity of greater than 80% for detecting clinically significant prostate cancer.[39–43] It is worth noting, however, that MR imaging suffers in terms of sensitivity for detecting low-volume lesions. Despite this limitation, MR imaging–targeted biopsy seems to offer improved sensitivity for detecting clinically significant prostate cancer compared with ultrasound-guided template biopsy.[44–46]

In the future, molecular imaging may be used to augment the ability of biopsy and MR imaging to determine the local extent of disease within the prostate gland. Early data with choline[47–50] and PSMA-targeted[51–54] PET suggest that these molecular imaging tests can provide added sensitivity when combined with multiparametric MR imaging. In our opinion, PSMA is particularly appealing for this application given the fact that expression of this protein has been shown to directly correlate with Gleason score[55–57] and thus can be potentially used to both locate and grade lesions within the prostate. One radiotracer targeting PSMA that is being explored for this purpose (albeit using single photon emission computed tomography) is the ^{99m}Tc-labeled MIP-1404 compound.[58,59] In a phase 2 study, uptake of this radiotracer was found to highly correlate with Gleason score in radical prostatectomy specimens.[60,61] Based on this observation, a phase 3 trial is currently underway to determine if ^{99}Tc-MIP-1404 SPECT/CT can be used to correctly identify appropriate active surveillance candidates.[62]

Guidance of Focal Therapy

In recent years there has been increasing interest in the use of focal therapy for the treatment of localized prostate cancer. Forms of focal therapy include cryotherapy,[63–65] high-intensity focused ultrasound[66–72] and interstitial laser.[73–76] When compared with whole gland treatments such as radiation and radical prostatectomy, these ablative approaches offer the promise of fewer side effects. A major concern of focal therapy, however, is that more than 80% of cases of prostate cancer are multifocal.[77–79] Thus, for these therapies to be successful, one must be able to locate and treat all areas of clinically significant prostate cancer. As in the selection of candidates for active surveillance, molecular imaging may aid in this regard.

IMAGING OF BIOCHEMICALLY RECURRENT PROSTATE CANCER

Despite appropriate initial therapy, 20% to 30% of men with localized prostate cancer will recur biochemically on the basis of an elevated/increasing PSA within 10 years of initial treatment.[4–7] For patients treated with radiation therapy, biochemical recurrence is defined as a PSA of $\geq$2 ng/mL above the postradiation nadir value.[80] For patients who have undergone a radical prostatectomy, biochemical recurrence is more simply defined as a PSA of $\geq$0.2 ng/mL.[81] Common to both of these definitions is the requirement that patients be without findings of metastatic disease on both bone scan and cross-sectional imaging.

Patients who experience a biochemical recurrence have several available management options. These include continued surveillance until progression to metastatic disease, salvage local treatment, and systemic therapy with androgen deprivation.[8,9] The reason for this range of treatment options is 2-fold. First, patients with biochemically recurrent prostate cancer are a heterogeneous group comprised of men with local, loco-regional, and distant disease. Treatment decisions for these men should ideally incorporate knowledge of both lesion location and extent of disease (eg, salvage radiation for a local recurrence and androgen deprivation for widespread disease). Unfortunately, these patients are without findings on conventional imaging, thus leaving clinicians to base decisions regarding the mode and timing of therapy on imperfect clinicopathologic parameters such as PSA doubling time, Gleason score, and surgical margins status.[82–86] A second reason for the variable range of treatment options for men with biochemically recurrent prostate cancer is that not all patients in this group will go on to develop overt metastatic disease.[4–7] For example, Pound and colleagues[87] found that approximately only half of all patients with an elevated PSA after radical prostatectomy went on to develop metastases, despite no patient receiving any additional therapy until metastatic progression. Thus, there is a group of patients with biochemically recurrent disease for whom salvage treatment is unwarranted.

Given the variable clinical trajectories of patients with biochemically recurrent prostate cancer, there is a significant need to help guide the management of this patient population. With the added sensitivity afforded by PET/CT when using an appropriately selected radiotracer, molecular imaging can potentially be used to help identify which patients are in need of treatment as well as to aid in the selection of the most appropriate mode of therapy.

IMAGING OF METASTATIC PROSTATE CANCER

The most common site of prostate cancer metastasis is bone, resulting in osteoblastic lesions that are readily detected with ^{99m}Tc-methylene diphosphonate bone scan. These lesions are also often visible on CT or MR imaging, thus confirming the diagnosis. Usually, patients with metastatic prostate cancer require treatment with systemic therapy. The first line of treatment for these patients is castration, most commonly with androgen deprivation therapy. However, data from 2 large clinical trials recently showed that a subset of men, in particular those with high-volume metastatic disease, will benefit from the early addition of docetaxel chemotherapy.[88,89] Conversely, emerging data from observational studies suggest that a subset of patients with a limited number of metastatic sites may benefit from metastasis-directed therapy with treatments such as surgical resection, cryotherapy, and stereotactic ablative radiation.[90,91] Molecular imaging can potentially be used to better define the extent of disease in patients presenting with metastatic prostate cancer, thus aiding in the selection of therapy. This is of course most likely to be relevant for patients who are thought, based on conventional imaging, to have oligometastatic disease and are being considered for metastasis-directed therapy.

Another area for the use of molecular imaging in the management of patients with metastatic prostate cancer is in the assessment of response to systemic therapy. Although PSA has proven in the castration-sensitive state to be an excellent surrogate of disease response, the accuracy of PSA for this purpose begins to decline as patients acquire castration resistance.[92,93] Moreover, conventional imaging, including bone scan, offers only limited information on the status of boney lesions owing to their osteoblastic nature and the long lag time required for lesion resolution. In contrast, molecular imaging offers the possibility of real-time functional assessment of tumor viability. In addition, given the quantitative nature of PET imaging, one can also measure whole body tumor volume. In fact, quantitative techniques have already been described to measure these parameters and are ripe to be applied to prostate cancer imaging.[94–97]

One final application of molecular imaging in patients with metastatic prostate cancer is to determine/measure the presence of a molecular therapeutic target. This druggable target can either be the same as, or more simply correlated with, the target of the imaging agent. An example of the former is the use of PSMA PET/CT to confirm the presence of this protein on metastatic lesions before administration of a therapeutic PSMA-targeted small molecule labeled with an α- or β-particle emitter. Recent experience with the PSMA-617 compound, which can be labeled with either ^{68}Ga for diagnostic imaging or ^{177}Lu for therapy, has shown outstanding early clinical results for this application.[98,99]

SUMMARY

Prostate cancer is a common malignancy with a number of varied clinical states for which there are a multitude of treatment options. In selecting an ideal mode of treatment for a given patient, it is critical to accurately determine the locations and extent of their disease. Molecular imaging offers the promise of improved sensitivity over conventional imaging and so may be used to more accurately stage disease. Additionally, molecular imaging may be used to determine functional information about a patient's disease, such as Gleason score or the abundance of a molecular theraputic target.

REFERENCES

1. Siegel RL, Miller KD, Jemal A. Cancer statistics, 2016. CA Cancer J Clin 2016;66(1):7–30.
2. Torre LA, Bray F, Siegel RL, et al. Global cancer statistics, 2012. CA Cancer J Clin 2015;65(2):87–108.
3. SEER stat fact sheets: prostate cancer. Available at: http://seer.cancer.gov/statfacts/html/prost.html. Accessed August 15, 2016.
4. Kessler B, Albertsen P. The natural history of prostate cancer. Urol Clin North Am 2003;30(2):219–26.
5. Rosenbaum E, Partin A, Eisenberger MA. Biochemical relapse after primary treatment for prostate cancer: studies on natural history and therapeutic considerations. J Natl Compr Canc Netw 2004;2(3):249–56.
6. Ward JF, Moul JW. Rising prostate-specific antigen after primary prostate cancer therapy. Nat Clin Pract Urol 2005;2(4):174–82.
7. Simmons MN, Stephenson AJ, Klein EA. Natural history of biochemical recurrence after radical prostatectomy: risk assessment for secondary therapy. Eur Urol 2007;51(5):1175–84.
8. Zaorsky NG, Raj GV, Trabulsi EJ, et al. The dilemma of a rising prostate-specific antigen level after local therapy: what are our options? Semin Oncol 2013;40(3):322–36.
9. Punnen S, Cooperberg MR, D'Amico AV, et al. Management of biochemical recurrence after primary treatment of prostate cancer: a systematic review of the literature. Eur Urol 2013;64(6):905–15.
10. Bishr M, Saad F. Overview of the latest treatments for castration-resistant prostate cancer. Nat Rev Urol 2013;10(9):522–8.
11. Sridhar SS, Freedland SJ, Gleave ME, et al. Castration-resistant prostate cancer: from new pathophysiology to new treatment. Eur Urol 2014;65(2):289–99.
12. Crawford ED, Higano CS, Shore ND, et al. Treating patients with metastatic castration resistant prostate cancer: a comprehensive review of available therapies. J Urol 2015;194(6):1537–47.
13. Miles KA, Williams RE. Warburg revisited: imaging tumour blood flow and metabolism. Cancer Imaging 2008;8:81–6.
14. Jadvar H. Imaging evaluation of prostate cancer with ^{18}F-fluorodeoxyglucose PET/CT: utility and limitations. Eur J Nucl Med Mol Imaging 2013;40(Suppl 1):S5–10.
15. Hoilund-Carlsen PF, Poulsen MH, Petersen H, et al. FDG in urologic malignancies. PET Clin 2014;9(4):457–68.
16. NCCN clinical practice guidelines in oncology, prostate cancer, Version 3.2016. Available at: https://www.nccn.org/professionals/physician_gls/pdf/prostate.pdf. Accessed August 15, 2016.
17. Tosoian JJ, Chappidi M, Feng Z, et al. Prediction of pathological stage based on clinical stage, serum prostate-specific antigen, and biopsy Gleason score: Partin Tables in the contemporary era. BJU Int 2016. [Epub ahead of print].
18. Briganti A, Larcher A, Abdollah F, et al. Updated nomogram predicting lymph node invasion in patients with prostate cancer undergoing extended pelvic lymph node dissection: the essential importance of percentage of positive cores. Eur Urol 2012;61(3):480–7.
19. Choosing Wisely. Available at: http://www.choosingwisely.org/clinician-lists. Accessed August 15, 2016.
20. Soloway MS, Soloway CT, Eldefrawy A, et al. Careful selection and close monitoring of low-risk prostate cancer patients on active surveillance minimizes the need for treatment. Eur Urol 2010;58(6):831–5.
21. Eggener SE, Mueller A, Berglund RK, et al. A multi-institutional evaluation of active surveillance for low risk prostate cancer. J Urol 2013;189(1):S19–25.
22. Selvadurai ED, Singhera M, Thomas K, et al. Medium-term outcomes of active surveillance for localised prostate cancer. Eur Urol 2013;64(6):981–7.

23. Klotz L, Vesprini D, Sethukavalan P, et al. Long-term follow-up of a large active surveillance cohort of patients with prostate cancer. J Clin Oncol 2015;33(3):272–7.
24. Tosoian JJ, Mamawala M, Epstein JI, et al. Intermediate and longer-term outcomes from a prospective active-surveillance program for favorable-risk prostate cancer. J Clin Oncol 2015;33(30):3379–85.
25. Bokhorst LP, Valdagni R, Rannikko A, et al. A decade of active surveillance in the PRIAS study: an update and evaluation of the criteria used to recommend a switch to active treatment. Eur Urol 2016;70(6):954–60.
26. Newcomb LF, Thompson IM, Boyer HD, et al. Outcomes of active surveillance for clinically localized prostate cancer in the prospective, multi-institutional Canary PASS Cohort. J Urol 2016; 195(2):313–20.
27. Budäus L, Leyh-Bannurah S, Salomon G, et al. Initial experience of ^{68}Ga-PSMA PET/CT imaging in high-risk prostate cancer patients prior to radical prostatectomy. Eur Urol 2016;69(3):393–6.
28. Maurer T, Gschwend J, Rauscher I, et al. Diagnostic efficacy of ^{68}Gallium-PSMA positron emission tomography compared to conventional imaging for lymph node staging of 130 consecutive patients with intermediate to high risk prostate cancer. J Urol 2016;195(5):1436–43.
29. Herlemann A, Wenter V, Kretschmer A, et al. ^{68}Ga-PSMA positron emission tomography/computed tomography provides accurate staging of lymph node regions prior to lymph node Dissection in patients with prostate cancer. Eur Urol 2016;70(4): 553–7.
30. van Leeuwen PJ, Emmett L, Ho B, et al. Prospective evaluation of 68Gallium-PSMA positron emission tomography/computerized tomography for preoperative lymph node staging in prostate cancer. BJU Int 2016. [Epub ahead of print].
31. Haseebuddin M, Dehdashti F, Siegel BA, et al. ^{11}C-acetate PET/CT before radical prostatectomy: nodal staging and treatment failure prediction. J Nucl Med 2013;54(5):699–706.
32. Epstein JI, Walsh PC, Carmichael M, et al. Pathologic and clinical findings to predict tumor extent of nonpalpable (stage T1c) prostate cancer. JAMA 1994;271(5):368–74.
33. Bastian PJ, Mangold LA, Epstein JI, et al. Characteristics of insignificant clinical T1c prostate tumors. A contemporary analysis. Cancer 2004;101(9):2001–5.
34. Isariyawongse BK, Sun L, Banez LL, et al. Significant discrepancies between diagnostic and pathologic Gleason sums in prostate cancer: the predictive role of age and prostate-specific antigen. Urology 2008;72(4):882–6.
35. Epstein JI, Feng Z, Trock BJ, et al. Upgrading and downgrading of prostate cancer from biopsy to radical prostatectomy: incidence and predictive factors using the modified Gleason grading system and factoring in tertiary grades. Eur Urol 2012;61(5):1019–24.
36. Raz O, Haider M, Trachtenberg J, et al. MRI for men undergoing active surveillance or with rising PSA and negative biopsies. Nat Rev Urol 2010;7(10):543–51.
37. Fascelli M, George AK, Frye T, et al. The role of MRI in active surveillance for prostate cancer. Curr Urol Rep 2015;16(6):42.
38. Scarpato KR, Barocas DA. Use of mpMRI in active surveillance for localized prostate cancer. Urol Oncol 2016;34(7):320–5.
39. Le JD, Tan N, Shkolyar E, et al. Multifocality and prostate cancer detection by multiparametric magnetic resonance imaging: correlation with whole-mount histopathology. Eur Urol 2015;67(3):569–76.
40. Tan N, Margolis DJ, Lu DY, et al. Characteristics of detected and missed prostate cancer foci on 3-T multiparametric MRI using an endorectal coil correlated with whole-mount thin-section histopathology. AJR Am J Roentgenol 2015;205(1):W87–92.
41. Borkowetz A, Platzek I, Toma M, et al. Direct comparison of multiparametric magnetic resonance imaging (MRI) results with final histopathology in patients with proven prostate cancer in MRI/ultrasonography-fusion biopsy. BJU Int 2016;118(2):213–20.
42. Russo F, Regge D, Armando E, et al. Detection of prostate cancer index lesions with multiparametric magnetic resonance imaging (mp-MRI) using whole-mount histological sections as the reference standard. BJU Int 2016;118(1):84–94.
43. Greer MD, Brown AM, Shih JH, et al. Accuracy and agreement of PIRADSv2 for prostate cancer mpMRI: a multireader study. J Magn Reson Imaging 2016. [Epub ahead of print].
44. Pokorny MR, de Rooij M, Duncan E, et al. Prospective study of diagnostic accuracy comparing prostate cancer detection by transrectal ultrasound-guided biopsy versus magnetic resonance (MR) imaging with subsequent MR-guided biopsy in men without previous prostate biopsies. Eur Urol 2014;66(1):22–9.
45. Mendhiratta N, Rosenkrantz AB, Meng X, et al. Magnetic resonance imaging-ultrasound fusion targeted prostate biopsy in a consecutive cohort of men with no previous biopsy: reduction of over detection through improved risk stratification. J Urol 2015; 194(6):1601–6.
46. Siddiqui MM, Rais-Bahrami S, Turkbey B, et al. Comparison of MR/ultrasound fusion-guided biopsy with ultrasound-guided biopsy for the diagnosis of prostate cancer. JAMA 2015;313(4):390–7.
47. Park H, Wood D, Hussain H, et al. Introducing parametric fusion PET/MRI of primary prostate cancer. J Nucl Med 2012;53(4):546–51.
48. Hartenbach M, Hartenbach S, Bechtloff W, et al. Combined PET/MRI improves diagnostic accuracy in patients with prostate cancer: a prospective diagnostic trial. Clin Cancer Res 2014;20(12):3244–53.

49. Kim Y, Cheon GJ, Paeng JC, et al. Usefulness of MRI-assisted metabolic volumetric parameters provided by simultaneous ^{18}F-fluorocholine PET/MRI for primary prostate cancer characterization. Eur J Nucl Med Mol Imaging 2015;42(8):1247–56.
50. Piert M, Montgomery J, Kunju LP, et al. ^{18}F-choline PET/MRI: the additional value of PET for MRI-guided transrectal prostate biopsies. J Nucl Med 2016;57(7):1065–70.
51. Rhee H, Thomas P, Shepherd B, et al. Prostate specific membrane antigen positron emission tomography may improve the diagnostic accuracy of multiparametric magnetic resonance imaging in localized prostate cancer as confirmed by whole mount histopathology. J Urol 2016;196(4):1261–7.
52. Rahbar K, Weckesser M, Huss S, et al. Correlation of intraprostatic tumor extent with ^{68}Ga-PSMA distribution in patients with prostate cancer. J Nucl Med 2016;57(4):563–7.
53. Eiber M, Weirich G, Holzapfel K, et al. Simultaneous ^{68}Ga-PSMA-HBED-CC PET/MRI improves the localization of primary prostate cancer. Eur Urol 2016;70(5):829–36.
54. Fendler WP, Schmidt DF, Wenter V, et al. ^{68}Ga-PSMA-HBED-CC PET/CT detects location and extent of primary prostate cancer. J Nucl Med 2016;57(11):1720–5.
55. Marchal C, Redondo M, Padilla M, et al. Expression of prostate specific membrane antigen (PSMA) in prostatic adenocarcinoma and prostatic intraepithelial neoplasia. Histol Histopathol 2004;19(3):715–8.
56. Perner S, Hofer MD, Kim R, et al. Prostate-specific membrane antigen expression as a predictor of prostate cancer progression. Hum Pathol 2007,38(5):696–701.
57. Kasperzyk JL, Finn SP, Flavin R, et al. Prostate-specific membrane antigen protein expression in tumor tissue and risk of lethal prostate cancer. Cancer Epidemiol Biomarkers Prev 2013;22(12):2354–63.
58. Hillier SM, Maresca KP, Lu G, et al. ^{99m}Tc-labeled small-molecule inhibitors of prostate-specific membrane antigen for molecular imaging of prostate cancer. J Nucl Med 2013;54(8):1369–76.
59. Vallabhajosula S, Nikolopoulou A, Babich JW, et al. ^{99m}Tc-labeled small-molecule inhibitors of prostate-specific membrane antigen: pharmacokinetics and biodistribution studies in healthy subjects and patients with metastatic prostate cancer. J Nucl Med 2014;55(11):1791–8.
60. Dabasi G, Barra M, Tenke P, et al. Correlation of Technetium Tc99m trofolastat chloride (MIP-1404) uptake using SPECT/CT with histopathology: a phase 2 study of prostate cancer (PCa) patients undergoing radical prostatectomy (RP) with extended lymph node dissection (ePLND). Eur J Nucl Med Mol Imaging 2014;41:S236–7.
61. Goffin K, Joniau S, Tenke P, et al. Upgrading and downgrading of prostate biopsy results in a phase 2 study of MIP-1404 SPECT/CT in men undergoing radical prostatectomy. Eur J Nucl Med Mol Imaging 2015;42:S33.
62. Study to evaluate 99mTc-MIP-1404 SPECT/CT imaging in men with biopsy proven low-grade rrostate cancer (proSPECT-AS). Available at: https://clinicaltrials.gov/ct2/show/NCT02615067. Accessed August 15, 2016.
63. Dhar N, Ward JF, Cher ML, et al. Primary full-gland prostate cryoablation in older men (> age of 75 years): results from 860 patients tracked with the COLD Registry. BJU Int 2011;108(4):508–12.
64. Ward JF, Jones JS. Focal cryotherapy for localized prostate cancer: a report from the national Cryo On-Line Database (COLD) Registry. BJU Int 2012;109(11):1648–54.
65. Tay KJ, Polascik TJ, Elshafei A, et al. Primary cryotherapy for high-grade clinically localized prostate cancer: oncologic and functional outcomes from the COLD registry. J Endourol 2016;30(1):43–8.
66. Ganzer R, Robertson CN, Ward JF, et al. Correlation of prostate-specific antigen nadir and biochemical failure after high-intensity focused ultrasound of localized prostate cancer based on the Stuttgart failure criteria - analysis from the @-Registry. BJU Int 2011;108(8):E196–201.
67. Blana A, Robertson CN, Brown SCW, et al. Complete high-intensity focused ultrasound in prostate cancer: outcome from the @-Registry. Prostate Cancer Prostatic Dis 2012;15(3):256–9.
68. Berge V, Dickinson L, McCartan N, et al. Morbidity associated with primary high intensity focused ultrasound and redo high intensity focused ultrasound for localized prostate cancer. J Urol 2014;191(6):1764–9.
69. Ahmed HU, Dickinson L, Charman S, et al. Focal ablation targeted to the index lesion in multifocal localised prostate cancer: a prospective development study. Eur Urol 2015;68(6):927–36.
70. van Velthoven R, Aoun F, Marcelis Q, et al. A prospective clinical trial of HIFU hemiablation for clinically localized prostate cancer. Prostate Cancer Prostatic Dis 2016;19(1):79–83.
71. Feijoo ER, Sivaraman A, Barret E, et al. Focal high-intensity focused ultrasound targeted hemiablation for unilateral prostate cancer: a prospective evaluation of oncologic and functional outcomes. Eur Urol 2016;69(2):214–20.
72. Dickinson L, Arya M, Afzal N, et al. Medium-term outcomes after whole-gland high-intensity focused ultrasound for the treatment of nonmetastatic prostate cancer from a multicentre registry cohort. Eur Urol 2016;70(4):668–74.
73. Lindner U, Weersink RA, Haider MA, et al. Image guided photothermal focal therapy for localized

prostate cancer: phase I trial. J Urol 2009;182(4): 1371–7.
74. Oto A, Sethi I, Karczmar G, et al. MR imaging-guided focal laser ablation for prostate cancer: phase I trial. Radiology 2013;267(3):932–40.
75. Lepor H, Llukani E, Sperling D, et al. Complications, recovery, and early functional outcomes and oncologic control following in-bore focal laser ablation of prostate cancer. Eur Urol 2015;68(6):924–6.
76. Natarajan S, Raman S, Priester AM, et al. Focal laser ablation of prostate cancer: phase I clinical trial. J Urol 2016;196(1):68–75.
77. Ruijter ET, van de Kaa CA, Schalken JA, et al. Histological grade heterogeneity in multifocal prostate cancer. Biological and clinical implications. J Pathol 1996;180(3):295–9.
78. Douglas TH, McLeod DG, Mostofi FK, et al. Prostate-specific antigen-detected prostate cancer (stage T1c): an analysis of whole-mount prostatectomy specimens. Prostate 1997;32(1):59–64.
79. Arora R, Koch MO, Eble JN, et al. Heterogeneity of Gleason grade in multifocal adenocarcinoma of the prostate. Cancer 2004;100(11):2362–6.
80. Roach M 3rd, Hanks G, Thames H Jr, et al. Defining biochemical failure following radiotherapy with or without hormonal therapy in men with clinically localized prostate cancer: recommendations of the RTOG-ASTRO Phoenix Consensus Conference. Int J Radiat Oncol Biol Phys 2006;65(4):965–74.
81. Cookson MS, Aus G, Burnett AL, et al. Variation in the definition of biochemical recurrence in patients treated for localized prostate cancer: the American Urological Association Prostate Guidelines for Localized Prostate Cancer Update Panel report and recommendations for a standard in the reporting of surgical outcomes. J Urol 2007;177(2):540–5.
82. Leventis AK, Shariat SF, Kattan MW, et al. Prediction of response to salvage radiation therapy in patients with prostate cancer recurrence after radical prostatectomy. J Clin Oncol 2001;19(4):1030–9.
83. D'Amico AV, Chen M, Roehl KA, et al. Identifying patients at risk for significant versus clinically insignificant postoperative prostate-specific antigen failure. J Clin Oncol 2005;23(22):4975–9.
84. Stephenson AJ, Scardino PT, Kattan MW, et al. Predicting the outcome of salvage radiation therapy for recurrent prostate cancer after radical prostatectomy. J Clin Oncol 2007;25(15):2035–41.
85. Trock BJ, Han M, Freedland SJ, et al. Prostate cancer-specific survival following salvage radiotherapy vs observation in men with biochemical recurrence after radical prostatectomy. JAMA 2008;299(23):2760–9.
86. Jackson W, Hamstra DA, Johnson S, et al. Gleason pattern 5 is the strongest pathologic predictor of recurrence, metastasis, and prostate cancer-specific death in patients receiving salvage radiation therapy following radical prostatectomy. Cancer 2013;119(18):3287–94.
87. Pound CR, Partin AW, Eisenberger MA, et al. Natural history of progression after PSA elevation following radical prostatectomy. JAMA 1999;281(17):1591–7.
88. Sweeney CJ, Chen YH, Carducci M, et al. Chemohormonal therapy in metastatic hormone-sensitive prostate cancer. N Engl J Med 2015;373(8):737–46.
89. James ND, Sydes MR, Clarke NW, et al. Addition of docetaxel, zoledronic acid, or both to first-line long-term hormone therapy in prostate cancer (STAMPEDE): survival results from an adaptive, multiarm, multistage, platform randomised controlled trial. Lancet 2016;387(10024):1163–77.
90. Reyes DK, Pienta KJ. The biology and treatment of oligometastatic cancer. Oncotarget 2015;6(11): 8491–524.
91. Ost P, Bossi A, Decaestecker K, et al. Metastasis-directed therapy of regional and distant recurrences after curative treatment of prostate cancer: a systematic review of the literature. Eur Urol 2015; 67(5):852–63.
92. Armstrong AJ, Febbo PG. Using surrogate biomarkers to predict clinical benefit in men with castration-resistant prostate cancer: an update and review of the literature. Oncologist 2009;14(8):816–27.
93. Colloca G. Prostate-specific antigen kinetics as a surrogate endpoint in clinical trials of metastatic castration-resistant prostate cancer: a review. Cancer Treat Rev 2012;38(8):1020–6.
94. Wahl RL, Jacene H, Kasamon Y, et al. From RECIST to PERCIST: evolving considerations for PET response criteria in solid tumors. J Nucl Med 2009; 50(Suppl 1):122S–50S.
95. Bi L, Kim J, Wen L, et al. Automated and robust PERCIST-based thresholding framework for whole body PET-CT studies. Conf Proc IEEE Eng Med Biol Soc 2012;2012:5335–8.
96. Son SH, Lee SW, Jeong SY, et al. Whole-body metabolic tumor volume, as determined by ^{18}F-FDG PET/CT, as a prognostic factor of outcome for patients with breast cancer who have distant metastasis. AJR Am J Roentgenol 2015;205(4):878–85.
97. Zhang H, Wroblewski K, Jiang Y, et al. A new PET/CT volumetric prognostic index for non-small cell lung cancer. Lung Cancer 2015;89(1):43–9.
98. Kratochwil C, Giesel FL, Stefanova M, et al. PSMA-targeted radionuclide therapy of metastatic castration-resistant prostate cancer with ^{177}Lu-Labeled PSMA-617. J Nucl Med 2016;57(8):1170–6.
99. Rahbar K, Schmidt M, Heinzel A, et al. Response and tolerability of a single dose of ^{177}Lu-PSMA-617 in patients with metastatic castration-resistant prostate cancer: a multicenter retrospective analysis. J Nucl Med 2016;57(9):1334–8.

Imaging of Prostate Cancer Using ^{64}Cu-Labeled Prostate-Specific Membrane Antigen Ligand

Aviral Singh, MD, MSc*, Harshad R. Kulkarni, MD, Richard P. Baum, MD, PhD

KEYWORDS

- Prostate cancer • Molecular imaging • ^{64}Cu-PSMA

KEY POINTS

- Several PET-based radiopharmaceuticals are currently available for imaging of prostate cancer, namely, ^{68}Ga-PSMA, ^{18}F-choline, ^{18}F-sodium fluoride, ^{18}F-FACBC, ^{18}F-FDG, and GRPR-antagonists, and several more are being researched.
- Recently ^{68}Ga-labeled PSMA-targeted PET imaging has demonstrated superior results in prostate cancer restaging compared with other modalities; nonetheless, ^{64}Cu has suitable properties for PET imaging and a relatively longer half-life compared with ^{68}Ga, rendering it lucrative from several logistical perspectives.
- ^{64}Cu-PSMA PET/CT could potentially become a suitable alternative for PET imaging of prostate cancer, offering a further possibility of radioligand therapy with the beta-emitting ^{67}Cu as a "theranostics pair."

INTRODUCTION

Prostate cancer is the most common noncutaneous cancer among men, and the leading cause of death from cancer in certain countries, including the United States[1] and Europe,[2] rendering the diagnosis and staging of this cancer of significant medical and public interest. Approximately 1 in 7 men are expected to develop prostate cancer in their lifetime, and this likelihood increases with age, and although prostate cancer can be slow growing, the disease nonetheless accounts for almost 10% of cancer-related deaths in men. The American Cancer Society estimates that 240,890 new cases of prostate cancer would be diagnosed in the United States in 2016 and that 26,120 men will die of the disease within this year.[1] For the past several decades, bone scintigraphy with ^{99m}Tc-labeled methylene diphosphonate (MDP) has been the standard for assessing potential bone metastases from prostate cancer in patients, but it suffers from a relatively low specificity.[3]

However, the current trend of moving toward personalized medicine warrants the development and standardization of more specialized and specific imaging techniques and biomarkers representing a more accurate picture of the extent of disease. In recent years, one of the most interesting developments in the application of nuclear oncology has been the development of novel diagnostic agents that are able to facilitate targeted therapies using the concept of theranostics.

The authors have nothing to disclose.
THERANOSTICS Center for Molecular Radiotherapy and Molecular Imaging (PET/CT), ENETS Center of Excellence, Zentralklinik Bad Berka, Robert-Koch-Allee 9, Bad Berka 99437, Germany
* Corresponding author.
E-mail address: aviral.singh@zentralklinik.de

PET Clin 12 (2017) 193–203
http://dx.doi.org/10.1016/j.cpet.2016.12.001

This review summarizes the current and emerging molecular imaging techniques for the investigation of patients with prostate cancer with emphasis on the potential of ^{64}Cu–prostate-specific membrane antigen (PSMA) PET/computed tomography (CT) in staging, restaging, and the application of theranostics.

CURRENT IMAGING TECHNIQUES

Conventional approaches for the morphologic imaging of prostate cancer include regular B-mode transperineal and transrectal ultrasound (TRUS), CT, and MR imaging. The use of TRUS, although limited, plays an essential role in guidance of interventions such as prostate biopsies, TRUS-guided brachytherapy, and also in the evaluation of recurrence after radical prostatectomy in patients with increasing serum prostate-specific antigen (PSA) levels.[4] Although CT is often used for the initial staging of intermediate to high-risk disease and the evaluation of pelvic and extraprostatic extension of nodal disease, its sensitivity is only 35%.[5] Multiparametric MR imaging, including diffusion-weighted imaging, dynamic contrast-enhanced MR imaging, and MR spectroscopy, have been reported to be more precise for detection and local staging of untreated prostate cancer or for detecting residual or local recurrent prostate cancer.[6,7]

CONVENTIONAL NUCLEAR MEDICINE IMAGING

Because prostate cancer mostly metastasizes to bones with predominantly osteoblastic (sclerotic) bone metastases, thus the mainstay of evaluating skeletal metastases has been whole-body planar with or without regional single-photon emission computed tomography (SPECT) bone scintigraphy using ^{99m}Tc-MDP. However, it suffers from a relatively low specificity and often requires correlation of the findings with other imaging modalities.[3] According to the joint European Association of Urology, European Society for Radiotherapy and Oncology, and International Society of Geriatric Oncology guidelines, suspicion of disease progression indicates the need for additional imaging modalities, guided by symptoms or possible subsequent treatments. In castration-resistant prostate cancer (CRPC), imaging must be individualized with the aim of maintaining the patient's quality of life.[8]

MOLECULAR IMAGING WITH PET

Although PET imaging is still considered less useful for establishing the initial diagnosis of prostate cancer, it plays an important role in the detection of biochemical relapse, recurrence, and extent of metastatic disease. Several radiopharmaceuticals are in use for this purpose. PET is usually combined with CT or MR imaging for the anatomic localization of the uptake of the radiotracers. However, the choice of the radiopharmaceutical is determined by tumor biology. Recent years have seen a surge in the variety of PET radiopharmaceuticals for the molecular imaging of prostate cancer.

Fluoride-18 Labeled Sodium Fluoride

Fluoride-18 labeled sodium fluoride (^{18}F-NaF) is a PET radiopharmaceutical that is used for identification of new bone formation with PET imaging. The uptake mechanism of NaF resembles that of MDP; however, with better pharmacokinetic characteristics, including very rapid blood clearance, which results in a high bone-to-background ratio with twofold higher uptake in bone compared with MDP,[9,10] and incorporation of bone findings from CT with ^{18}F-fluoride PET/CT results in improved specificity.[11]

^{18}F-Fluorodeoxyglucose

^{18}F-fluorodeoxyglucose (^{18}F-FDG) PET is an analog of glucose that reflects local rates of glucose consumption by tissues, and shows increased trapping by tumor cells due to increased metabolism and thus glycolytic activity of tumors.[12] Although widely used in cancer imaging, its use is limited in primary prostate cancer detection, due to slow growth and low glucose metabolism in low grade disease and nonspecific uptake in prostatitis and benign prostatic hypertrophy (BPH).[13] However, certain studies have indicated its role in more advanced prostate cancer states for evaluating lymph node and bone metastases, thus suggesting use for restaging after PSA relapse and for assessment of treatment response in aggresive CRPC.[12,14–16]

^{11}C-/^{18}F-Choline

Prostate cancer cells rely more on fatty acid metabolism than glycolysis with upregulation and increased activity of lipogenic enzymes.[17] The ^{11}C/18F choline-based (^{11}C/^{18}F-choline) and ^{11}C-acetate agents are lipid-metabolism PET agents that have been associated with overexpression of choline kinase[18,19] and fatty acid synthase,[20] respectively. ^{11}C/^{18}F-choline are taken up in prostate cancer cells through choline transporters and phosphorylated intracellularly by choline kinase.[21] The role of these agents in initial staging is not well established, because of false positives in prostatitis and BPH and false negatives in small (<5 mm) or necrotic tumors.[22,23] However, they have promising results for restaging after PSA relapse, with high sensitivity for local recurrence, nodal metastases, and bone metastases.[24–26]

^{18}F-Fluorocyclobutane-1-Carboxylic Acid

Amino acids, such as leucine, methionine, and glutamine, are effectively taken up by many tumors because of increased amino acid transport and metabolism. The most promising of these agents for prostate cancer imaging is anti-1-amino-3-^{18}F-fluorocyclobutane-1-carboxylic acid (anti-^{18}F-FACBC or ^{18}F-FACBC), a synthetic alicyclic alpha-amino acid. It is preferentially taken up by prostate cancer cells by transporters such as LAT-1 and ASCT2, which are upregulated in prostate cancer cells. This agent was approved in May 2016 for PET imaging in men with suspected prostate cancer recurrence,[27,28] based on a comparative trial with ^{11}C-choline. Sensitivities for ^{11}C-choline and ^{18}F-fluciclovine were 32% versus 37%, specificities 40% versus 67%, accuracies 32% versus 38%, and positive predictive values 90% versus 97%, respectively.[29]

Gastrin-Releasing Peptide Receptor–Based Radiopharmaceuticals

Gastrin-releasing peptide receptor (GRPR) is physiologically expressed in the gastrointestinal tract and the central nervous system. It is overexpressed in different malignant tumors, particularly in prostate cancer, and is thus considered a suitable target for prostate cancer imaging.[30] The superior pharmacokinetics of GRPR radioantagonists over their agonist counterparts in combination with their higher inherent biosafety has shifted current research toward the design of new improved GRPR radioantagonist candidates with clear potential for clinical translation.[30–33] A multicenter European collaboration, including our group, initially reported the first experience of excellent pharmacokinetics of ^{67}Ga-labeled GRPR antagonist (SB3) in PC-3 tumor–bearing mice, whereas ^{68}Ga-SB3 PET/CT visualized lesions in approximately 50% of patients with advanced and metastasized prostate and breast cancer.[34] Another combined preclinical and clinical study with the GRPR-antagonist NeoBOMB1 showed a comparable behavior in prostate cancer models with successful visualization of prostate cancer lesions in humans using ^{68}Ga-NeoBOMB1 PET/CT imaging.[35] In a pilot study in 4 patients with prostate cancer, Wieser and colleagues demonstrated the favorable biodistribution and high tumor uptake of the GRPR antagonist ^{64}Cu-CB-TE2A-AR06 ([^{64}Cu-4,11-bis(carboxymethyl)-1,4,8,11-tetraazabicyclo (6.6.2)hexadecane]-PEG4-D-Phe-Gln-Trp-Ala-Val-Gly-His-Sta-Leu-NH2), associated with a rapid clearance from normal physiologic tissue.[30]

PROSTATE-SPECIFIC MEMBRANE ANTIGEN: BIOLOGICAL PROPERTIES

PSMA is a type II transmembrane protein with an extensive extracellular domain, a transmembrane segment, and an intracellular domain that is overexpressed in prostate cancer, including androgen-independent, advanced, and metastatic disease.[36–38] It is also located on the luminal side of the brush border cells in the jejunum, where it is known as folate hydrolase I, and cleaves ϒ-linked glutamates from folates.[39] PSMA expression and localization in the normal human prostate is associated with the cytoplasm and apical side of the epithelium surrounding prostatic ducts but not basal epithelium, neuroendocrine, or stromal cells.[40] Following substrate binding, small-molecule antagonist or specific antibody binding, PSMA-bound ligands are internalized within the cell and are either retained in lysosomal compartments along with the degrading PSMA receptor,[37] or bound ligands may be released to distribute within the cell or diffuse out of the cell as labile metabolites.[41,42]

Because PSMA is a well-characterized target for prostate cancer and its elevated expression is associated with metastasis,[43] androgen independence,[44] and disease recurrence,[45] and generally increases with increasing Gleason score,[46] it has become a valuable focus for the development of new imaging agents, particularly for PET radiopharmaceuticals.

PROSTATE-SPECIFIC MEMBRANE ANTIGEN–BASED IMAGING OF PROSTATE CANCER

Over the past 2 decades, researchers have made efforts to target specific regions of the intracellular or extracellular domain of PSMA with monoclonal antibodies labeled with different radioisotopes. Thus far, only the In-111 radiolabeled anti-PSMA antibody 7E11 (ProstaScint) had been approved by the Food and Drug Administration.[47] It acts by recognizing the intracellular portion of PSMA and offers the potential to detect recurrent disease in patients with rising serum PSA levels after primary therapy.[48] Unfortunately, it has several logistical limitations and a low diagnostic sensitivity.[49,50]

The identification of the active substrate recognition site of PSMA with its structural and functional homology to glutamate carboxypeptidase 2 (also known as *N*-acetylated-α-linked acidic dipeptidase I) promoted the development of small molecules as PSMA ligands or inhibitors.[51,52] PSMA inhibitors fall into 3 categories: phosphorous-based, thiol-based, and urea-based. Urea-based inhibitors have a high affinity and specificity for PSMA with fast and efficient internalization in LNCaP (androgen-sensitive human prostate adenocarcinoma) cells.[53]

The first radiolabeled, low-molecular-weight imaging agent targeting PSMA was *N*-[*N*-[(*S*)-1,3-dicarboxypropyl]carbamoyl]-*S*-[^{11}C]methyl-L-cysteine (^{11}C-DCMC), which demonstrated the proof-of-principle for radiolabeled ureas to be used as PSMA-targeted agents for PET imaging.[54,55]

Eder and colleagues[53] initially described the PSMA inhibitor Glu-NH-CO-NH-Lys(Ahx)-HBED-CC (^{68}Ga-PSMA-HBED-CC), which has been extensively used in clinical practice for the evaluation of recurrent prostate cancer, for selection of patients for ^{177}Lu-PSMA radioligand therapy and assessment of response to therapy.[56] PET/CT using ^{68}Ga-labeled PSMA-HBED-CC has been proven to better detect prostate cancer relapse and metastases as compared with ^{18}F-choline PET/CT.[57] In another study of 130 patients with intermediate to high-risk prostate cancer, preoperative lymph node staging with ^{68}Ga-PSMA-PET proved to be superior to standard routine imaging using CT and MR imaging.[58] ^{68}Ga-PSMA has also been recently shown to be useful for the restaging of prostate cancer in patients being considered for salvage radiotherapy even at PSA levels less than 0.5 ng/mL.[59] Other recently developed ^{68}Ga-labeled PSMA ligands include ^{68}Ga-DOTAGA-ffk(Sub-KuE) (^{68}Ga-PSMA imaging and therapy [I&T])[60] and PSMA-DKFZ-617,[61] both of which have been used for the imaging of prostate cancer, ^{177}Lu-based PSMA-targeted radioligand therapy, and response assessment to PSMA inhibitor radioligand therapy with very encouraging clinical results, at our and other centers.[62–64]

Theranostics of metastatic CRPC (mCRPC) is fast gaining worldwide attention, whereby PSMA ligands are preferentially radiolabeled with ^{68}Ga for whole-body PET imaging followed by targeted therapy with beta-emitting (^{177}Lu) or alpha-emitting (^{225}Ac and ^{213}Bi) radionuclides. However, the widespread use of PET/CT imaging using ^{68}Ga-PSMA can be limited by the unavailability of an onsite ^{68}Ge/^{68}Ga generator. Therefore, newer radiopharmaceuticals are being investigated to overcome the shortcomings of ^{68}Ga as a radionuclide. One such option could potentially be PSMA-labeled ^{64}Cu PET imaging.

COPPER-64: GENERAL AND PHYSICAL PROPERTIES FOR PET IMAGING

Copper (Cu) is a transition metal with atomic number 29, and an important trace element for most organisms. In humans, copper plays a role as a cofactor for numerous enzymes, such as Cu/Zn-superoxide dismutase, cytochrome-c oxidase, tyrosinase, ceruloplasmin, and other proteins, crucial for respiration, iron transport and metabolism, cell growth, and hemostasis.[65,66] For widespread use in medicine of any radioisotope, 2 factors are essential: availability of the isotope and a stable and effective mode of binding with an appropriate chemical carrier.[67] Selection of the proper radionuclide in radiopharmaceutical design is critical and depends on several factors, including the half-life of the radionuclide, which should allow sufficient uptake and distribution to yield considerable contrast and quality images. The energies of the radionuclide emission should be appropriate for proper detection by the equipment, whereas cost and availability are also important considerations.[68] Natural copper comprises 2 stable isotopes, ^{63}Cu (69.17%) and ^{65}Cu (30.83%), and 27 known radioisotopes; 5 of them are particularly interesting for molecular imaging applications (^{60}Cu, ^{61}Cu, ^{62}Cu, and ^{64}Cu), and in vivo targeted radionuclide therapy (^{64}Cu and ^{67}Cu).[67]

^{64}Cu-labeled molecules are promising imaging agents for PET due to the favorable nuclear characteristics of the isotope (half-life = 12.7 hours, $\beta+$ 17.8%, maximum energy (Emax) = 0.655 MeV, $\beta-$ 38.4%, Emax = 0.573 MeV) and its availability in high specific activity.[68] The longer physical half-life of ^{64}Cu compared to ^{68}Ga (68.73 h) (**Table 1**), ^{11}C (20 minutes) and ^{18}F (110 minutes) enables imaging at delayed time points, which allows sufficient time for clearance from background tissues, resulting in increased image contrast, particularly for targeting agents that demonstrate long circulation times, such as antibodies and nanoparticles.[69]

PRODUCTION OF COPPER 64

^{64}Cu is a highly unusual isotope because it decays by 3 processes, namely, positron, electron capture, and beta decays. This property allows either cyclotron or reactor production.[70] At present, the most common production method for ^{64}Cu uses the ^{64}Ni(p,n) ^{64}Cu reaction.[71,72]

The production of noncarrier-added ^{64}Cu via the ^{64}Ni(p,n)^{64}Cu reaction on a biomedical cyclotron was proposed by Szelecsenyi and colleagues.[73] Subsequent studies by McCarthy and colleagues[71] were performed, and this method is

Table 1
Decay characteristics of copper-64 and copper-67 in comparison to gallium-68

Isotope	Half-Life	β^- keV (%)	β^+ keV (%)	EC (%)	γ keV (%)
^{64}Cu	12.7 h	573 (38.4)	655 (17.8)	43.8	511 (35.6)
^{68}Ga	67.83 min	1899 (87.8) 822 (1.2)	88.88 (41) —	41 —	511 (178) 1077 (3.2)
^{67}Cu	61.83 h	395 (45) 484 (35) 577 (20)	—	—	184 (40) — —

now used to provide ^{64}Cu for research. Another method of ^{64}Cu production is the ^{64}Zn(n,p)^{64}Cu reaction in a nuclear reactor.[74] Smith and colleagues[75] separated large amounts of ^{64}Cu by-product from cyclotron production of ^{67}Ga via the ^{68}Zn(p,2n)^{67}Ga reaction at the National Medical Cyclotron, Sydney, Australia; this method of production has the advantage of being economical and allows for the production of large amounts (>111 GBq [>3 Ci]) of reasonably high specific activity material (~31.8 TBq/mmol [~860 Ci/mmol]). However, the on-demand production would be problematic, because most of the produced radionuclide is long lived ^{67}Ga (half-life = 72 hours). Although the proton-induced reaction on enriched ^{64}Ni plays a key role for practical production; recently the deuteron-induced reactions are also intensively studied and seem promising.[76]

PRECLINICAL IMAGING WITH COPPER 64–LABELED PROSTATE-SPECIFIC MEMBRANE ANTIGEN

The well-established coordination chemistry of Cu allows for its reaction with a wide variety of chelator systems that can potentially be linked to antibodies, proteins, peptides, and other biologically relevant small molecules.[68]

All Cu radioisotopes are currently investigated for clinical applications, but ^{64}Cu, particularly its form $^{64}CuCl_2$, is the most widely studied isotope for its potential role in PET imaging and therapy; it has been bound to several carriers that can be applied to monitor copper metabolism status and guide personalized copper chelator treatment in patients with cancer.[77] In a study to determine whether human prostate cancer xenografts in mice can be localized by PET using $^{64}CuCl_2$, Peng and colleagues[78] subjected athymic mice bearing human prostate cancer xenografts to ^{64}Cu PET, followed by quantitative analysis of the tracer concentrations and immunohistochemistry study of human copper transporter 1 expression in the tumor tissues. As a result, the human prostate cancer xenografts expressing high levels of human copper transporter 1 were well visualized on PET images obtained 24 hours after injection, but not on the images obtained 1 hour after injection. PET quantitative analysis demonstrated a high concentration of $^{64}CuCl_2$ in the tumors in comparison with that in the corresponding normal tissue at 24 hours after injection, concluding that locally recurrent prostate cancer might be localized with ^{64}Cu PET using $^{64}CuCl_2$ as a probe.[78]

The first radiolabeled, low-molecular-weight imaging agent targeting PSMA was *N*-[*N*-[(*S*)-1,3-dicarboxypropyl]carbamoyl]-*S*-[^{11}C]methyl-L-cysteine (^{11}C-DCMC) 6, and was described by the group of Pomper.[54,55] Banerjee and colleagues,[69] of the same group, described 5 new low-molecular-weight, urea-based, ^{64}Cu-labeled, PSMA-targeted radiotracers that incorporated well-established chelating agents. All compounds demonstrated high tumor uptake and retention, with the choice of chelator having a profound effect on pharmacokinetics, revealing that ^{64}Cu, which uses the CB-TE2A chelator, demonstrated improved biodistribution with rapid clearance from normal tissues, including kidney, resulting in significantly improved image contrast. Accordingly, it provides a potentially clinically viable imaging agent for PSMA-expressing tissues, particularly if delayed imaging is required, which is obtainable with ^{64}Cu.[69]

Nedrow and colleagues[79] evaluated the PET imaging agent, [^{64}Cu]ABN-1, for selective uptake both in vitro and in vivo in PSMA-positive cells of varying expression levels in a panel of prostate tumor–bearing mouse models. [^{64}Cu]ABN-1 demonstrated excellent uptake in PSMA-positive cells in vitro, with approximately 80% internalization at 4 hours for each PSMA-positive cell line with uptake (fmol/mg) correlating to PSMA expression levels. The imaging data indicated significant tumor uptake in all models. The biodistribution for late-passage LNCaP cell lines with the highest PSMA expression demonstrated the highest specific uptake of [^{64}Cu]ABN-1 with tumor-to-muscle and tumor-to-blood ratios of 30 ± 11 and 21 ± 7, respectively, at 24 hours postinjection. [^{64}Cu]ABN-1 cleared through all tissues except for PSMA-positive kidneys, thus suggesting that [^{64}Cu]ABN-1 will selectively target and image PSMA expression and in the future will serve as a noninvasive method to follow the progression of prostate cancer in men.[79]

Recently, the group from Paul Scherer Institut, Villigen, Switzerland, reported the synthesis of a novel albumin-binding folate conjugate (rf42).[80] Based on this concept, the same group studied the in vitro stability and binding properties and folate receptor–specific uptake and internalization into folate receptor–positive KB (cervical carcinoma cell line) tumor cells, with subsequent in vivo assessment of the biodistribution of ^{64}Cu-labeled and ^{68}Ga-labeled NODAGA-folates on PET/CT studies using these KB-tumor–bearing mice. The study revealed that the novel albumin-binding NODAGA-folate was suitable for labeling with ^{64}Cu and ^{68}Ga in high radiochemical yields, with both ^{64}Cu-rf42 and ^{68}Ga-rf42 exhibiting excellent in vitro properties, and favorable in vivo pharmacokinetics with regard to tumor uptake and reduced retention in the kidneys. However, eventually ^{64}Cu-labeled rf42 was recommended as the most promising compound for PET imaging due to the resulting favorable tumor-to-kidney ratios, and the novel NODAGA-folate rf42 was proposed to be investigated further using the matched pair ^{64}Cu/^{67}Cu for theranostic applications.[81]

COPPER 64–PROSTATE-SPECIFIC MEMBRANE ANTIGEN-BASED MOLECULAR IMAGING OF PROSTATE CANCER

Despite extensive preclinical studies performed over the past decades, not much work has yet been reported in relation to the clinical imaging of prostate cancer.

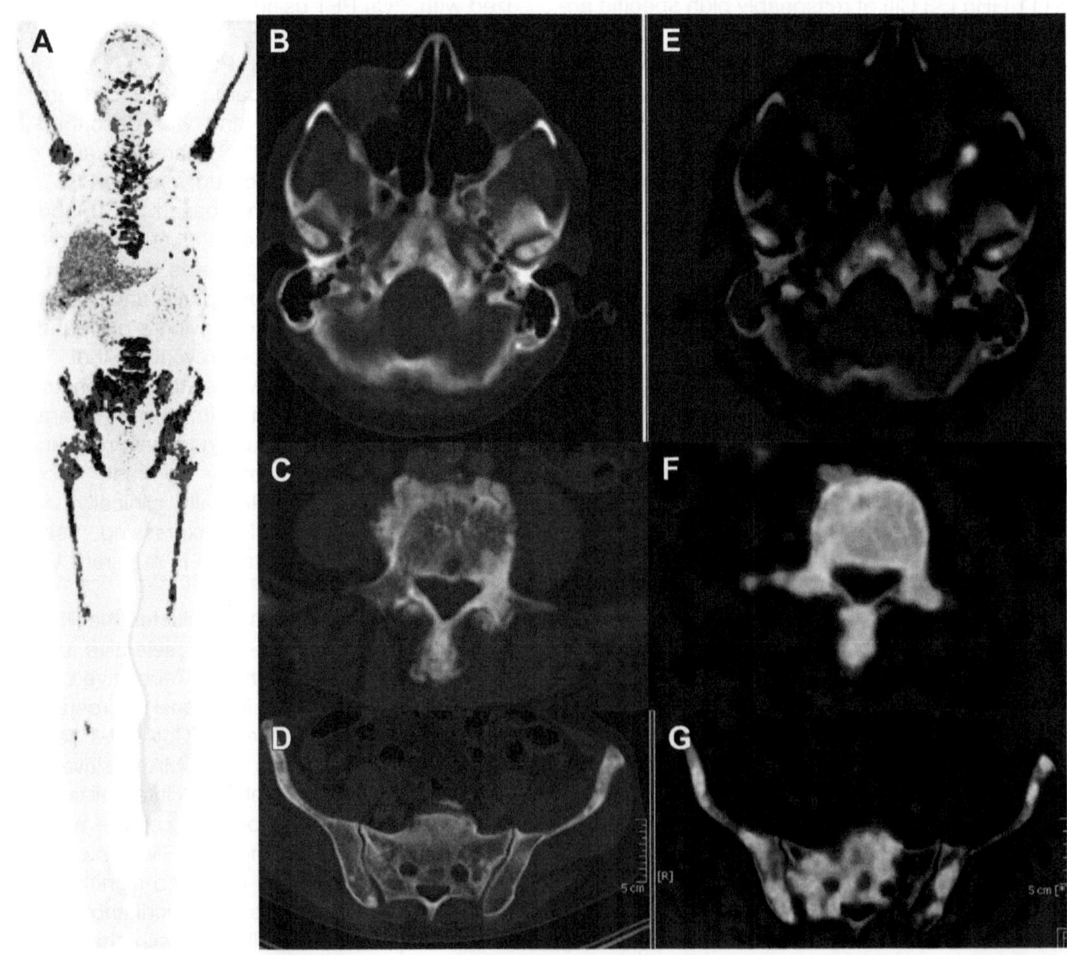

Fig. 1. ^{64}Cu-PSMA PET/CT demonstrates extensive axial and appendicular skeletal metastases. (*A*) MIP image. (*B–D*) Serial axial CT. (*E–G*) Corresponding PET/CT fusion images.

The first-in-human study using the urea-based PSMA ligand labeled with ^{64}Cu (^{64}Cu-PSMA-617) PET (n = 21) and PET/CT (n = 8) for molecular imaging of prostate cancer was performed simultaneously at the Institute of Nuclear Medicine and PET-Center, Wilhelminenspital, Vienna, Austria, and Theranostics Center for Radiotherapy and Molecular Imaging, Zentralklinik Bad Berka, Germany. Dosimetry performed on 3 patients according to Medical Internal Radiation Dose scheme using the OLINDA/EXM software (Vanderbilt University, Nashville, TN), based on images acquired up to 24 hours following the injection of ^{64}Cu-PSMA-617, revealed a total body dose of 0.014 mGy/MBq. In this study, patients that were imaged with ^{64}Cu-PSMA PET alone, demonstrated local recurrence of prostate cancer in 5 (24%) of 21, and detected lymph node metastases in 9 (43%) of 21 and skeletal metastases in 6 (29%) of 21 patients. Overall, 17 (81%) of 21 cases were found positive on ^{64}Cu-PSMA-617 PET. The patients who underwent restaging with ^{64}Cu-PSMA-617 PET/CT demonstrated positive uptake in the prostate bed in 2 (25%) of 8, within lymph node and skeletal metastases in 4 (50%) of 8 patients each. Overall, 6 (75%) of 8 studies demonstrated positive uptake of ^{64}Cu-PSMA-617.[82]

Based on previously described extensive experience with ^{68}Ga-PSMA PET/CT imaging and ^{177}Lu-PSMA radioligand therapy,[56] the updated results of the initial clinical application of ^{64}Cu-PSMA PET/CT in theranostics of prostate cancer in 9 patients were reported by our group, where 2 (22.2%) of 9 patients demonstrated uptake in the prostate bed, suggestive of local recurrent disease; and lymph node and skeletal metastases were detected in 5 (55.5%) of 9 and 4 (44.4%) of 9 patients, respectively (**Figs. 1–3**). The clinical implication of the ^{64}Cu-based PSMA-617 inhibitor ligand PET/CT molecular imaging was evaluated, and progressive disease was observed in 4 (44.4%) of 9 patients. Based on the principle of theranostics, 3 of these patients received ^{177}Lu-PSMA radioligand therapy. No adverse effects to the administration of ^{64}Cu-PSMA-617 were reported in these patients.[83]

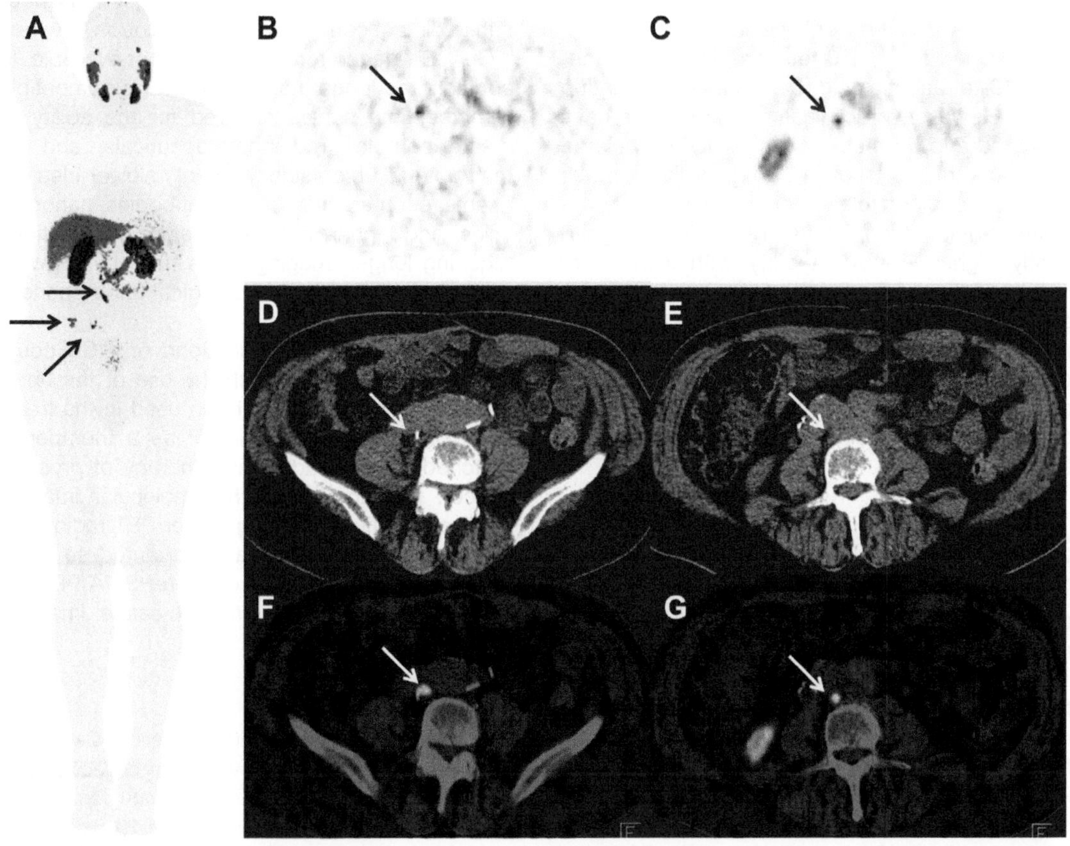

Fig. 2. Patient restaged with progressive disease. ^{64}Cu-PSMA PET/CT demonstrates multiple abdominopelvic lymph node metastases. (*A*) MIP image. (*B, C*) Axial PET images. (*D, E*) Corresponding CT. (*F, G*) PET/CT fusion images. Arrows indicate positive findings.

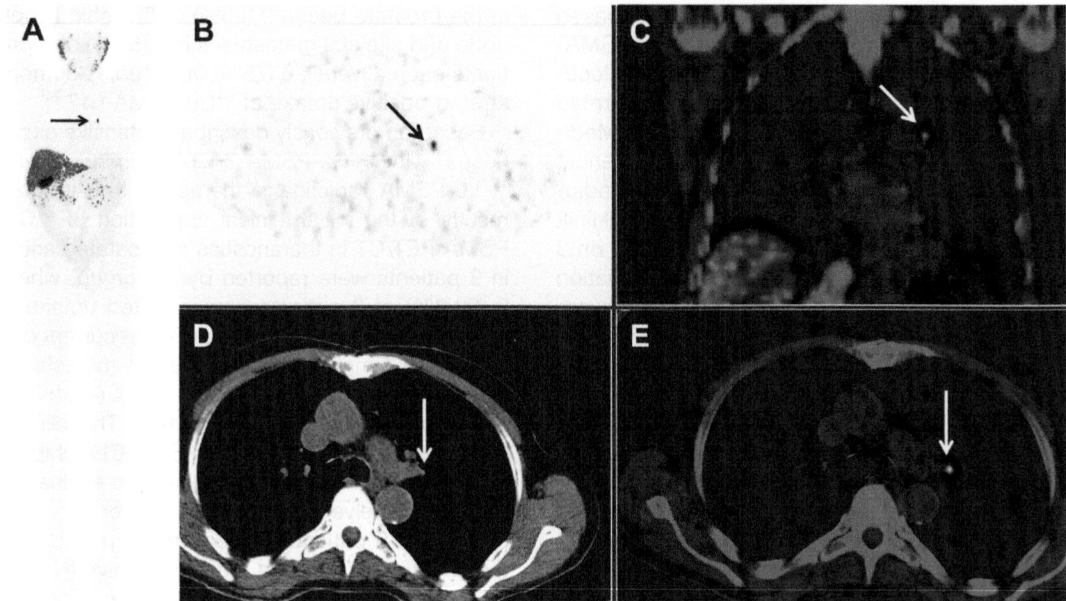

Fig. 3. Patient restaged due to increasing serum PSA. ^{64}Cu-PSMA PET/CT demonstrates multiple lymph node metastases. (*A*) MIP image. (*B*) Axial PET image; (*D*) corresponding axial CT and (*E*) PET/CT fusion image. (*C*) Coronal fusion PET/CT image. Arrows indicate positive findings.

The synthesis of ^{64}Cu-PSMA-617 was performed at Advanced Center Oncology Maserata, Italy, using 1,4,7,10-tetraazacyclododecane-1,4,7,10-tetraacetic acid (DOTA) as the chelating agent. However, preclinical animal studies have indicated a lower stability of the DOTA-chelated ^{64}Cu radiotracers, showing a higher liver uptake and slower blood clearance, indicative of free Cu(II) sequestration in the liver, and a significantly higher in vivo stability with lower liver uptake of the 1,4,7-triazacyclononane-1,4,7-tris-acetic acid (NOTA)- and CB2-TE2A-conjugated radiotracers.[69] This certainly warrants the application of other proposed chelators in the radiochemistry of labeling ^{64}Cu with PSMA to enhance the molecular imaging results of prostate cancer.

SUMMARY

^{64}Cu-based radiopharmaceuticals aim to establish a “one-stop-shop” for the diagnosis, staging, restaging, and prognostication of prostate cancer. The emerging evidence holds great promise for the future of ^{64}Cu-based radiopharmaceuticals. Initial clinical studies demonstrate that high-quality images can be obtained using ^{64}Cu-PSMA PET/CT. The longer half-life of ^{64}Cu, compared with that of ^{68}Ga, provides the significant advantage of late imaging up to 24 hours after administration of the radiopharmaceutical, and the possibility of centralized production of the radiopharmaceutical and subsequent distribution to distant centers lacking a cyclotron or where ^{68}Ge/^{68}Ga-generator facilities are not available. In addition, the longer half-life of ^{64}Cu is compatible with the time scales required for the ability to create complex radiopharmaceuticals, and for the optimal biodistribution of slower-clearing agents, such as monoclonal antibodies, nanoparticles, and higher-molecular-weight polypeptides requiring longer imaging times, thereby allowing several applications in oncological and nononcological fields.[84]

Future diagnostic applications of ^{64}Cu could possibly be enhanced with the use of the beta-emitting ^{67}Cu, which has been used in the treatment of other malignancies,[85] as a therapeutic matched pair for radioligand therapy of prostate cancer. Nonetheless, further molecular imaging studies directly comparing newer PET radiopharmaceuticals, ^{18}F-PSMA, are warranted so as to establish the specific role of ^{64}Cu-PSMA PET imaging in the algorithm of prostate cancer imaging.

REFERENCES

1. Cancer Facts & Figures 2016. American Cancer Society. Available at: http://www.cancer.org/acs/groups/content/@research/documents/document/acspc-047079.pdf. Accessed September 9, 2016.
2. Arnold M, Karim-Kos HE, Coebergh JW, et al. Recent trends in incidence of five common cancers in 26 European countries since 1988: analysis of the

European Cancer Observatory. Eur J Cancer 2015; 51:1164.

3. Langsteger W, Haim S, Knauer M, et al. Imaging of bone metastases in prostate cancer: an update. Q J Nucl Med Mol Imaging 2012;56(5):447–58.
4. Shinohara K, Wheeler TM, Scardino PT. The appearance of prostate cancer on transrectal ultrasonography: correlation of imaging and pathological examinations. J Urol 1989;142(1):76–82.
5. Hricak H, Choyke PL, Eberhardt SC, et al. Imaging prostate cancer: a multidisciplinary perspective. Radiology 2007;243(1):28–53.
6. Bonekamp D, Jacobs MA, El-Khouli R, et al. Advancements in MR imaging of the prostate: from diagnosis to interventions. Radiographics 2011; 31(3):677–703.
7. Pepe P, Garufi A, Priolo G, et al. Can MRI/TRUS fusion targeted biopsy replace saturation prostate biopsy in the re-evaluation of men in active surveillance? World J Urol 2016;34(9):1249–53.
8. Available at: http://uroweb.org/guideline/prostate-cancer/. Accessed August 8, 2016.
9. Segall G, Delbeke D, Stabin MG, et al. SNM practice guideline for sodium 18F-fluoride PET/CT bone scans 1.0. J Nucl Med 2010;51(11):1813–20.
10. Grant FD, Fahey FH, Packard AB, et al. Skeletal PET with 18F-fluoride: applying new technology to an old tracer. J Nucl Med 2008;49(1):68–78.
11. Even-Sapir E, Metser U, Mishani E, et al. The detection of bone metastases in patients with high-risk prostate cancer: 99mTc-MDP planar bone scintigraphy, single- and multi-field-of-view SPECT, 18F-fluoride PET, and 18F-fluoride PET/CT. J Nucl Med 2006;47(2):287–97.
12. Fox JJ, Schöder H, Larson SM. Molecular imaging of prostate cancer. Curr Opin Urol 2012; 22(4):320–7.
13. Hofer C, Laubenbacher C, Block T, et al. Fluorine-18-fluorodeoxyglucose positron emission tomography is useless for the detection of local recurrence after radical prostatectomy. Eur Urol 1999;36(1): 31–5.
14. Morris MJ, Akhurst T, Larson SM, et al. Fluorodeoxyglucose positron emission tomography as an outcome measure for castrate metastatic prostate cancer treated with antimicrotubule chemotherapy. Clin Cancer Res 2005;11(9):3210–6.
15. Chang CH, Wu HC, Tsai JJ, et al. Detecting metastatic pelvic lymph nodes by ^{18}F-2-deoxyglucose positron emission tomography in patients with prostate-specific antigen relapse after treatment for localized prostate cancer. Urol Int 2003;70(4):311–5.
16. Schöder H, Herrmann K, Gönen M, et al. 2-[18F]fluoro-2-deoxyglucose positron emission tomography for the detection of disease in patients with prostate-specific antigen relapse after radical prostatectomy. Clin Cancer Res 2005;11(13):4761–9.
17. Zadra G, Photopoulos C, Loda M. The fat side of prostate cancer. Biochim Biophys Acta 2013; 1831(10):1518–32.
18. Contractor K, Challapalli A, Barwick T, et al. Use of [11C]choline PET-CT as a noninvasive method for detecting pelvic lymph node status from prostate cancer and relationship with choline kinase expression. Clin Cancer Res 2011;17(24): 7673–83.
19. Henriksen G, Herz M, Hauser A, et al. Synthesis and preclinical evaluation of the choline transport tracer deshydroxy-[18F]fluorocholine ([18F]dOC). Nucl Med Biol 2004;31(7):851–8.
20. Vavere AL, Kridel SJ, Wheeler FB, et al. 1-11C-acetate as a PET radiopharmaceutical for imaging fatty acid synthase expression in prostate cancer. J Nucl Med 2008;49(2):327–34.
21. Beheshti M, Haim S, Zakavi R, et al. Impact of 18F-choline PET/CT in prostate cancer patients with biochemical recurrence: influence of androgen deprivation therapy and correlation with PSA kinetics. J Nucl Med 2013;54(6):833–40.
22. Souvatzoglou M, Weirich G, Schwarzenboeck S, et al. The sensitivity of [11C]choline PET/CT to localize prostate cancer depends on the tumor configuration. Clin Cancer Res 2011;17(11):3751–9.
23. Umbehr MH, Müntener M, Hany T, et al. The role of 11C-choline and 18F-fluorocholine positron emission tomography (PET) and PET/CT in prostate cancer: a systematic review and meta-analysis. Eur Urol 2013;64(1):106–17.
24. Castellucci P, Fuccio C, Nanni C, et al. Influence of trigger PSA and PSA kinetics on ^{11}C-choline PET/CT detection rate in patients with biochemical relapse after radical prostatectomy. J Nucl Med 2009;50(9):1394–400.
25. Picchio M, Castellucci P. Clinical indications of C-choline PET/CT in prostate cancer patients with biochemical relapse. Theranostics 2012;2(3):313–7.
26. Picchio M, Spinapolice EG, Fallanca F, et al. [11C] choline PET/CT detection of bone metastases in patients with PSA progression after primary treatment for prostate cancer: comparison with bone scintigraphy. Eur J Nucl Med Mol Imaging 2012;39(1): 13–26.
27. Okudaira H, Shikano N, Nishii R, et al. Putative transport mechanism and intracellular fate of trans-1-amino-3-18F-fluorocyclobutanecarboxylic acid in human prostate cancer. J Nucl Med 2011;52(5): 822–9.
28. Oka S, Hattori R, Kurosaki F, et al. A preliminary study of anti-1-amino-3-18F-fluorocyclobutyl-1-carboxylic acid for the detection of prostate cancer. J Nucl Med 2007;48(1):46–55.
29. Nanni C, Zanoni L, Pultrone C, et al. (18)F-FACBC (anti1-amino-3-(18)F-fluorocyclobutane-1-carboxylic acid) versus (11)C-choline PET/CT in prostate

cancer relapse: results of a prospective trial. Eur J Nucl Med Mol Imaging 2016;43(9):1601–10.

30. Wieser G, Mansi R, Grosu AL, et al. Positron emission tomography (PET) imaging of prostate cancer with a gastrin releasing peptide receptor antagonist – from mice to men. Theranostics 2014;4(4):412–9.
31. Mansi R, Abiraj K, Wang X, et al. Evaluation of three different families of bombesin receptor radioantagonists for targeted imaging and therapy of gastrin releasing peptide receptor (GRP-R) positive tumors. J Med Chem 2015;58:682–91.
32. Marsouvanidis PJ, Nock BA, Hajjaj B, et al. Gastrin releasing peptide receptor-directed radioligands based on a bombesin antagonist: synthesis, 111In-labeling, and preclinical profile. J Med Chem 2013; 56:2374–84.
33. Chatalic KL, Konijnenberg M, Nonnekens J, et al. In vivo stabilization of a gastrin- releasing peptide receptor antagonist enhances PET imaging and radionuclide therapy of prostate cancer in preclinical studies. Theranostics 2016;6:104–17.
34. Maina T, Bergsma H, Kulkarni HR, et al. Preclinical and first clinical experience with the gastrin-releasing peptide receptor-antagonist [68Ga]SB3 and PET/CT. Eur J Nucl Med Mol Imaging 2016;43: 964–73.
35. Nock BA, Kaloudi A, Lymperis E, et al. Theranostic perspectives in prostate cancer with the GRPR-antagonist NeoBOMB1 – preclinical and first clinical results. J Nucl Med 2017;58(1):75–80.
36. Antunes AA, Leite KR, Sousa-Canavez JM, et al. The role of prostate specific membrane antigen and pepsinogen C tissue expression as an adjunctive method to prostate cancer diagnosis. J Urol 2009; 181:594–600.
37. Ghosh A, Heston WD. Tumor target prostate specific membrane antigen (PSMA) and its regulation in prostate cancer. J Cell Biochem 2004;91(3): 528–39.
38. Silver DA, Pellicer L, Fair WR, et al. Prostate-specific membrane antigen expression in normal and malignant human tissues. Clin Cancer Res 1997;3:81–5.
39. Halsted CH. The intestinal absorption of folates. Am J Clin Nutr 1979;32:846–55.
40. DeMarzo AM, Nelson WG, Isaacs WB, et al. Pathological and molecular aspects of prostate cancer. Lancet 2003;361:955–64.
41. Carrasquillo J. Imaging and dosimetry determinations using radio-labeled antibodies. Cancer Treat Res 1993;68:65–97.
42. Commandeur LC, Parsons JR. Degradation of halogenated aromatic compounds. Biodegradation 1990;1:207–20.
43. Chang SS, Reuter VE, Heston WD, et al. Comparison of anti-prostate-specific membrane antigen antibodies and other immunomarkers in metastatic prostate carcinoma. Urology 2001;57:1179–83.
44. Wright GL Jr, Grob BM, Haley C, et al. Upregulation of prostate-specific membrane antigen after androgen-deprivation therapy. Urology 1996;48: 326–34.
45. Ross JS, Sheehan CE, Fisher HA, et al. Correlation of primary tumor prostate-specific membrane antigen expression with disease recurrence in prostate cancer. Clin Cancer Res 2003;9(17):6357–62.
46. Birtle AJ, Freeman A, Masters JR, et al. Tumour markers for managing men who present with metastatic prostate cancer and serum prostate-specific antigen levels of <10 ng/mL. BJU. Int 2005;96: 303–7.
47. Marko J, Gould CF, Bonavia GH, et al. State-of-the-art imaging of prostate cancer. Urol Oncol 2016; 34(3):134–46.
48. Taneja SS. ProstaScint(R) scan: contemporary use in clinical practice. Rev Urol 2004;6(Suppl 10): S19–28.
49. Haseman MK, Rosenthal SA, Polascik TJ. Capromab pendetide imaging of prostate cancer. Cancer Biother Radiopharm 2000;15:131–40.
50. Seo Y, Aparici CM, Cooperberg MR, et al. In vivo tumor grading of prostate cancer using quantitative ^{111}In-capromab pendetide SPECT/CT. J Nucl Med 2010;51:31–6.
51. Luthi-Carter R, Barczak AK, Speno H, et al. Molecular characterization of human brain N-acetylated α-linked acidic dipeptidase (NAALADase). J Pharmacol Exp Ther 1998;286:1020–5.
52. Tiffany CW, Lapidus RG, Merion A, et al. Characterization of the enzymatic activity of PSM: comparison with brain NAALADase. Prostate 1999;39:28–35.
53. Eder M, Schäfer M, Bauder-Wüst U, et al. ^{68}Ga-complex lipophilicity and the targeting property of a urea-based PSMA inhibitor for PET imaging. Bioconjug Chem 2012;23:688–97.
54. Pomper MG, Musachio JL, Zhang J, et al. 11C-MCG: synthesis, uptake selectivity, and primate PET of a probe for glutamate carboxypeptidase II (NAALADase). Mol Imaging 2002;1:96–101.
55. Foss CA, Mease RC, Fan H, et al. Radiolabeled small-molecule ligands for prostate-specific membrane antigen: in vivo imaging in experimental models of prostate cancer. Clin Cancer Res 2005; 11:4022–8.
56. Baum RP, Kulkarni HR, Schuchardt C, et al. Lutetium-177 PSMA radioligand therapy of metastatic castration resistant prostate cancer: safety and efficacy. J Nucl Med 2016;57(7):1006–13.
57. Afshar-Oromieh A, Zechmann CM, Malcher A, et al. Comparison of PET imaging with a (68)Ga-labelled PSMA ligand and (18)F-choline-based PET/CT for the diagnosis of recurrent prostate cancer. Eur J Nucl Med Mol Imaging 2014;41(1):11–20.
58. Maurer T, Gschwend JE, Rauscher I, et al. Diagnostic efficacy of (68)Gallium-PSMA positron

emission tomography compared to conventional imaging for lymph node staging of 130 consecutive patients with intermediate to high risk prostate cancer. J Urol 2016;195(5):1436–43.

59. van Leeuwen PJ, Stricker P, Hruby G, et al. ^{68}Ga-PSMA has high detection rate of prostate cancer recurrence outside the prostatic fossa in patients being considered for salvage radiation treatment. BJU Int 2016;117(5):732–9.
60. Weineisen M, Simicek J, Schottelius M, et al. Synthesis and preclinical evaluation of DOTAGA-conjugated PSMA ligands for functional imaging and endoradiotherapy of prostate cancer. EJNMMI Res 2014;4:63.
61. Afshar-oromieh A, Kratochwil C, Benesova M, et al. The novel PSMA ligand DKFZ-617 in the diagnosis of prostate cancer: biodistribution in humans and first evaluation of tumor lesions. J Nucl Med 2015; 56(Suppl 3):398.
62. Weineisen M, Schottelius M, Simecek J, et al. ^{68}Ga- and ^{177}Lu-labeled PSMA I&T: optimization of a PSMA-targeted theranostic concept and first proof-of-concept human studies. J Nucl Med 2015;56: 1169–76.
63. Kulkarni H, Singh A, Niepsch K, et al. PSMA radioligand therapy of metastatic castration-resistant prostate cancer: first results using the PSMA Inhibitor 617. J Nucl Med 2016;57(2):139.
64. Kulkarni HR, Singh A, Baum RP. Response assessment to treatment with Lu-177 PSMA inhibitor in patients with metastatic castration-resistant prostate cancer: differential response of bone versus lymph node lesions. J Nucl Med 2016;57(2):1547.
65. Puig S, Thiele DJ. Molecular mechanisms of copper uptake and distribution. Curr Opin Chem Biol 2002; 6(2):171–80.
66. Bertini I, Cavallaro G, McGreevy KS. Cellular copper management—a draft user's guide. Coord Chem Rev 2010;254(5–6):506–24.
67. Szymánski P, Frączek T, Markowicz M, et al. Development of copper based drugs, radiopharmaceuticals and medical materials. Biometals 2012;25:1089–112.
68. Wadas TJ, Wong EH, Weisman GR, et al. Copper chelation chemistry and its role in copper radiopharmaceuticals. Curr Pharm Des 2007;13(1):3–16.
69. Banerjee SR, Pullambhatla M, Foss CA, et al. ^{64}Cu-labeled inhibitors of prostate-specific membrane antigen for PET imaging of prostate cancer. J Med Chem 2014;57:2657–69.
70. Williams HA, Robinson S, Julyan P, et al. A comparison of PET imaging characteristics of various copper radioisotopes. Eur J Nucl Med Mol Imaging 2005;32(12):1473–80.
71. McCarthy DW, Shefer RE, Klinkowstein RE, et al. Efficient production of high-specific-activity 64Cu using a biomedical cyclotron. Nucl Med Biol 1997;24(1): 35–43.
72. Alliot C, Michel N, Bonraisin A-C, et al. One step purification process for no-carrier-added ^{64}Cu produced using enriched nickel target. Radiochim Acta 2011;99(10):627–30.
73. Szelecsenyi F, Blessing G, Qaim SM. Excitation functions of proton induced nuclear reactions on enriched ^{61}Ni and ^{64}Ni: possibility of production of No-carrier-added ^{61}Cu and ^{64}Cu at a small cyclotron. Appl Radiat Isot 1993;44(3):575–80.
74. Zinn KR, Chaudhuri TR, Cheng T-P, et al. Production of no-carrier-added ^{64}Cu from zinc metal irradiated under boron shielding. Cancer 1994;73:774–8.
75. Smith SV, Waters DJ, di Bartolo N. Separation of 64Cu from ^{67}Ga waste products using anion exchange and low acid aqueous/organic mixtures. Radiochimica Acta 1996;75(2):65–8.
76. Kozempel PJ, Abbas K, Simonelli F, et al. Preparation of ^{67}Cu via deuteron irradiation of ^{70}Zn. Radiochimica Acta 2012;100:419–23.
77. Hancock CN, Stockwin LH, Han B, et al. A copper chelate of thiosemicarbazone NSC 689534 induces oxidative/ER stress and inhibits tumor growth in vitro and in vivo. Free Radic Biol Med 2011; 50(1):110–21.
78. Peng F, Lu X, Janisse J, et al. PET of human prostate cancer xenografts in mice with increased uptake of $^{64}CuCl_2$. J Nucl Med 2006;47(10):1649–52.
79. Nedrow JR, Latoche JD, Day KE, et al. Targeting PSMA with a Cu-64 labeled phosphoramidate inhibitor for PET/CT imaging of variant PSMA-expressing xenografts in mouse models of prostate cancer. Mol Imaging Biol 2015;18(3):402–10.
80. Müller C, Struthers H, Winiger C, et al. DOTA conjugate with an albumin-binding entity enables the first folic acid-targeted ^{177}Lu-radionuclide tumor therapy in mice. J Nucl Med 2013;54(1):124–31.
81. Farkas R, Siwowska K, Ametamey SM, et al. 64Cu- and 68Ga-based PET imaging of folate receptor-positive tumors: development and evaluation of an albumin-binding NODAGA-folate. Mol Pharm 2016; 13(6):1979–87.
82. Grubmüller B, Baum RP, Capasso E, et al. ^{64}Cu-PSMA-617 PET/CT imaging of prostate adenocarcinoma: first in-human studies. Cancer Biother Radiopharm 2016;31(8):277–86.
83. Singh A, Kulkarni H, Klette I, et al. Clinical application of ^{64}Cu PSMA PET/CT in theranostics of prostate cancer. J Nucl Med 2016;57(Suppl 2):1538.
84. Niccoli AA, Cascini GL, Altini C, et al. The copper radioisotopes: a systematic review with special interest to ^{64}Cu. Biomed Res Int 2014;2014:786463.
85. DeNardo GL, Kukis DL, Shen S, et al. ^{67}Cu- versus ^{131}I-Labeled lym-1 antibody: comparative pharmacokinetics and dosimetry in patients with non-Hodgkin's lymphoma. Clin Cancer Res 1998; 5:533–41.

From Bench to Bed

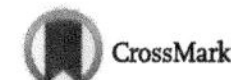

New Gastrin-Releasing Peptide Receptor-Directed Radioligands and Their Use in Prostate Cancer

Theodosia Maina, PhD*, Berthold A. Nock, PhD

KEYWORDS

• Gastrin-releasing peptide receptor targeting • Prostate cancer • Preclinical design • Clinical translation • Theranostics

KEY POINTS

- Gastrin-releasing peptide receptors (GRPRs) are overexpressed in prostate cancer and may serve as molecular targets for diagnosis and therapy with GRPR-directed radiolabeled peptide probes.
- The amphibian bombesin and the mammalian gastrin-releasing peptide have served as motifs for the development of GRPR-directed diagnostic and therapeutic radiolabeled analogs.
- A shift of paradigm from internalizing radiolabeled GRPR-agonists to GRPR-radioantagonists has occurred owing to the higher biosafety and superior pharmacokinetics of the latter.
- Peptide chain, spacer, and chelator play a critical role in the final performance of GRPR antagonists labeled with medically relevant radiometals in mice and in humans.
- Translational studies have revealed the diagnostic value of GRPR-radioantagonists in prostate cancer; their role versus PSMA-based agents needs to be accurately evaluated.

INTRODUCTION

The gastrin-releasing peptide receptor (GRPR) has been widely regarded as an attractive molecular target for tumor diagnosis and therapy with radiolabeled peptide analogs, owing to its upregulation in major human cancers.[1–3] Thus, high-density expression of GRPR has been documented in primary prostate cancer as opposed to lack of expression in surrounding healthy or hyperplastic prostate tissue, thereby offering the opportunity for diagnosis of early neoplastic events in the prostate.[4,5] In most cases, disease infiltrated to adjacent lymph nodes still retains a high GRPR expression, allowing follow-up of metastatic spread. In advanced prostate cancer, GRPR expression seems to decline, especially in osseous metastases[6]; however, more and more thorough clinical studies are needed to fully understand the molecular background affecting GRPR expression in advanced states of the disease.

On the other hand, standard imaging modalities, such as MRI, computed tomography (CT), and ultrasound, as well as conventional nuclear medicine techniques (eg, PET with fluorodeoxyglucose F-18 [^{18}F]FDG/PET]) have shown low specificity that compromises their diagnostic value in prostate cancer.[7] Currently, reliable diagnosis and staging of the disease relies almost exclusively on biopsy; yet, the high number of inconclusive biopsies, which are associated with much patient discomfort and anxiety, as well as with an increase in health care costs, demonstrates the urgent

Disclosure: The authors participate in a contract for the commercialization of NeoBOMB1 and are co-inventors in a patent of AAA.
Molecular Radiopharmacy, INRASTES, NCSR "Demokritos", Agia Paraskevi, Attikis, Athens 15310, Greece
* Corresponding author.
E-mail address: maina_thea@hotmail.com

PET Clin 12 (2017) 205–217
http://dx.doi.org/10.1016/j.cpet.2016.12.002
1556-8598/17/

clinical need for a noninvasive and accurate molecular diagnostic tool in prostate cancer.[8]

For molecular diagnosis and radionuclide therapy of GRPR-positive cancer, a wide array of suitably modified peptide analogs have been developed over the past 2 decades. Initial studies have involved tracers based on the amphibian tetradecapeptide bombesin (BBN) and its C-terminal octapeptide and nonapeptide fragments retaining full affinity for the GRPR.[9–11] Coupling of a variety of chelators on the N-terminus of such BBN-peptides, either directly or via different-length and hydrophilicity spacers, has allowed for labeling with a wide range of radiometals, suitable for SPECT (^{99m}Tc, ^{111}In, ^{67}Ga) or PET (^{68}Ga, ^{64}Cu) imaging, as well as for radionuclide therapy (^{177}Lu, ^{90}Y, ^{213}Bi). Preclinical evaluation in prostate cancer cells and animal models have demonstrated the impact of peptide chain, linker, chelator, and radiometal applied on the pharmacologic and pharmacokinetic profiles of resulting radioligands and has revealed analogs of interest for translation in humans.

Unlike BBN, which binds with high affinity to both the GRPR and the neuromedin B receptor (NMBR), the mammalian gastrin-releasing peptide (GRP) and neuromedin C (**Fig. 1**) are GRPR-preferring.[12] Therefore, more selective GRP-based radioligands have recently been introduced for diagnosis of GRPR-expressing cancer, with the aim to reduce background activity by evading NMBR-binding sites expressed in physiologic tissues in addition to GRPRs.[13] On the other hand, a search toward pan-BBN radioligands has been pursued as well, based on the rationale that NMBRs and/or BBN subtype 3 receptors (BB_3R) coexpressed in cancer together with GRPRs would enhance the clinical indications of GRPR-preferring radioligands.[14] Interestingly, research has recently shifted toward GRPR-antagonist–based radiopeptides,[15] following the successful shift of paradigm in the field of somatostatin receptor subtype 2 (sst_2)-radiotracers from agonists to antagonists.[16] Radioantagonists have often displayed faster background clearance and higher tumor localization in animal models and in humans.[17,18] In the case of GRPR-radioantagonists, an extra benefit in their use is associated to their inherent higher biosafety for human intravenous administration.

Exhaustive research in all these fronts has facilitated accumulation of crucial structure-activity relationships data that have synergistically fostered the design of improved radioligands and the selection of candidates for clinical translation. Clinical proof-of-principle studies have established the validity of this approach in patients with prostate cancer and have contributed in our better understanding of biological and biochemical GRPR-related processes during propagation of the disease. More extended clinical studies are now needed to evaluate the diagnostic and potentially also therapeutic value of radiolabeled GRPR-directed peptide probes in early and advanced stages of prostate cancer.

RADIOPEPTIDES BASED ON BOMBESIN

As already mentioned, frog BBN and its C-terminus fragments retaining full binding affinity for the GRPR have served as motifs for the development of peptide radioligands able to specifically localize in cancer-associated GRPR-sites. The first analogs were produced by replacing Arg[3] by Lys[3] in the full BBN sequence and subsequent coupling of the diaminedithiolate group in its lateral primary amine via different linkers to enable ^{99m}Tc labeling (**Table 1**).[19] Owing to the high lipophilicity of the ^{99m}Tc chelate, however, the resulting ^{99m}Tc radiotracers displayed high hepatobiliary excretion and hence unfavorably high accumulation in the abdomen. Subsequent introduction of a "built-in" diethylenetriaminepentaacetic acid (DTPA) hydrophilic modifier that replaced N-terminal Pyr[1] resulted in impressive reduction of abdominal accumulation and good targeting of prostate cancer xenografts in mouse models.[20,21]

Following a similar trend, coupling of DTPA or 1,4,7,10-tetraazacyclododecane-1,4,7,10-tetraacetic acid (DOTA) on either Lys[3] or Pro[1] of full-length BBN analogs (see **Table 1**) allowed for labeling with ^{111}In.[22–24] Formation of potent and hydrophilic radiotracers with excellent tumor-to-background ratios in the abdomen was achieved. These analogs exhibited clear agonistic activity at the GRPR

BBN pGlu-Gln-Arg-Leu-**Gly-Asn**-Gln-**Trp-Ala-Val-Gly-His-Leu-Met**-NH_2

GRP 27mer Val-Pro-Leu-Pro-Ala-Gly-Gly-Gly-Thr-Val-Leu-Thr-Lys-Met-Tyr-Pro-Arg-**Gly-Asn**-His-**Trp-Ala-Val-Gly-His-Leu-Met**-NH_2

NMC: GRP(18–27) **Gly-Asn**-His-**Trp-Ala-Val-Gly-His-Leu-Met**-NH_2

Fig. 1. Amino acid sequences of amphibian tetradecapeptide BBN showing high affinity for GRPR and NMBR. The native human 27mer GRP and its C-terminal decapeptide fragment NMC, both GRPR-preferring, are also shown underneath with amino acids preserved across species highlighted in red.

Table 1
Representative peptide analogs based on amphibian BBN sequences coupled to different metal chelators

Peptide		Position No. from BBN N-Terminus 1	2	3	4	5	6	7	8	9	10	11	12	13	14	References
BBN		pGlu	Gln	Arg	Leu	Gly	Asn	Gln	Trp	Ala	Val	Gly	His	Leu	Met-NH_2	
		(DTPA)		*Lys-X-DADT*	Leu	Gly	Asn	Gln	Trp	Ala	Val	Gly	His	Leu	Met-NH_2	19–21
DTPA-BBN	*DTPA*	*Pro*	Gln	Arg	*Tyr*	Gly	Asn	Gln	Trp	Ala	Val	Gly	His	Leu	Met-NH_2	22–24
Demobesin 4	*N_4*	*Pro*	Gln	Arg	*Tyr*	Gly	Asn	Gln	Trp	Ala	Val	Gly	His	Leu	*Nle-NH_2*	25,26
RP527					*Dmg-Ser-Cys*	Gly	*5Ava*	Gln	Trp	Ala	Val	Gly	His	Leu	Met-NH_2	27,28
AMBA					*DOTA*	Gly	*PABA*	Gln	Trp	Ala	Val	Gly	His	Leu	Met-NH_2	34–36,43
DOTA-Pesin						*DOTA*	*$dPEG_4$*	Gln	Trp	Ala	Val	Gly	His	Leu	Met-NH_2	44,45
BZH3					*DOTA*	*$dPEG_2$*	*dTyr*	Gln	Trp	Ala	Val	*βAla*	His	*Thi*	Met-NH_2	14,48

Additions/replacements in the native sequence are highlighted in italic.

Abbreviations: 5Ava, 5-aminovaleric acid; BBN, bombesin; DADT, diaminedithiol; Dmg, N,N-dimethylglycine; DOTA, 1,4,7,10-tetraazacyclododecane-1,4,7,10-tetraacetic acid; $dPEG_2$, 8-amino-3,6-dioxaoctanoic acid; $dPEG_4$, 15-amino-4,7,10,13-tetraoxapentadecanoic acid; DTPA, diethylenetriaminepentaacetic acid; N_4, 6-carboxy-1,4,8,11-tetraazaundecane; PABA, p-aminobenzoic acid; Thi, 3-(2-thienyl)-L-alanine.

and excellent internalization in GRPR-expressing cells. In contrast, radiolabeled GRPR antagonists included for comparison purposes in these studies were abandoned as noninternalizing and therefore unsuitable for in vivo targeting of GRPR-expressing tumors (vide infra). Later on, coupling of an acyclic tetraamine moiety on N-terminal Pro of (Pro[1],Tyr[4],Nle[14]-NH_2)BBN afforded Demobesin 4 suitable for ^{99m}Tc-labeling in high yield and specific activity. The resulting radiotracer ^{99m}Tc-Demobesin 4 specifically and efficiently accumulated in prostate cancer xenografts in mice showing an attractive pharmacokinetic profile with fast clearance from background tissues via the kidneys.[25] Favorable pharmacokinetics were recently confirmed as well in a small group of patients with prostate cancer in whom the tracer was able to target early prostate-confined cancer, lymph-node metastases, and approximately 50% of bone metastases in cases with advanced disease.[26]

Another early developed ^{99m}Tc radiotracer showing localization in GRPR-expressing lesions in patients is ^{99m}Tc-RP527.[27] Labeling with ^{99m}Tc is achieved by a Dmg-Ser-Cys tripeptide unit introduced at the N-terminus of the BBN(7–14) octapeptide fragment via a Gly-5Ava linker (see **Table 1**). Although the high ^{99m}Tc-chelate lipophilicity resulted in excessive abdominal accumulation, ^{99m}Tc-RP527 was still able to specifically localize in GRPR-positive cancer lesions in patients demonstrating for the first time the feasibility of GRPR-targeted diagnostic imaging in prostate cancer.[28] Thereafter, a wide range of chelators suitable for labeling with ^{99m}Tc or with trivalent radiometals were coupled via different linkers to the N-terminus of either BBN(6–14) nonapeptide or BBN(7–14) octapeptide that retain full binding capacity for the GRPR. As shown in several structure-activity-relationships studies, chelator, radiometal, as well as length and type of linker had a great impact on most pharmacologic properties of end-radiotracers, including receptor affinity and internalization rate. Moreover, they strongly influenced in vivo profiles, affecting tumor uptake and retention as well as background clearance.[9,10,29–32]

It is interesting to observe how this concise research effort has shaped a theranostic approach for prostate cancer management over the years, especially with the advent of peptide analogs conjugated to the universal chelator DOTA. According to this concept, a diagnostic or a therapeutic radiopeptide-pair can be alternatively applied by merely switching the radiometal tagged to the same peptide-conjugate. Hence, using the diagnostic radiometal detection, staging, stratification, and dosimetry of patients is possible for subsequent radionuclide therapy using the therapeutic radiometal counterpart. On the other hand, by applying again the initial diagnostic radiometal monitoring of therapy response and follow-up of disease become feasible.

Following the paradigm of ^{177}Lu-labeled somatostatin octapeptide analogs clinically applied in the treatment of sst_2-expressing neuroendocrine tumors,[33] ^{177}LuAMBA was developed and proposed for the GRPR-targeted treatment of prostate cancer.[34–36] It should be noted that very soon crucial differences in the implementation of these two methods in the clinic became apparent, related to biosafety, stability, and pharmacokinetic issues. First, unlike somatostatin analogs, BBN-like peptides elicit strong adverse effects after intravenous injection in humans following binding to GRPR and NMBR sites physiologically expressed in the pancreas, stomach, and intestinal mucosa.[37–41] These gastrointestinal system effects are further intensified during radionuclide therapy, whereby higher peptide doses are administered to patients. Second, unlike the in vivo robust cyclic octapeptide somatostatin analogs, the linear ^{177}LuAMBA peptide-radioligand showed suboptimal in vivo stability, compromising efficient supply and uptake to tumor sites and consequently therapeutic efficacy. The rapid in vivo degradation of ^{177}LuAMBA has been predominantly attributed to the action of neutral endopeptidase (NEP).[42] Finally, the observed high accumulation and prolonged retention of radioactivity in tissues physiologically expressing the GRPR (and the NMBR), such as the pancreas and the gastrointestinal tract, presents dosimetric challenges and further restricts the therapeutic applicability of ^{177}LuAMBA.[36] Despite these limitations, however, ^{177}LuAMBA has served as an invaluable model-compound to explore the strengths and pitfalls of GRPR-targeted therapy using BBN-like agonist radioligands. Furthermore, labeling with the PET radionuclide ^{68}Ga theranostic perspectives were also explored in prostate cancer.[43] Representative whole-body images and sections of high ^{68}Ga-AMBA uptake on a femoral head metastasis and a large pelvic lymph-node metastasis from a poorly differentiated prostate adenocarcinoma on PET/CT are included in **Fig. 2**.

Following a parallel development, theranostic approaches in prostate cancer with DOTA-Pesin radioligands (see **Table 1**)[44] based on ^{68}Ga (PET), ^{177}Lu, and for the first time the alpha emitter ^{213}Bi have been studied in prostate cancer animal models.[45] Of particular interest is the higher therapeutic efficacy of alpha therapy (^{213}Bi-DOTA-Pesin

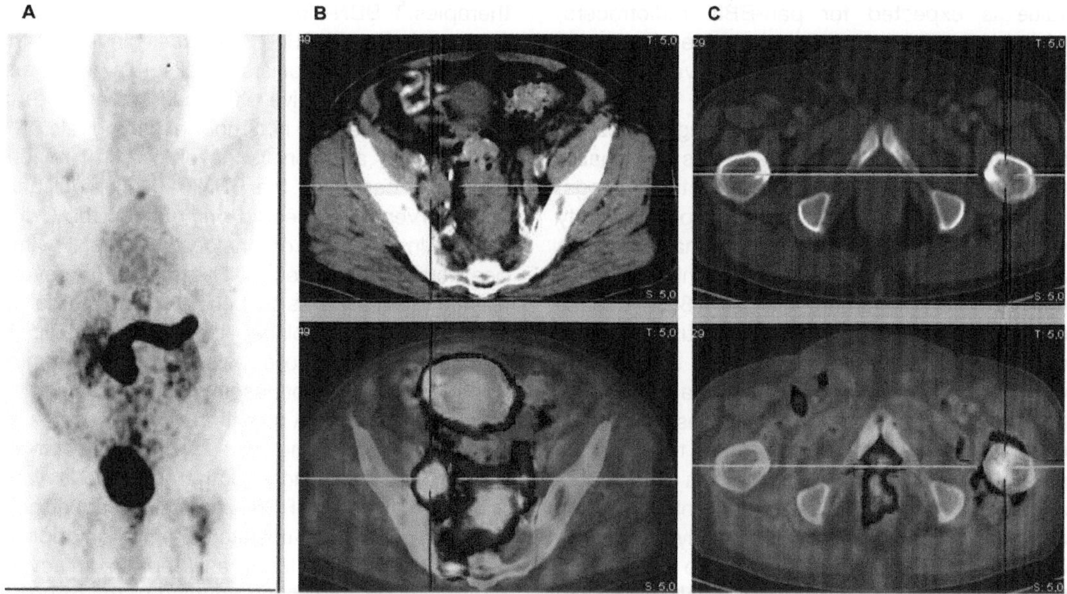

Fig. 2. PET/CT with ^{68}Ga-AMBA in a patient with poorly differentiated prostate adenocarcinoma, Gleason 9 (4 + 5). (*A*) Whole-body view. (*B*) Section showing intensive uptake in a large pelvic lymph-node metastasis. (*C*) Section showing intensive uptake in a left femoral head metastasis. (*Courtesy of* Dr A. Singh and Prof Dr R.P. Baum, Bad Berka, Germany.)

and ^{213}Bi-AMBA) over beta therapy (^{177}Lu-DOTA-Pesin) in a PC-3 tumor model xenografted in mice. Additional benefits in the use of ^{213}Bi are its short physical half-life, appearing to harmonize especially well with fast-localizing and clearing (radio)peptides, as well as its accompanying 440-keV gamma-emission that could serve for quantification and imaging. Moreover, in a head-to-head comparison, ^{213}Bi-DOTA-Pesin demonstrated higher biosafety compared with ^{213}Bi-AMBA. As a result, ^{213}Bi-DOTA-Pesin was proposed for the treatment of recurrent prostate cancer in men. Nevertheless, toxicology and dosimetry risks have to be competently addressed first before clinical translation.

BOMBESIN RECEPTOR SUBTYPE SELECTIVITY: RADIOPEPTIDES BASED ON PAN-BOMBESIN OR ON HUMAN GASTRIN-RELEASING PEPTIDE

As already mentioned, BBN interacts with both GRPR and NMBR acting as a receptor agonist, but not with the "orphan" BBN subtype 3-receptor (BB_3R) also found in mammalian tissues.[2,3,12] Initially, the radioiodinated pan-BBN analog ^{125}I-(dTyr^6,βAla^{11},Phe^{13},Nle^{14}-NH$_2$)BBN(6–14) was developed for in vitro BBN subtype receptor studies including the BB_3R,[46,47] for which the native hormone has no binding affinity. Coupling of DOTA to (dTyr^6,βAla^{11},Thi^{13},Nle^{14}-NH$_2$)BBN(6–14) via different linkers, led to the pan-BBN BZH series amenable to labeling with trivalent radiometals that displayed good pharmacokinetics in mouse models.[14] During a clinical evaluation in 17 patients with gastrointestinal stromal tumors, ^{68}Ga-BZH3 (see **Table 1**) missed most of the lesions, showing less diagnostic accuracy compared with ^{18}F-FDG PET.[48] It should be noted that a similar ^{111}In-pan-BBN tracer ([^{111}In-DOTA-dTyr^6,βAla^{11},Phe^{13},Nle^{14}-NH$_2$]BBN[6–14]) was shown to rapidly degrade after intravenous injection in mice, displaying low localization in GRPR-positive prostate cancer xenografts in mice.[49] Coinjection of the NEP inhibitor phosphoramidon resulted in marked stabilization of the radiotracer in peripheral blood that translated into a more than fivefold increase of tumor uptake. This finding implicating NEP in the fast in vivo degradation of linear pan-BBN radioligands confirms previous observations on the in vivo metabolic fate of ^{177}LuAMBA.[42]

The search for pan-BBN radiotracers seems to have followed a similar trend as in the field of somatostatin. Based on molecular evidence that sst_{1-5} can be expressed alone and/or in different combinations in several of human tumors, radiolabeled pan-somatostatins were aimed to expand the clinical indications and the diagnostic sensitivity of sst_2-preferring radioligands.[50,51] This rationale, however, cannot be applied in the case of BBN, because the NMBR and BB_3R are expressed in quite rare tumors.[47] Accordingly, little added value is expected for pan-BBN radiotracers, whereas the risk for more severe side effects and higher background activity after intravenous injection in humans is enhanced.[38,40,41]

Because GRPR is the prevailing molecular target for BBN-like radiotracers, it is reasonable to assume that by using GRPR-selective analogs, side effects and physiologic background activity will be reduced. Following this rationale, a series of different-length C-terminal fragments of the human GRP, as for example, the GRP(18–27) decapeptide neuromedin C (NMC), were functionalized with acyclic tetraamines or DOTA for labeling with ^{99m}Tc or trivalent radiometals, respectively.[13,52,53] Although in vivo profiles, especially background clearance, appeared to improve, several radiotracer attributes, such as GRPR-affinity, internalization rate, metabolic stability, and tumor uptake, were found largely dependent on peptide chain length and/or amino acid substitutions in the sequence potentially masking GRPR-selectivity effects. Further comparative studies are therefore required to clearly establish potential benefits of GRPR-selective radioligands versus their BBN-like and pan-BBN counterparts.

GASTRIN-RELEASING PEPTIDE RECEPTOR-ANTAGONIST RADIOLIGANDS

A shift of paradigm has recently occurred in the field of somatostatin radioligands from sst_2-agonists to sst_2-antagonists owing to accumulating evidence that radioantagonists exhibit a superior pharmacokinetic profile in animal models and, most significantly, in humans.[16–18] Despite their inability to internalize in target cancer cells, radioantagonists were shown in vitro to bind to more receptor conformations present on cancer cells and in vivo to clear more rapidly from background tissues, including sst_2-rich physiologic organs. This surprising finding had a direct impact on BBN-based radioligands and has triggered the development of radiolabeled GRPR antagonists for application in prostate cancer and other GRPR-expressing tumors.[15,54] Interest in this direction has been further stimulated by the fact that GRPR antagonists do not activate the receptor upon binding. Consequently, GRPR-radioantagonists are not expected to elicit acute pharmacologic effects after intravenous administration in humans as opposed to BBN-agonist based radioligands, such as ^{177}LuAMBA.

It is interesting to note that a great number of GRPR antagonists have been made available in the preceding decades as molecular tools for studies on the BBN receptor system, but also as candidates for anticancer GRPR-targeted therapies.[55] BBN-like peptides act as proliferative factors via the GRPR.[56–58] Hence, binding of the receptors by antagonists blocks this route and has an antiproliferative effect, as shown both at the cellular level and in tumor animal models.[58–60] Most GRPR antagonists developed in previous years are based on the BBN(6/7–14) motif after key interventions directed primarily on the C-terminus. In one set of analogs, Met^{14}-NH$_2$ has been omitted with Leu^{13}-NH$_2$ modified to several alkylamides, such as to Leu^{13}-NHEt, whereas in addition Asn^6 is replaced by dPhe^6 or dTyr^6 to confer higher metabolic resistance of the forming peptide to aminopeptidases.[61,62]

By coupling DTPA to either dTyr^6 or dPhe^6 via a Tyr-linker, labeling with ^{111}In was allowed (**Table 2**). Interestingly, both radioligands were not internalized in GRPR-expressing cancer cells and thus considered unsuitable for in vivo application.[22–24] In contrast to this assumption, an acyclic tetraamine unit was soon coupled to the dPhe^6 of the same peptide chain via a linker (see **Table 2**) affording ^{99m}Tc-Demobesin 1 in excellent yields and specific activities. This agent showed high affinity and selectivity for the GRPR and high uptake in a prostate cancer xenograft in mice.[63] Most importantly, ^{99m}Tc-Demobesin 1 washed out from the GRPR-rich pancreas much faster than from the tumor and was later fully characterized as a GRPR antagonist.[15]

Further modification of the same peptide chain with DOTA in SB3 (see **Table 2**) allowed labeling with ^{68}Ga and other trivalent metals, like ^{111}In and ^{177}Lu. Based on the favorable in vivo profile of ^{68}Ga-SB3 in prostate cancer xenografts in mice, its diagnostic value was first explored in a group of patients with prostate or breast cancer applying PET/CT.[64] The tracer successfully localized in early-stage lesions, but in patients with more advanced stages of prostate cancer and/or patients previously subjected to different therapies, it was less successful in visualizing all the lesions. These results confirmed previous reports on the GRPR-expression levels during prostate cancer propagation and its relation to androgens.[4,6,65] Therefore, in a subsequent study only patients with primary and therapy-naïve prostate cancer were included. Furthermore, intensity of tumor uptake was related to GRPR expression, determined in surgically excised biopsy material from patients. Although this study is still ongoing, diagnostic efficacy appears to be higher thus far.[66] On the other hand, the theranostic perspectives of ^{68}Ga/^{111}In/^{177}Lu-SB3 have also been investigated in mice. Surprisingly, ^{111}In-SB3 and ^{177}Lu-SB3 showed lower in vivo stability and inferior uptake in prostate cancer xenografts in mice compared

Table 2
Representative gastrin-releasing peptide receptor antagonist sequences coupled to different metal chelators

	Position No. from BBN N-Terminus														
Peptide	**1**	**2**	**3**	**4**	**5**	**6**	**7**	**8**	**9**	**10**	**11**	**12**	**13**	**14**	**References**
BBN	pGlu	Gln	Arg	Leu	Gly	Asn	Gln	Trp	Ala	Val	Gly	His	Leu	Met-NH_2	
				DTPA	*Tyr*	*dPhe*	Gln	Trp	Ala	Val	Gly	His	*Leu-NHEt*		14–22
Demobesin 1				*N_4'*	*Dig*	*dPhe*	Gln	Trp	Ala	Val	Gly	His	*Leu-NHEt*		15,63
SB3			*DOTA*	*Aba*	*Dig*	*dPhe*	Gln	Trp	Ala	Val	Gly	His	*Leu-NHEt*		64,66,67
RM2				*DOTA*	*Acp*	*dPhe*	Gln	Trp	Ala	Val	Gly	His	*Sta*	*Leu-NH_2*	69,73,76
JMV4168			*DOTA*	*βAla*	*βAla*	*dPhe*	Gln	Trp	Ala	Val	Gly	His	*Sta*	*Leu-NH_2*	70,71
NeoBOMB1			*DOTA*	*Aba*	*Dig*	*dPhe*	Gln	Trp	Ala	Val	Gly	*His-NHCH[$CH_2CH(CH_3)_2$]$_2$*			79–81

Additions/replacements in the native sequence are highlighted in italic.

Abbreviations: Aba, 4-aminobenzylamine; Acp, 4-amino-1-carboxymethylpiperidine; BBN, bombesin; Dig, diglycolic acid; DOTA, 1,4,7,10-tetraazacyclododecane-1,4,7,10-tetraacetic acid; DTPA, diethylenetriaminepentaacetic acid; N_4', 6-[(4-aminophenyl)methyl]-1,4,8,11-tetraazaundecane; Sta, statine, (3S,4S)-4-amino-3-hydroxy-6-methylheptanoic acid.

with ^{68}Ga-SB3. By coinjection of phosphoramidon, however, both radioligands achieved comparable to ^{68}Ga-SB3 tumor uptake in mice,[67] as previously observed in the case of BBN-like agonists.[49]

A second class of GRPR antagonists is generated by replacement of the Leu^{13}-Met^{14}-NH$_2$ C-terminal dipeptide of BBN(6–14) by Sta^{13}-Leu^{14}-NH$_2$. Further Asn^6-substitution by dPhe^6 yields the GRPR antagonist JMV594.[68] Recently, various chelators have been attached at the N-terminus of JMV594 via a great variety of linkers and after labeling with radiometals attractive for PET and SPECT imaging as well as for radionuclide therapy were evaluated in prostate cancer mice models and in humans.[54,69–75] Among these analogs, ^{68}Ga-RM2 produced after coupling DOTA to the N-terminal dPhe^6 of JMV594 via a 4-amino-1-carboxymethyl-piperidine linker (see **Table 2**) and labeling with ^{68}Ga, has attracted considerable attention. Owing to its excellent pharmacokinetic profile and efficient in vivo localization in prostate cancer xenografts in mice, ^{68}Ga-RM2 was further tested in a small group of patients with prostate cancer.[69,73] The new PET-tracer showed high diagnostic accuracy in primary prostate cancer, with the sensitivity slightly declining in infiltrating disease. Interestingly, its ability to visualize all distant bone lesions in advanced spread disease was found compromised, confirming previous findings with other GRPR-targeting radioligands. The new radioantagonist (also known as BAY86–7548) is currently under clinical evaluation sponsored by industry as a candidate PET-tracer in the accurate detection of early prostate cancer and in restaging of recurrent disease.

In view of the expected higher biosafety and better tolerability of radiolabeled GRPR antagonists confirmed during recent clinical studies, the interest in radionuclide therapy of prostate cancer in a theranostic approach is revived. Recent studies with ^{177}Lu-RM2[76] and other JMV594-derived radioligands, such as ^{177}Lu-JMV4168 (^{177}Lu-DOTA-[βAla]$_2$-JMV594)[71] and ^{90}Y-AR (^{90}Y-DOTA-PEG4-JMV594),[77] in animal models have shown the feasibility of this approach. Metabolic stability in peripheral blood of mice was recently shown to affect therapeutic efficacy of ^{177}Lu-JMV4168 in preclinical models, whereby phosphoramidon coinjection enhanced therapy outcome. In addition, differences in the in vivo profiles of ^{68}Ga-labeled and ^{177}Lu-labeled antagonists became once more apparent, most probably caused by the different coordination properties of these radiometals to DOTA.[67,71] A promising alternative in this respect is offered by the use of $^{64/67}$Cu-analogs (see Aviral Singh and colleagues' article, "Imaging of Prostate Cancer Using ^{64}Cu-labeled Prostate-Specific Membrane Antigen Ligand," elsewhere in this issue).

Based on yet another modification, the Leu^{26}-Met^{27}-NH$_2$ C-terminal dipeptide of GRP(20–27) has been altogether omitted and the His^{25} alkylamidated to yield the highly potent and metabolically stable Ac-His-Trp-Ala-Val-Gly-His-NH-CH(CH$_2$CH[CH$_3$]$_2$)$_2$ GRPR antagonist.[78] Elongation with dPhe and coupling of DOTA via a known linker[64] yielded NeoBOMB1 (see **Table 2**), suitable for labeling with trivalent radiometals of interest.[79] Remarkably, ($^{67/68}$Ga/^{111}In/^{177}Lu)NeoBOMB1 radioligands were recently shown to have indistinguishable low-nanomolar affinity for the human GRPR, high metabolic stability in peripheral mouse blood, and excellent localization in prostate cancer xenografts in mice, thereby showing convincing perspectives for theranostic application in prostate cancer. Furthermore, tuning of peptide dose turned out to be effective in reducing the radioactivity uptake in physiological GRPR-rich tissues and to greatly improve dosimetry, further supporting therapeutic options.[80] In a recent study in 4 patients with prostate cancer, (^{68}Ga)NeoBOMB1 was successful in visualizing prostate-confined cancer as well as distant soft tissue and osseous metastases.[79,81] Representative PET/CT scans of a primary prostate adenocarcinoma later confirmed by biopsy shows high (^{68}Ga)NeoBOMB1 uptake in the lower left prostate lobe (**Fig. 3**). High (^{68}Ga)NeoBOMB1 uptake is also shown by PET/CT in a focal liver metastasis from a cribriform prostate adenocarcinoma (**Fig. 4**), confirming first results. Although the number of patients is still too small and further studies will establish the diagnostic efficacy and eventually also the theranostic value of the new agent, results have attracted attention by the private sector.

CONCLUDING REMARKS: FUTURE PERSPECTIVES

The search for effective molecular tools for prostate cancer has been quite intensive in the past few years, responding to an urgent clinical need for state-of-the art theranostic approaches, although much interest is also attracted in diagnostic ^{18}F-labeled GRPR-specific PET-tracers (not discussed in this article). Molecular probes to deliver diagnostic or therapeutic radiometals to GRPR-expressing cancer have evolved from BBN-based agonists to GRPR antagonists. The higher biosafety of the latter along with their better pharmacokinetic profile, including faster background clearance, has raised hopes for

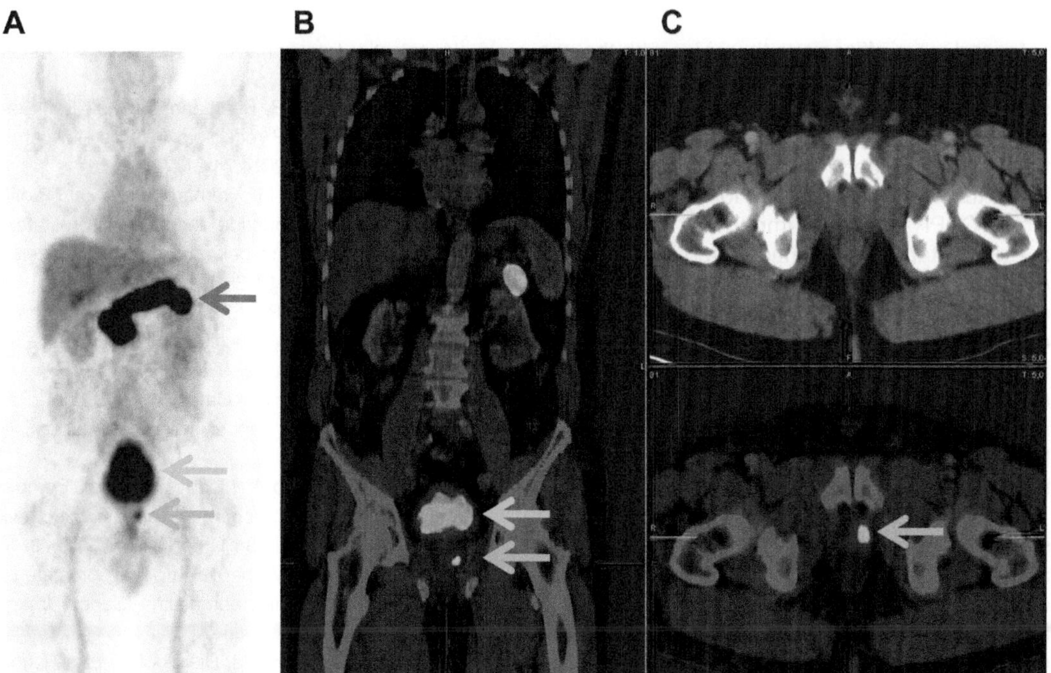

Fig. 3. PET/CT with ^{68}Ga-NeoBOMB1 in a patient with a primary prostate adenocarcinoma, Gleason 6 (3 + 3) and PSA 10.6 ng/mL at the time of imaging and 3 previous negative biopsies and 4th biopsy after ^{68}Ga-NeoBOMB1 visualized pathologic uptake in the prostate cancer on PET/CT. (*A, B*) Whole-body images with dark blue arrow showing physiologic uptake in pancreas, light blue arrows showing tracer excreted in urinary bladder, and green arrow revealing also in (*C*) intensive focal uptake in the left lower prostate lobe. (*Courtesy of* Dr A. Singh and Prof Dr R.P. Baum, Bad Berka, Germany).

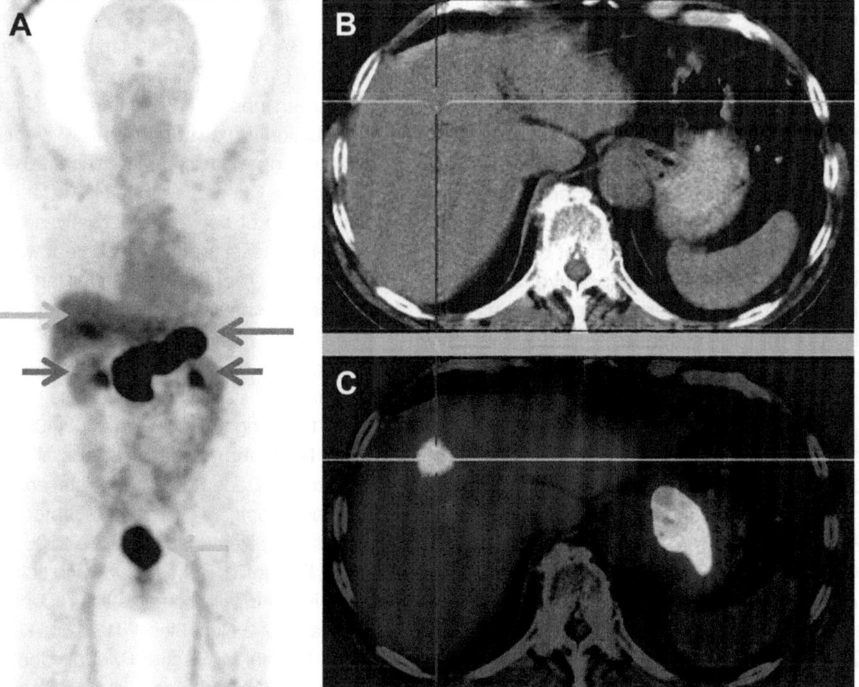

Fig. 4. PET/CT with ^{68}Ga-NeoBOMB1 in a patient with cribriform prostate adenocarcinoma. (*A*) Whole-body image with focal metastasis in segment 5 of liver shown with the green arrow; blue arrow corresponds to physiologic uptake in pancreas, orange arrows depict tracer drainage in renal pelvices, and light blue arrow tracer excretion in urinary bladder. (*B*) Liver section on CT and (*C*) on PET/CT revealing intensive uptake in the lesion. (*Courtesy of* Dr A. Singh and Prof Dr R.P. Baum, Bad Berka, Germany.)

safer and more efficacious therapies with the use of therapeutic radionuclides. Nevertheless, several antagonist-related issues need to be clarified first. Receptor affinity is not enough to ensure prolonged retention of a radioantagonist on tumor cells, but ability for sustained binding to GRPR is equally important. The issue of in vivo stability is critical too, given that maximum supply to tumor sites is needed to deliver a maximum radiotoxic load on tumor cells. Eventually, the lack of radioantagonist internalization in tumor cells may prevent their use for effective radionuclide therapy in combination with α-emitters compared with agonists. Research on these topics is expected to intensify in the coming years.

Moreover, the upregulation of GRPR in early stages of prostate cancer is altered in more advanced stages of the disease. In the latter case, the biochemical and molecular parameters affecting GRPR expression need to be better understood. Recent clinical studies in small groups of patients have to be expanded to include more patient cohorts, and imaging findings should be correlated with histology, androgen receptor status, and other factors. We still do not understand the molecular basis for the high GRPR expression in some bone metastases versus the total lack of expression in others. In addition, GRPR-targeting radioligands should be compared with other molecular tools, as for example, radiolabeled prostate-specific membrane antigen inhibitors.[82] Comparative head-to-head studies are instrumental for gaining better knowledge of the disease as it propagates in humans and for exploiting that knowledge to the maximum for the benefit of our patients. In this respect, the availability of different molecular targets and the development of suitable radiolabeled analogs of the respective vectors may provide invaluable synergy opportunities to successfully combat the disease.

REFERENCES

1. Reubi JC. Peptide receptors as molecular targets for cancer diagnosis and therapy. Endocr Rev 2003;24: 389–427.
2. Kroog GS, Jensen RT, Battey JF. Mammalian bombesin receptors. Med Res Rev 1995;15:389–417.
3. Gonzalez N, Moody TW, Igarashi H, et al. Bombesin-related peptides and their receptors: recent advances in their role in physiology and disease states. Curr Opin Endocrinol Diabetes Obes 2008; 15:58–64.
4. Markwalder R, Reubi JC. Gastrin-releasing peptide receptors in the human prostate: relation to neoplastic transformation. Cancer Res 1999;59: 1152–9.
5. Körner M, Waser B, Rehmann R, et al. Early overexpression of GRP receptors in prostatic carcinogenesis. Prostate 2014;74:217–24.
6. Beer M, Montani M, Gerhardt J, et al. Profiling gastrin-releasing peptide receptor in prostate tissues: clinical implications and molecular correlates. Prostate 2012;72:318–25.
7. Hricak H, Choyke PL, Eberhardt SC, et al. Imaging prostate cancer: a multidisciplinary perspective. Radiology 2007;243:28–53.
8. Roehl KA, Antenor JA, Catalona WJ. Serial biopsy results in prostate cancer screening study. J Urol 2002;167:2435–9.
9. Sancho V, Di Florio A, Moody TW, et al. Bombesin receptor-mediated imaging and cytotoxicity: review and current status. Curr Drug Deliv 2011;8:79–134.
10. Maina T, Nock B, Mather S. Targeting prostate cancer with radiolabelled bombesins. Cancer Imaging 2006;6:153–7.
11. Ananias HJ, de Jong IJ, Dierckx RA, et al. Nuclear imaging of prostate cancer with gastrin-releasing-peptide-receptor targeted radiopharmaceuticals. Curr Pharm Des 2008;14:3033–47.
12. Uehara H, Gonzalez N, Sancho V, et al. Pharmacology and selectivity of various natural and synthetic bombesin related peptide agonists for human and rat bombesin receptors differs. Peptides 2011;32:1685–99.
13. Nock BA, Cescato R, Ketani E, et al. [^{99m}Tc]demomedin C, a radioligand based on human gastrin releasing peptide(18-27): synthesis and preclinical evaluation in gastrin releasing peptide receptor-expressing models. J Med Chem 2012;55:8364–74.
14. Zhang H, Chen J, Waldherr C, et al. Synthesis and evaluation of bombesin derivatives on the basis of pan-bombesin peptides labeled with indium-111, lutetium-177, and yttrium-90 for targeting bombesin receptor-expressing tumors. Cancer Res 2004;64: 6707–15.
15. Cescato R, Maina T, Nock B, et al. Bombesin receptor antagonists may be preferable to agonists for tumor targeting. J Nucl Med 2008;49:318–26.
16. Ginj M, Zhang H, Waser B, et al. Radiolabeled somatostatin receptor antagonists are preferable to agonists for in vivo peptide receptor targeting of tumors. Proc Natl Acad Sci U S A 2006;103:16436–41.
17. Wild D, Fani M, Béhé M, et al. First clinical evidence that imaging with somatostatin receptor antagonists is feasible. J Nucl Med 2011;52:1412–7.
18. Wild D, Fani M, Fischer R, et al. Comparison of somatostatin receptor agonist and antagonist for peptide receptor radionuclide therapy: a pilot study. J Nucl Med 2014;55:1248–52.
19. Baidoo KE, Lin KS, Zhan Y, et al. Design, synthesis, and initial evaluation of high-affinity technetium

bombesin analogues. Bioconjug Chem 1998;9: 218–25.
20. Lin KS, Luu A, Baidoo KE, et al. A new high affinity technetium analogue of bombesin containing DTPA as a pharmacokinetic modifier. Bioconjug Chem 2004;15:1416–23.
21. Lin KS, Luu A, Baidoo KE, et al. A new high affinity technetium-99m-bombesin analogue with low abdominal accumulation. Bioconjug Chem 2005; 16:43–50.
22. Breeman WA, De Jong M, Bernard BF, et al. Pre-clinical evaluation of [^{111}In-DTPA-Pro^{1},Tyr^{4}]bombesin, a new radioligand for bombesin-receptor scintigraphy. Int J Cancer 1999;83:657–63.
23. Breeman WA, Hofland LJ, de Jong M, et al. Evaluation of radiolabelled bombesin analogues for receptor-targeted scintigraphy and radiotherapy. Int J Cancer 1999;81:658–65.
24. Breeman WA, de Jong M, Erion JL, et al. Preclinical comparison of ^{111}In-labeled DTPA- or DOTA-bombesin analogs for receptor-targeted scintigraphy and radionuclide therapy. J Nucl Med 2002; 43:1650–6.
25. Nock BA, Nikolopoulou A, Galanis A, et al. Potent bombesin-like peptides for GRP-receptor targeting of tumors with ^{99m}Tc: a preclinical study. J Med Chem 2005;48:100–10.
26. Mather SJ, Nock BA, Maina T, et al. GRP receptor imaging of prostate cancer using [^{99m}Tc]Demobesin 4: a first-in-man study. Mol Imaging Biol 2014;16: 888–95.
27. Van de Wiele C, Dumont F, Vanden Broecke R, et al. Technetium-99m RP527, a GRP analogue for visualisation of GRP receptor-expressing malignancies: a feasibility study. Eur J Nucl Med 2000; 27:1694–9.
28. Van de Wiele C, Dumont F, Dierckx RA, et al. Biodistribution and dosimetry of ^{99m}Tc-RP527, a gastrin-releasing peptide (GRP) agonist for the visualization of GRP receptor-expressing malignancies. J Nucl Med 2001;42:1722–7.
29. Smith CJ, Gali H, Sieckman GL, et al. Radiochemical investigations of ^{99m}Tc-N_3S-X-BBN[7-14]NH_2: an in vitro/in vivo structure-activity relationship study where X = 0-, 3-, 5-, 8-, and 11-carbon tethering moieties. Bioconjug Chem 2003;14:93–102.
30. Hoffman TJ, Gali H, Smith CJ, et al. Novel series of ^{111}In-labeled bombesin analogs as potential radiopharmaceuticals for specific targeting of gastrin-releasing peptide receptors expressed on human prostate cancer cells. J Nucl Med 2003;44:823–31.
31. Smith CJ, Sieckman GL, Owen NK, et al. Radiochemical investigations of gastrin-releasing peptide receptor-specific [^{99m}Tc(X)$(CO)_3$-Dpr-Ser-Ser-Ser-Gln-Trp-Ala-Val-Gly-His-Leu-Met-NH_2] in PC-3, tumor-bearing, rodent models: syntheses, radiolabeling, and in vitro/in vivo studies where Dpr = 2,3-diaminopropionic acid and X = H_2O or $P(CH_2OH)_3$. Cancer Res 2003;63:4082–8.
32. Smith CJ, Volkert WA, Hoffman TJ. Gastrin releasing peptide (GRP) receptor targeted radiopharmaceuticals: a concise update. Nucl Med Biol 2003;30: 861–8.
33. van Vliet EI, Hermans JJ, de Ridder MA, et al. Tumor response assessment to treatment with [^{177}Lu-DOTA^{0},Tyr^{3}]octreotate in patients with gastroentero-pancreatic and bronchial neuroendocrine tumors: differential response of bone versus soft-tissue lesions. J Nucl Med 2012;53:1359–66.
34. Lantry LE, Cappelletti E, Maddalena ME, et al. ^{177}Lu-AMBA: synthesis and characterization of a selective ^{177}Lu-labeled GRP-R agonist for systemic radiotherapy of prostate cancer. J Nucl Med 2006;47: 1144–52.
35. Maddalena ME, Fox J, Chen J, et al. ^{177}Lu-AMBA biodistribution, radiotherapeutic efficacy, imaging, and autoradiography in prostate cancer models with low GRP-R expression. J Nucl Med 2009;50: 2017–24.
36. Panigone S, Nunn AD. Lutetium-177-labeled gastrin releasing peptide receptor binding analogs: a novel approach to radionuclide therapy. Q J Nucl Med Mol Imaging 2006;50:310–21.
37. Waser B, Eltschinger V, Linder K, et al. Selective in vitro targeting of GRP and NMB receptors in human tumours with the new bombesin tracer ^{177}Lu-AMBA. Eur J Nucl Med Mol Imaging 2007; 34:95–100.
38. Delle Fave G, Annibale B, de Magistris L, et al. Bombesin effects on human GI functions. Peptides 1985;6(Suppl 3):113–6.
39. Bruzzone R, Tamburrano G, Lala A, et al. Effect of bombesin on plasma insulin, pancreatic glucagon, and gut glucagon in man. J Clin Endocrinol Metab 1983;56:643–7.
40. Severi C, Jensen RT, Erspamer V, et al. Different receptors mediate the action of bombesin-related peptides on gastric smooth muscle cells. Am J Physiol 1991;260:G683–90.
41. Bodei L, Ferrari M, Nunn A, et al. ^{177}Lu-AMBA bombesin analogue in hormone refractory prostate cancer patients: a phase I escalation study with single-cycle administrations. Eur J Nucl Med Mol Imaging 2007;34:S221.
42. Linder KE, Metcalfe E, Arunachalam T, et al. In vitro and in vivo metabolism of Lu-AMBA, a GRP-receptor binding compound, and the synthesis and characterization of its metabolites. Bioconjug Chem 2009; 20:1171–8.
43. Cagnolini A, Chen J, Ramos K, et al. Automated synthesis, characterization and biological evaluation of [^{68}Ga]Ga-AMBA, and the synthesis and characterization of ^{nat}Ga-AMBA and [^{67}Ga]Ga-AMBA. Appl Radiat Isot 2010;68:2285–92.

44. Zhang H, Schuhmacher J, Waser B, et al. DOTA-PESIN, a DOTA-conjugated bombesin derivative designed for the imaging and targeted radionuclide treatment of bombesin receptor-positive tumours. Eur J Nucl Med Mol Imaging 2007;34:1198–208.
45. Wild D, Frischknecht M, Zhang H, et al. Alpha- versus beta-particle radiopeptide therapy in a human prostate cancer model (^{213}Bi-DOTA-PESIN and ^{213}Bi-AMBA versus ^{177}Lu-DOTA-PESIN). Cancer Res 2011;71:1009–18.
46. Pradhan TK, Katsuno T, Taylor JE, et al. Identification of a unique ligand which has high affinity for all four bombesin receptor subtypes. Eur J Pharmacol 1998;343:275–87.
47. Reubi JC, Wenger S, Schmuckli-Maurer J, et al. Bombesin receptor subtypes in human cancers: detection with the universal radioligand ^{125}I-[D-Tyr^{6},-beta-Ala^{11},Phe^{13},Nle^{14}]bombesin(6-14). Clin Cancer Res 2002;8:1139–46.
48. Dimitrakopoulou-Strauss A, Hohenberger P, Haberkorn U, et al. ^{68}Ga-labeled bombesin studies in patients with gastrointestinal stromal tumors: comparison with ^{18}F-FDG. J Nucl Med 2007;48: 1245–50.
49. Nock BA, Maina T, Krenning EP, et al. "To serve and protect": enzyme inhibitors as radiopeptide escorts promote tumor targeting. J Nucl Med 2014;55:121–7.
50. Reubi JC, Eisenwiener KP, Rink H, et al. A new peptidic somatostatin agonist with high affinity to all five somatostatin receptors. Eur J Pharmacol 2002;456:45–9.
51. Maina T, Cescato R, Waser B, et al. [^{111}In-DOTA]LTT-SS28, a first pansomatostatin radioligand for in vivo targeting of somatostatin receptor-positive tumors. J Med Chem 2014;57:6564–71.
52. Marsouvanidis PJ, Maina T, Sallegger W, et al. ^{99m}Tc-Radiotracers based on human GRP(18-27): synthesis and comparative evaluation. J Nucl Med 2013;54(10):1797–803.
53. Marsouvanidis PJ, Maina T, Sallegger W, et al. Tumor diagnosis with new ^{111}In-radioligands based on truncated human gastrin releasing peptide sequences: synthesis and preclinical comparison. J Med Chem 2013;56:8579–87.
54. Mansi R, Wang X, Forrer F, et al. Evaluation of a 1,4,7,10-tetraazacyclododecane-1,4,7,10-tetraacetic acid-conjugated bombesin-based radioantagonist for the labeling with single-photon emission computed tomography, positron emission tomography, and therapeutic radionuclides. Clin Cancer Res 2009;15:5240–9.
55. de Castiglione R, Gozzini L. Bombesin receptor antagonists. Crit Rev Oncol Hematol 1996;24:117–51.
56. Preston SR, Miller GV, Primrose JN. Bombesin-like peptides and cancer. Crit Rev Oncol Hematol 1996;23:225–38.
57. Rozengurt E. Bombesin stimulation of mitogenesis. Specific receptors, signal transduction, and early events. Am Rev Respir Dis 1990;142:S11–5.
58. Pinski J, Schally AV, Halmos G, et al. Effect of somatostatin analog RC-160 and bombesin/gastrin releasing peptide antagonist RC-3095 on growth of PC-3 human prostate-cancer xenografts in nude mice. Int J Cancer 1993;55:963–7.
59. Milovanovic SR, Radulovic S, Groot K, et al. Inhibition of growth of PC-82 human prostate cancer line xenografts in nude mice by bombesin antagonist RC-3095 or combination of agonist [D-Trp^{6}]-luteinizing hormone-releasing hormone and somatostatin analog RC-160. Prostate 1992;20:269–80.
60. Woll PJ, Rozengurt E. A neuropeptide antagonist that inhibits the growth of small cell lung cancer in vitro. Cancer Res 1990;50:3968–73.
61. Wang LH, Coy DH, Taylor JE, et al. Desmethionine alkylamide bombesin analogues: a new class of bombesin receptor antagonists with potent antisecretory activity in pancreatic acini and antimitotic activity in Swiss 3T3 cells. Biochemistry 1990;29:616–22.
62. Wang LH, Coy DH, Taylor JE, et al. *des*-Met carboxyl-terminally modified analogues of bombesin function as potent bombesin receptor antagonists, partial agonists, or agonists. J Biol Chem 1990; 265:15695–703.
63. Nock B, Nikolopoulou A, Chiotellis E, et al. [^{99m}Tc] Demobesin 1, a novel potent bombesin analogue for GRP receptor-targeted tumour imaging. Eur J Nucl Med Mol Imaging 2003;30:247–58.
64. Maina T, Bergsma H, Kulkarni HR, et al. Preclinical and first clinical experience with the gastrin-releasing peptide receptor-antagonist [^{68}Ga]SB3 and PET/CT. Eur J Nucl Med Mol Imaging 2016;43: 964–73.
65. Schroeder RP, de Visser M, van Weerden WM, et al. Androgen-regulated gastrin-releasing peptide receptor expression in androgen-dependent human prostate tumor xenografts. Int J Cancer 2010;126: 2826–34.
66. Bakker IL, Fröberg A, Busstra M, et al. PET imaging of therapy-naïve primary prostate cancer patients using the GRPr-targeting ligand Sarabesin 3. Eur Urol Suppl 2016;15:e567.
67. Lymperis E, Maina T, Kaloudi A, et al. Transient in vivo NEP inhibition enhances the theranostic potential of the new GRPR-antagonist [^{111}In/^{177}Lu] SB3. Eur J Nucl Med Mol Imaging 2014;41:S319.
68. Azay J, Nagain C, Llinares M, et al. Comparative study of in vitro and in vivo activities of bombesin pseudopeptide analogs modified on the C-terminal dipeptide fragment. Peptides 1998;19:57–63.
69. Mansi R, Wang X, Forrer F, et al. Development of a potent DOTA-conjugated bombesin antagonist for targeting GRPr-positive tumours. Eur J Nucl Med Mol Imaging 2011;38:97–107.

70. Marsouvanidis PJ, Nock BA, Hajjaj B, et al. Gastrin releasing peptide receptor-directed radioligands based on a bombesin antagonist: synthesis, ^{111}In-labeling, and preclinical profile. J Med Chem 2013; 56:2374–84.
71. Chatalic KL, Konijnenberg M, Nonnekens J, et al. In vivo stabilization of a gastrin-releasing peptide receptor antagonist enhances PET imaging and radionuclide therapy of prostate cancer in preclinical studies. Theranostics 2016;6:104–17.
72. Mansi R, Fleischmann A, Macke HR, et al. Targeting GRPR in urological cancers–from basic research to clinical application. Nat Rev Urol 2013;10:235–44.
73. Kähkönen E, Jambor I, Kemppainen J, et al. In vivo imaging of prostate cancer using [^{68}Ga]-labeled bombesin analog BAY86-7548. Clin Cancer Res 2013;19(19):5434–43.
74. Varasteh Z, Rosenstrom U, Velikyan I, et al. The effect of mini-PEG-based spacer length on binding and pharmacokinetic properties of a ^{68}Ga-labeled NOTA-conjugated antagonistic analog of bombesin. Molecules 2014;19:10455–72.
75. Varasteh Z, Mitran B, Rosenstrom U, et al. The effect of macrocyclic chelators on the targeting properties of the ^{68}Ga-labeled gastrin releasing peptide receptor antagonist PEG2-RM26. Nucl Med Biol 2015;42: 446–54.
76. Dumont RA, Tamma M, Braun F, et al. Targeted radiotherapy of prostate cancer with a gastrin-releasing peptide receptor antagonist is effective as monotherapy and in combination with rapamycin. J Nucl Med 2013;54:762–9.
77. Lohrmann C, Zhang H, Thorek DL, et al. Cerenkov luminescence imaging for radiation dose calculation of a ^{90}Y-labeled gastrin-releasing peptide receptor antagonist. J Nucl Med 2015;56:805–11.
78. Heimbrook DC, Saari WS, Balishin NL, et al. Gastrin releasing peptide antagonists with improved potency and stability. J Med Chem 1991;34:2102–7.
79. Nock BA, Kaloudi A, Lymperis E, et al. Theranostic perspectives in prostate cancer with the GRPR-antagonist NeoBOMB1 – preclinical and first clinical results. J Nucl Med 2017;58(1):75–80.
80. Dalm S, Bakker I, de Blois E, et al. ^{68}Ga/^{177}Lu-NeoBOMB1, a novel radiolabeled GRPR antagonist for theranostic use. J Nucl Med 2016;57:331.
81. Nock BA, Kaloudi A, Lymperis E, et al. [^{68}Ga]NeoBomb1, a new potent GRPR-antagonist for PET imaging—preclinical and first clinical evaluation in prostate cancer. J Nucl Med 2016;57:583.
82. Minamimoto R, Hancock S, Schneider B, et al. Pilot comparison of ^{68}Ga-RM2 PET and ^{68}Ga-PSMA-11 PET in patients with biochemically recurrent prostate cancer. J Nucl Med 2016;57:557–62.

Gallium-68 Prostate-Specific Membrane Antigen PET Imaging

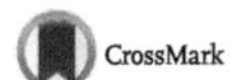

Michael S. Hofman, MBBS, FRACP, FAANMS[a,b,*],
Amir Iravani, MD, FRACP[a]

KEYWORDS

• Prostate cancer • Prostate-specific membrane antigen • PET • ^{68}Ga-PSMA • ^{68}Ga-PSMA PET

KEY POINTS

- Gallium-68 (^{68}Ga) prostate-specific membrane antigen (^{68}Ga-PSMA) imaging has superior accuracy to conventional imaging modalities, including choline PET/computed tomography (CT).
- ^{68}Ga-PSMA imaging can be used in the context of high-risk localized prostate cancer (PCa), by defining the extent of primary, regional, and distant metastases; prostate-specific antigen (PSA) recurrence; the location of PCa lesion even in the low level of PSA; and of oligometastatic disease and by determining the extent of disease to guide the therapy.
- Imaging specialists need to familiarize themselves with physiologic ^{68}Ga-PSMA uptake, common variants, pattern of locoregional and distant spread of PCa, and its inherent pitfalls; they should also educate the clinicians about the capabilities and limitations of this imaging modality.

INTRODUCTION

Prostate cancer (PCa) is one the most common malignancies in men worldwide and leads to substantial morbidity and mortality. Imaging of PCa is indicated for primary diagnosis, staging, and restaging as well as for localization of recurrent disease. Currently, conventional imaging modalities, including ultrasound, bone scintigraphy, CT, and MR imaging, are used to detect primary and metastatic PCa for staging and risk stratification. Despite significant efforts, conventional imaging of PCa does not contribute to patient management as much as imaging performed in patients with other common cancers.

The main limitation of conventional imaging modalities is their low sensitivity in detecting metastases in primary diagnosis or in recurrent PCa, in particular with low PSA levels when disease is often small in volume. In a meta-analysis of 24 studies, the pooled sensitivity and specificity of CT for lymph node diagnosis were 42% and 82%, respectively. For MR imaging, this review reported the pooled sensitivity and specificity of 39% and 82%, respectively.[1] Although functional assessment of the disease with additional MR sequences, such as diffusion-weighted MR imaging or dynamic contrast-enhanced MR imaging, are increasingly used for imaging of PCa, these

Disclosure Statement: The authors have nothing to disclose.
[a] Department of Cancer Imaging, Centre for Molecular Imaging, Peter MacCallum Cancer Centre, 305 Grattan Street, Melbourne, Victoria 3000, Australia; [b] University of Melbourne, Melbourne, Victoria 3000, Australia
* Corresponding author. Department of Cancer Imaging, Peter MacCallum Cancer Centre, 305 Grattan Street, Melbourne, Victoria 3000, Australia.
E-mail address: Michael.hofman@petermac.org

PET Clin 12 (2017) 219–234
http://dx.doi.org/10.1016/j.cpet.2016.12.004

imaging techniques suffer from nontumor specificity and a lack of high-level evidence for their utility.

Molecular imaging with PET using an increasing list of biologically relevant radiotracers is facilitating the precision and personalized medicine in PCa.[2] PSMA has received a resurgence of attention over the past few years as a useful biomarker in the imaging of PCa. Among the available tracers and ligands available to image PSMA-expressing tumors, Glu-NH-CO-NH-Lys-(Ahx)-[^{68}Ga(HBED-CC)], also known as ^{68}Ga-PSMA HBED-CC or ^{68}Ga-PSMA-11, developed by the Heidelberg group in Germany, became one of the most successful and promising PSMA radioligands and demonstrated a rapid spread across many countries.[3–5]

RADIOLABELED PROSTATE-SPECIFIC MEMBRANE ANTIGEN LIGANDS

PSMA is a type II, integral membrane glycoprotein that was first detected on the human prostatic carcinoma cell line LNCaP.[6] It consists of 750 amino acid integral membrane glycoprotein (100–120 kDa), with a 19–amino acid intracellular component, a 24–amino acid intramembrane segment, and a large 707–amino acid extracellular domain.[7] It has several enzymatic functions and is known to be up-regulated in castrate-resistant and metastatic PCa.[8] PSMA is not specific to the prostate gland and is expressed in other normal tissues, including salivary glands, duodenal mucosa, proximal renal tubular cells, and subpopulation of neuroendocrine cells in the colonic crypts. In PCa, PSMA is overexpressed approximately 100 times to 1000 times compared with normal prostate tissue.[9] It is also overexpressed in multiple other neoplasms (eg, subtypes of transitional cell carcinoma, renal cell carcinoma, colon carcinoma, and peritumoral and endotumoral endothelial cell of neovasculature).[10] There is no known natural ligand for PSMA and the reasons for its up-regulation in PCa remains unclear. PSMA undergoes constitutive internalization and as such can serve not only as an imaging biomarker but also for targeted therapy – in other words, PSMA may be useful as a target for theranostic agents.[11]

In malignant tissue, PSMA has been suggested as involved in angiogenesis, because increased PSMA expression was found expressed in the stroma adjacent to neovasculature of solid tumors.[12] Due to its selective overexpression in 90% to 100% of local PCa lesions, as well as in cancerous lymph nodes and bone metastases,[13–15] PSMA is a reliable tissue marker for PCa and is considered an ideal target for theranostic applications.[16–19]

Increased PSMA expression is correlated with an increase in tumor grade, pathologic stage, aneuploidy, and biochemical recurrence. Of clinical importance is that PSMA expression is up-regulated when tumors become androgen independent and also after antiandrogen therapy (ADT) in most cases.[20] This characteristic makes PSMA particularly valuable, because it has potential as an early indicator of tumor progression after ADT and could play a role as a prognostic factor for disease recurrence.[21]

One of the first imaging probes specifically targeting PSMA was indium-111 (^{111}In) capromab pendetide (ProstaScint), a ^{111}In-labeled anti-PSMA antibody.[22] An important limitation of capromab pendetide is that it binds to an intracellular epitope of the transmembrane PSMA glcyoprotein. Therefore, capromab pendetide either binds to viable tumor cells after internalization or to dying cells with disrupted cellular membranes. Furthermore, slow plasma clearance of the antibody results in poor tumor-to-background contrast, the application of ^{111}In–capromab pendetide for imaging prostatic malignancies remained limited.[23,24]

Subsequently, high-affinity antibodies directed against extracellular epitopes of PSMA have been developed, such as J415, J533, and J591.[25] It was shown that ^{111}In-J591 accurately targets bone and soft tissue metastatic PCa lesions[26] and that lutetium-177 (^{177}Lu)-labeled J591 can be used safely in radioimmunotherapy directed against micrometastatic PCa.[27] Major disadvantages limiting the use of radiolabeled monoclonal antibodies as theranostic radiopharmaceuticals are their long circulatory half-life (3–4 days), poor tumor penetration, and low tumor-to-normal tissue ratios, especially at early time points. Small molecules, in contrast, exhibit rapid extravasation, rapid diffusion in the extravascular space, and faster blood clearance. This could result in high tumor-to-normal tissue contrast early after injection of the tracer.

In search for PSMA tracers with such favorable characteristics, modified forms of N-acetylated-a-linked acidic dipeptidase (NAALAdase) inhibitors, which were originally developed for possible neuroprotective effects in neurologic disorders, such as amyotrophic lateral sclerosis,[28] have been evaluated for their potential to diagnose and treat PCa. A series of preclinical studies evaluated the role of radiolabeled small-molecule PSMA-inhibiting ligands for imaging of human PCa using various radionuclides, such as carbon-11 (^{11}C),[29] fluorine-18 (^{18}F),[30] iodine-123 (^{123}I),[31] technetium-99m (^{99m}Tc),[32,33] and ^{68}Ga.[34,35] Overall, the PSMAs tested in these preclinical studies showed high tumor uptake peaking at 0.5 hour to 1 hour in mice with

PSMA-expressing tumors. At earlier time points, the contrast was impaired due to high blood levels. For imaging purposes, this time frame matches best with radionuclides with half-lives of 1 hour to 2 hours (ie, ^{68}Ga or ^{18}F). In some of these preclinical studies, remarkable changes in affinity and tumor uptake were observed on changes in the radiolabel, chelator, and linker. First of all, it has been suggested that a spacer is required between the PSMA binding motif and the chelator. Chen and colleagues[36] have compared PSMAs with different linker lengths and showed that an increased linker length enhanced the affinity for PSMA and increased tumor uptake.

Since 2012, the number of clinical studies using urea-based PSMAs, such as $^{123/124/131}$IMIP-1072/-1095,[37] ^{99m}Tc-MIP-1404/-1405,[38] ^{68}Ga-HBED-PSMA, ^{18}F-DCFBC,[39] and ^{18}F-DCFPyl, exponentially increased.[4,40–42] Among these agents, the ^{68}G-lableled and ^{18}F-labeled compounds have attracted the most attention, because these compounds can be used for PET/CT imaging. The availability of ^{123}I or ^{99m}Tc, however, allows single-photon emission CT (SPECT)/CT imaging in centers without facilities for PET.

PET/COMPUTED TOMOGRAPHY IMAGING WITH GALLIUM-68 PROSTATE-SPECIFIC MEMBRANE ANTIGEN

During the past few years, the application of ^{68}Ga-labeled peptides has attracted considerable interest for cancer imaging due to the physical characteristics of ^{68}Ga (half-life of 68 minutes, beta decay of 1899 keV)[43] and the availability of reliable germanium-68 (^{68}Ge)/^{68}Ga generators. This enabled ^{68}Ga-DOTATATE PET/CT imaging of neuroendocrine tumors,[44,45] owing to the rapid binding and cellular uptake of DOTATATE, and this is now widely recognized as the new gold standard for imaging these tumors. Moreover, the half-life of ^{68}Ga is suitable for the pharmacokinetics of the small PSMA-inhibiting peptides, which have rapid binding and cellular uptake. Among the first PSMA inhibitors available for labeling with ^{68}Ga and PET imaging of PCa were 1,4,7,10-tetraazacyclododecane-1,4,7,10-tetraacetic acid (DOTA) conjugated urea-based PSMA inhibitors, developed and tested preclinically by Banerjee and colleagues.[34] Eder and colleagues[46] prepared the ^{68}Ga-PSMA inhibitor Glu-NH-CO-NHLys(Ahx)-HBED-CC using the chelator N,N'-bis[2–hydroxy-5-(carboxyethyl)-benzyl]ethylene diamineN,N'-diacetic acid (HBED-CC). Potentially, HBED is a more attractive chelator for ^{68}Ga than DOTA because it forms a more thermodynamically stable complex with ^{68}Ga, even at room temperature.[47] Eder and colleagues[46] compared Glu-NH-CO-NHLys(Ahx)-HBED-CC with Glu-NH-CO-NH-Lys-DOTA and demonstrated that the HBED-CC conjugated compound had more favorable properties for PCa imaging than the DOTA analog. ^{68}Ga-labeled Glu-NH-CO-NH-Lys(Ahx)-HBED-CC (^{68}Ga-PSMA) showed fast blood clearance, low liver uptake, and high specific uptake in PSMA-expressing tissues and tumor (tumor uptake 7.7% $\pm$ 1.5% injected dose (ID)/g for the HBED-CC conjugate, which was 2.6-fold higher compared with the DOTA compound). In addition, liver uptake of the HBED-CC conjugated ligand was 5.7-fold lower (**Fig. 1**).

Based on the promising preclinical results, the German Cancer Research Center in Heidelberg performed the first clinical investigation of the ^{68}Ga-PSMA in a cohort of 37 patients. In 84% of the patients, PCa lesions were identified.

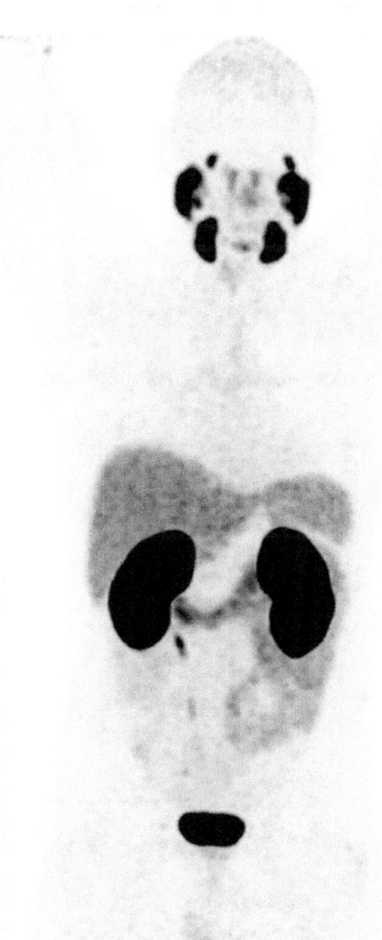

Fig. 1. Maximum intensity projection image demonstrates physiologic distribution of ^{68}Ga-PSMA with highest intensity of uptake in the kidneys, excreted urine in the bladder and salivary glands.

PCa lesions were found in 60% of the patients with PSA levels less than 2.2 ng/mL, whereas at PSA levels of greater than 2.2 ng/mL, PCa lesions were found in all patients. Thus, even at low blood PSA levels, ^{68}Ga-PSMA PET/CT identified lesions with high tumor-to-background ratios. Tumor uptake of ^{68}Ga-PSMA was stable between 1 hour and 3 hours, whereas in normal tissue, uptake slightly decreased between 1 hour and 3 hours. As a result, late scans exhibited higher tumor-to-background ratios, which might be useful when lesions remain unclear in an early scan.[4] In a more recent study by this group, imaging with ^{68}Ga-PSMA PET/CT was performed at 5 minutes, 1 hour, 2 hours, 3 hours, 4 hours, and 5 hours after injection in patients with recurrent PCa. Most of tumor lesions were visible at 3 hours post injection, whereas at all other time points many were not qualitatively present; therefore, they concluded that this time point would be optimal for imaging.[48] Since this study, there has been increasing number of studies investigating ^{68}Ga-PSMA in the different aspects of PCa.

Gallium-68 Prostate-Specific Membrane Antigen in Biochemical Recurrence After Radical Treatment of Prostate Cancer

Biochemical relapse after radical prostatectomy or radiotherapy occurs in up to half of patients with PCa.[49] More than a quarter of patients with biochemical recurrence eventually develop clinical recurrence in approximately 7 years to 8 years.[49] Detection of the sites of recurrent disease is of paramount importance because this avoids futile localized treatment in cases and systemic recurrence and avoids the side effects of systemic treatments in cases of localized recurrence (**Fig. 2**). One of the major drivers in detecting very low volume disease in the recurrent setting is the feasibility of treating oligometastatic disease with technologies, such as stereotactic radiotherapy, and in doing so potentially obtaining a further clinical/biochemical remission.[50] Whether this approach improves long-term patient outcomes, however, is yet to be established.

The diagnostic yield of conventional imaging modalities for local recurrence and lymph node and bone metastasis after radical prostatectomy

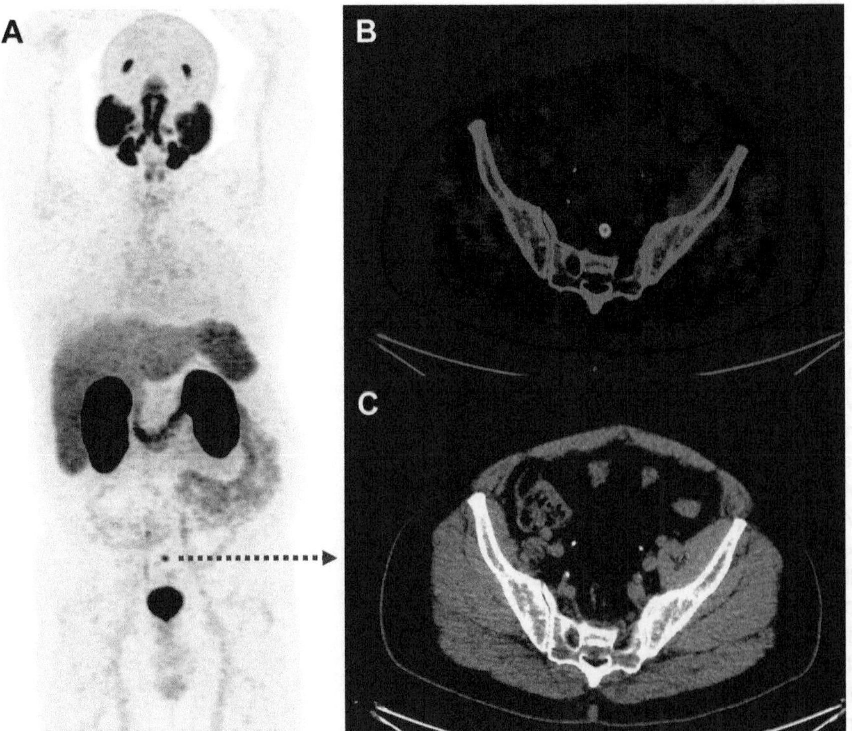

Fig. 2. PSMA PET maximum intensity projection image (*A*) of a patient with biochemical recurrence after radical prostatectomy with PSA of 0.34 ng/mL, demonstrates focal uptake in the pelvis (*arrow*). PET/CT images (*B, C*) show uptake in a small presacral lymph node.

is low. Bone scan (BS) has detection rate of less than 5% for PSA values of less than 7 ng/mL.[49] Similarly CT has low sensitivity (11%–14%) in predicting lymph node and local recurrence in this cohort of patients.[49] ^{68}Ga-PSMA PET imaging has had its most promising outcomes in patients with recurrent PCa and its ability to detect metastatic disease at very low volume disease and low PSA levels.

Gallium-68 prostate-specific membrane antigen detection rate and its relation to prostate-specific antigen level

Afshar-Oromieh and colleagues[51] retrospectively investigated the diagnostic value of ^{68}Ga–HBED-CC–PSMA PET/CT in 319 patients with PCa. ^{68}Ga-PSMA PET/CT detected PCa in 83% of the patients suspected recurrent PCa (264 of 319 patients). In addition, the tracer is highly specific for PCa: histologic analysis demonstrated that tracer accumulation in tumor lesions correlated with manifestations of PCa in virtually all cases without false-positive lesions. Eiber and colleagues[52] reported the diagnostic accuracy of ^{68}Ga–HBED-CC–PSMA PET/CT in 248 patients with biochemical recurrence after radical prostatectomy. In this study, 222 patients (89.5%) showed pathologic findings in ^{68}Ga–HBED-CC–PSMA PET/CT. Positive correlation was found between the PSA level and PSMA PET/CT detection rate. The detection rates were 96.8%, 93%, 72.7%, and 57.9% in patients with serum PSA-levels of greater than or equal to 2.1 ng/mL, less than 2.0 ng/mL to 1.0 ng/mL, less than 1.0 ng/mL to 0.5 ng/mL, and less than 0.5 ng/mL to 0.2 ng/mL, respectively.[52]

In a meta-analysis performed by Perera and colleagues,[53] including 16 articles and 1309 patients, the overall percentage of positive ^{68}Ga-PSMA PET was 76% for biochemical recurrence. The detection rate for the PSA categories 0 to 0.2, 0.2 to 1, 1 to 2, and greater than 2 ng/mL were 42%, 58%, 76%, and 95% scans, respectively. On per-patient analysis, the sensitivity and specificity of ^{68}Ga-PSMA PET were both 86% whereas on per-lesion analysis, the sensitivity and specificity were 80% and 97%, respectively.[53]

Comparison between gallium-68 prostate-specific membrane antigen and radiolabeled choline PET

^{68}Ga-PSMA showed substantially higher detection rates compared with choline ligand PET/CTs with the detection rates between 34% and 88% for ^{11}C-choline, 43% to 79% for ^{18}F-choline, and 59% to 80% for ^{11}C-acetate.[54] Bluemel and colleagues[55] investigated the value of ^{68}Ga-PSMA PET/CT in biochemically recurring PCa patients with negative ^{18}F-choline PET/CT. With the sequential imaging approach, Ga-PSMA PET identified sites of recurrent disease in 43.8% of the patients with negative F-choline PET scans. Subgroup analysis of Ga-PSMA PET in ^{18}F-choline–negative patients revealed detection rates of 28.6%, 45.5%, and 71.4% for PSA levels of 0.2 ng/mL to 1 ng/mL, 1 ng/mL to 2 ng/mL, and greater than 2 ng/mL, respectively.[55]

Comparison between gallium-68 prostate-specific membrane antigen and histologic assessment and morphologic imaging

There is a paucity of data comparing between ^{68}Ga-PSMA findings and histologic assessment. Rauscher and colleagues[56] investigated the accuracy of the ^{68}Ga-PSMA PET/CT compared with morphologic imaging (CT or MR imaging) in 48 patients with biochemical recurrence of PCa who underwent salvage lymphadenectomy. The specificity of ^{68}Ga-PSMA PET was 97% compared with 99% morphologic imaging. PET, however, detected 78% of histopathologic proved lymph node, whereas morphologic imaging was positive in only 27%. Diagnostic accuracy of ^{68}Ga-PSMA PET imaging was, therefore, 90% and for morphologic imaging 72%. The mean short axis size of ^{68}Ga suspicious lymph node on PET was 8.3 mm $\pm$ 4.3 mm compared with 13.0 mm $\pm$ 4.9 mm for suspicious nodes identified on morphologic imaging alone. Histopathologic assessment of false-negative lymph node fields in ^{68}Ga-PSMA HBED-CC PET revealed a mean lesion size of 4.7 $\pm$ 3.4 mm (range: 0.5–11 mm).[56] In another study performed by Giesel and colleagues[57] comparing the lymph node detection rates between ^{68}Ga-PSMA-based PET/CT imaging and 3-D CT volumetric lymph node assessment in 21 patients with intermediate-risk and high-risk PCa patients who had biochemical recurrence after radical prostatectomy,^{68}Ga-PSMA PET/CT was more sensitive than volume-based CT evaluation of lymph node recurrence, with PET detecting nodal recurrence in two-thirds of patients who would have otherwise been missed by CT evaluation.

Afshar-Oromieh and colleagues[40] reported initial experience of ^{68}Ga-PSMA PET/CT compared with PET/MR imaging. In this study, 20 patients were scanned with PET/CT and PET/MR imaging sequentially. Of the 75 lesions that were characterized further, 4 lesions unclear in PET/CT could be established as PCa lesions in PET/MR imaging. Pathologic lesions visible on PET often correlated with signals on MR imaging, offering a considerable advantage for

PET/MR imaging. Overall, PCa was detected more easily and more accurately with ^{68}Ga-PSMA PET/MR imaging than with PET/CT. A potential disadvantage of PET/MR imaging, however, was the appearance of halo artifacts around the bladder and kidneys, resulting in a reduced PET signal, potentially making lesions in their vicinity undetectable.[40]

Factors affecting gallium-68 prostate-specific membrane antigen detection rate

Although it has been shown that the diagnostic value of ^{68}Ga-PSMA PET/CT in patients with PCa is high, even in patients with low PSA serum levels and compared with other tracers, such as radiolabeled choline, approximately 40% of the patients with PSA levels of less than 0.5 ng/mL showed negative ^{68}Ga-PSMA PET/CT results.[51] Therefore, Ceci and colleagues[58] evaluated which factors are associated with the ^{68}Ga-PSMA PET/CT tumor lesion detection rate. In this study, 70 patients with recurrent PCa underwent ^{68}Ga-PSMA PET/CT and were retrospectively evaluated regarding their previous therapies, serum PSA levels, PSA doubling times, and PSA velocity. A serum PSA level of 0.83 ng/mL and a PSA doubling time of 6.5 months were found valuable cutoff values for predicting, with high probability a positive or negative scan result. In particular, 85% of patients with short PSA doubling times who were candidates for radiotherapy to the prostate bed (early phase of biochemical recurrence with low PSA levels) showed positive findings on PET/CT, whereas only 18.7% of patients with similar low PSA levels but with long PSA doubling time were PET positive.[58]

Gallium-68 Prostate-Specific Membrane Antigen in the Lymph Node Staging Prior to Radical Prostatectomy

Due to the low accuracy of current imaging modalities for lymph node staging, clinicians are reliant on preoperative models using PSA levels, Gleason score (GS), and T stage to dictate lymphadenectomy protocols.[59] Lymphadenectomy may add significant morbidity to the radical prostatectomy procedure and more accurate staging may enable management change. The evidence favoring ^{68}Ga-PSMA PET imaging for detection of lymph node metastasis in this cohort of patients is evolving. Eiber and colleagues[60] prospectively evaluated ^{68}Ga-PSMA PET imaging for preoperative lymph node staging in 37 intermediate-risk and high-risk patients undergoing radical prostatectomy and extended pelvic lymph node dissection. In the PET-positive cohort (33/37), on patient-based analysis, sensitivity and specificity were 75% and 96%, respectively. On field-based analysis, the sensitivity and specificity were 65% and 98%, respectively.[60] In the PET-negative patients (4/37), 2 patients had false-negative results. In a recent retrospective series, Budaus and colleagues[61] reported less promising results with overall sensitivity, specificity, positive predictive value, and negative predictive value of ^{68}Ga-PSMA PET/CT for lymph node metastasis detection of 33%, 100%, 100%, and 69%, respectively. This group hypothesized that in primary staging a significant proportion of the PSMA is taken up by the prostate, as a result limiting its availability in the lymph nodes.[61] Other suggestions for the less impressive outcomes were restricted perfusion in lymph node metastasis due to a critical size or vascularization threshold, variable expertise, and small sample size.[61]

Gallium-68 Prostate-Specific Membrane Antigen in Local Staging of the Prostate Cancer

There are few data on the role of ^{68}Ga-PSMA PET imaging in primary local staging of PCa. PCa patient risk is determined by considering several factors, including PSA level and GS. Various imaging techniques have been used for local staging and biopsy guidance. In particular, multiparametric MR imaging shows promising results for localizing PCa and improving accuracy of transrectal ultrasound biopsy.[62,63] Despite significant effort in standardization of reporting, the major drawback of MR imaging remains significant interobserver variability resulting in heterogeneous reported accuracy in the literature.[64] Furthermore, MR imaging performance in low-volume disease and identifying extraprostatic extension of cancer is less impressive.[65] Additional molecular information and higher tumor-to-background ratio, however, provided by ^{68}Ga-PSMA PET could potentially overcome this inadequacy and further refine the targeting of lesions[66] (**Fig. 3**).

In a recent study, Fendler and colleagues[67] evaluated the accuracy of ^{68}Ga-PSMA PET/CT in localizing PCa at initial diagnosis in 21 patients. This study demonstrates promising accuracy with high positive predictive value in excess of 95%. On segment-based analysis, however, the sensitivity of PSMA PET was moderate (67%), which still was higher than pooled sensitivity (54%–66%) of various MR imaging protocols in a systematic review.[68] Furthermore, ^{68}Ga-PSMA PET had high (86%) accuracy for the detection of seminal vesicle involvement.[67]

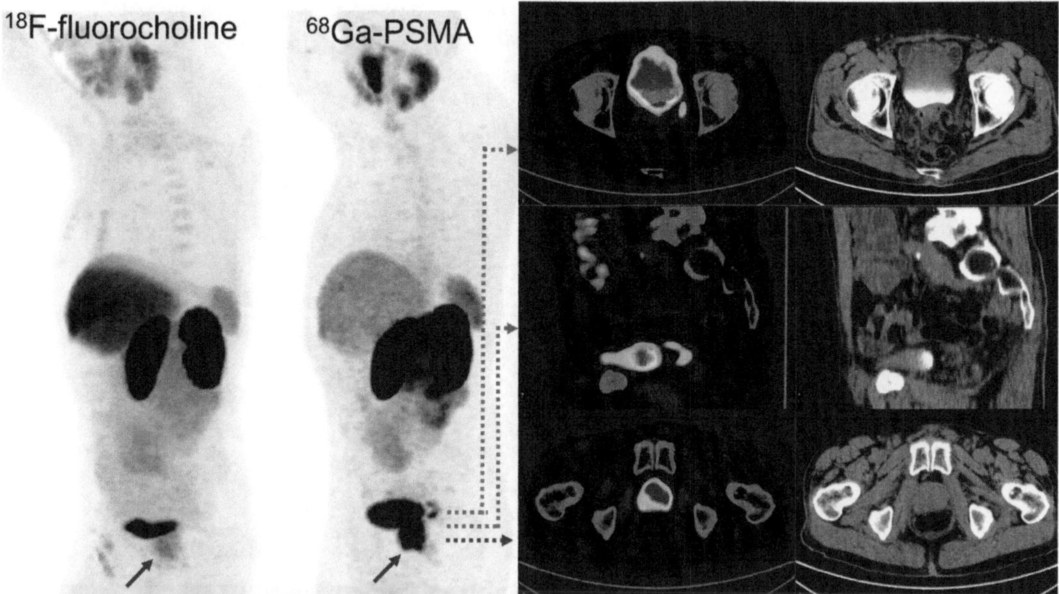

Fig. 3. (*Left*) Fluorocholine PET MIP (oblique projection) image of a 70-year-old man with GS 9 PCa and PSA of 100 ng/mL demonstrates mildly avid primary prostate cancer (*solid red arrow*). (*Right*) PSMA PET MIP image and corresponding PET/CT images show intensely PSMA expressing locally advanced prostate cancer (*dashed red arrow*) with extension of tumor along the seminal vesicle (*dashed blue arrow*) and vas deference (*dashed orange arrow*).

Gallium-68 Prostate-Specific Membrane Antigen PET and Response Assessment

Response assessment in metastatic PCa is often suboptimal due to limited applicability of Response Evaluation Criteria in Solid Tumors version 1.1 criteria due to nontarget lymph nodes and frequently presents sclerotic bone metastases. Evaluation with BS is also remains a challenge to reliably prove therapy response due to frequently seen flare phenomenon. Despite efforts in standardization by Prostate Cancer Clinical Trials Working Group consensus recommendations[69] and European Organization for Research and Treatment[70] cancer imaging group, response assessment in metastatic PCa poses a significant challenge to clinicians in the clinical trials. Radiolabeled choline PET imaging has had promising results in predicting the response to treatment modalities, such as ADTs.[71] Early experience suggests that PSMA PET/CT may be more robust and reliable than choline PET/CT or conventional imaging but there are currently no data available to support its use, and research is required to validate this as a new biomarker (**Figs. 4** and **5**). Assessment of response by molecular imaging incorporating PSMA and other tracers, such as fluorodeoxyglucose (FDG), may potentially pave the way to address the heterogeneity of response to treatment in particular in the advanced stages of the PCa.

Interpretation and Pitfalls

Clinical studies so far convincingly demonstrate that ^{68}Ga-PSMA is a promising tracer for both staging high-risk patients and detection of biochemical recurrence. The experience with ^{68}Ga-PSMA PET/CT in clinical practice, however, continues to evolve and several pitfalls have become apparent.

Physiologic distribution of gallium-68 prostate-specific membrane antigen

Any focal uptake of ^{68}Ga-PSMA higher than the surrounding background, in particular in the typical lymphatic drainage of the prostate, has to be considered malignant. To provide an accurate interpretation of ^{68}Ga-PSMA, however, nuclear medicine specialists and radiologists should be familiar with physiologic PSMA distribution, common variants, artifacts, pattern of locoregional and distant spread of PCa, and its inherent pitfalls.

The physiologic PSMA uptake can be observed in the following tissues: lacrimal gland, parotid gland, submandibular gland, liver, spleen, small intestine, colon, and kidney (see **Fig. 1**). Depending on the type of PSMA used in the imaging, however, there is slight variability in the distribution of and intensity of uptake in these organs. Nonetheless, kidneys, urinary collecting system, and salivary glands are consistently demonstrating the highest radiotracer uptake.

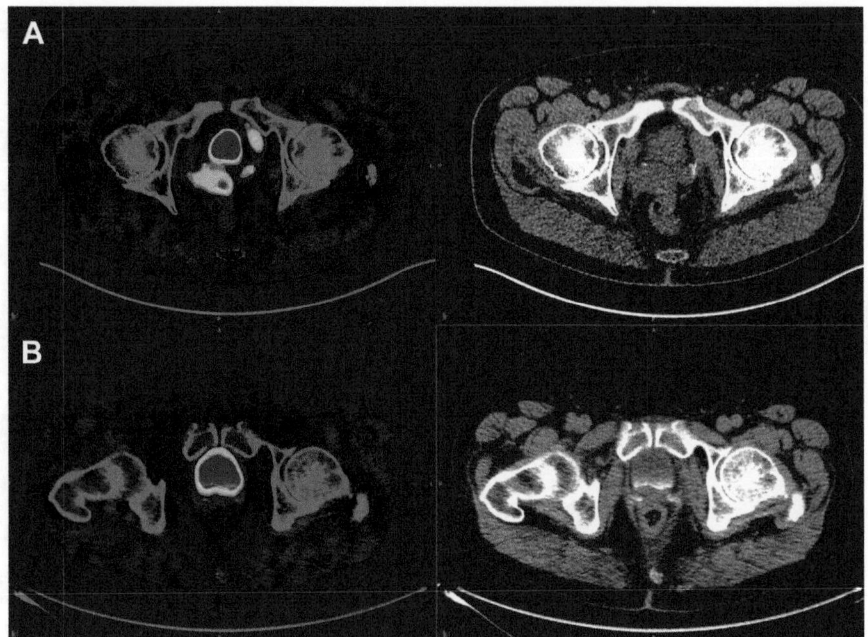

Fig. 4. Top row (*A*). PSMA PET/CT (*left*) and CT (*right*) images demonstrate intensely PSMA avid soft tissue in the prostatic fossa and left pelvis (not shown). Bottom row (*B*). PET/CT (*left*) and CT (*right*) show resolution of uptake and soft tissue lesion after chemotherapy consistent with complete response. Urinary activity is seen in the partially enhanced bladder.

Local recurrence and nodal metastases

The most common pattern of nodal spread in PCa is through pelvic and retroperitoneal nodes. Care should be taken, however, not to mistake a celiac ganglion with a small lymph node. It is known that celiac ganglia show a relevant ^{68}Ga-PSMA uptake. In a study by Krohn and colleagues,[72] at least 1 ganglion with tracer uptake was found in 76 of 85

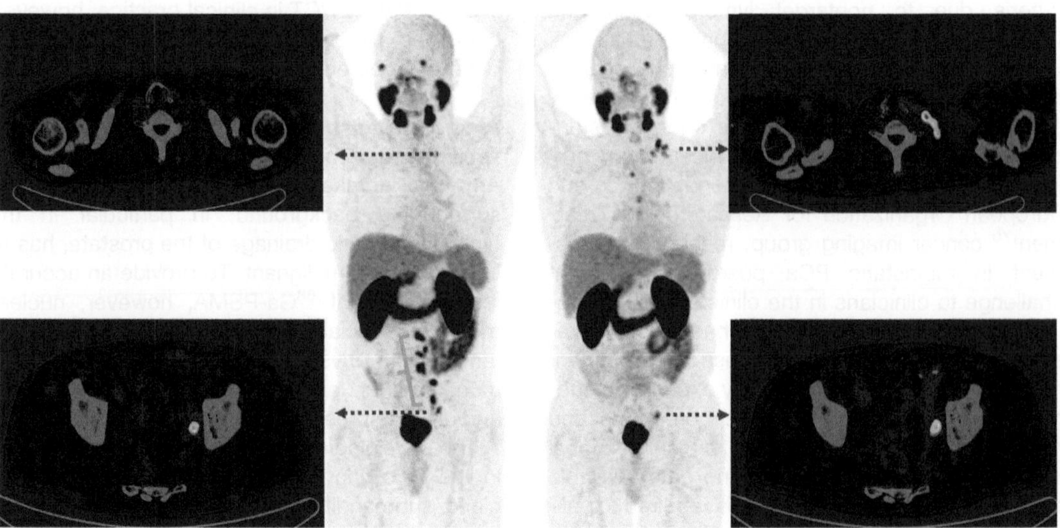

Fig. 5. (*Left*) A 68 year old with biochemical relapse with retroperitoneal nodal disease (*parenthesis*) on baseline PSMA PET MIP and corresponding PET/CT images of the pelvis (*dashed arrow, bottom left*) with no evidence of disease in the supraclavicular region (*dashed arrow, top left*). (*Right*) Four months after retroperitoneal nodal dissection with rising PSA from 1.4 ng/mL to 3.4 ng/mL in 1 month. PSMA PET MIP image shows resolution of retroperitoneal lymph nodes except one lymph node (*dashed arrow, bottom right*) and development of new nodal disease caudal to the surgical bed in the retroperitoneum, in the mediastinum and left supraclavicular region (*dashed arrow, top right*) as well as multiple osseous metastases.

patients (89.4%) undergoing ^{68}Ga-PSMA PET/CT examination, which may mimic lymph node metastases in this area. Typical location of celiac ganglia at the level between the origins of the celiac and superior mesenteric arteries and symmetric uptake on both sides should assist in delineating these organs. Similarly, PSMA uptake in the colonic ganglia and stellate ganglia has been observed.[73]

Due to significant radiotracer excretion from kidneys and accumulation in ureters and the urinary bladder, small lymph nodes in the proximity of the ureters could potentially be obscured. Several approaches have been used to address this issue. Kabasakal and colleagues[74] performed early (at 5 minutes) and delayed (at 45–60 minutes) pelvic images. No difference was found in the number of lesions detected within the field of view. In early pelvic images, the assessment of the primary tumor and local lesions was easier because of lack of accumulated bladder activity. The intensity of uptake was significantly lower in early images, however, compared with late pelvic images. Rauscher and colleagues[75] described their departmental protocol where intravenous diuretic at the time of tracer injection is used to enhance the diuresis. This was used to improve image quality by reducing artifacts due to high activity of tracer in the bladder and the urinary collection system. They have also suggested that this would be more relevant when PET/MR imaging is used by avoiding the commonly seen halo artifact around the areas of the urine collection.[40] In a retrospective study at the authors' institution, intravenous contrast media was administered and delayed time point CT in the urogram phase was acquired as part of PET/CT protocol. Of 50 patients who were imaged, CT urogram was helpful in final interpretation of 60% of the cases and in 50% of patients with high clinical impact by either delineating or excluding the solitary site of local or nodal recurrence[76] (**Fig. 6**). The authors propose this method as a 1-stop imaging procedure for ^{68}Ga-PSMA without the need to perform multiple time-point imaging in particular in busy nuclear medicine departments.

Osseous metastases

BS provides a whole-body overview evaluating the presence of bone metastases. Preliminary data indicate, however, that the detection rate of ^{68}Ga-PSMA PET/CT is clearly superior to the BS.[77] Pyka and colleagues,[78] in a study of 126 patients with PCa, have shown the higher diagnostic performance of ^{68}Ga-PSMA PET compared with the BS. In this study, PSMA PET sensitivity and specificity of the overall bone involvement were 98.7% to 100% and 88.2% to 100% for PET

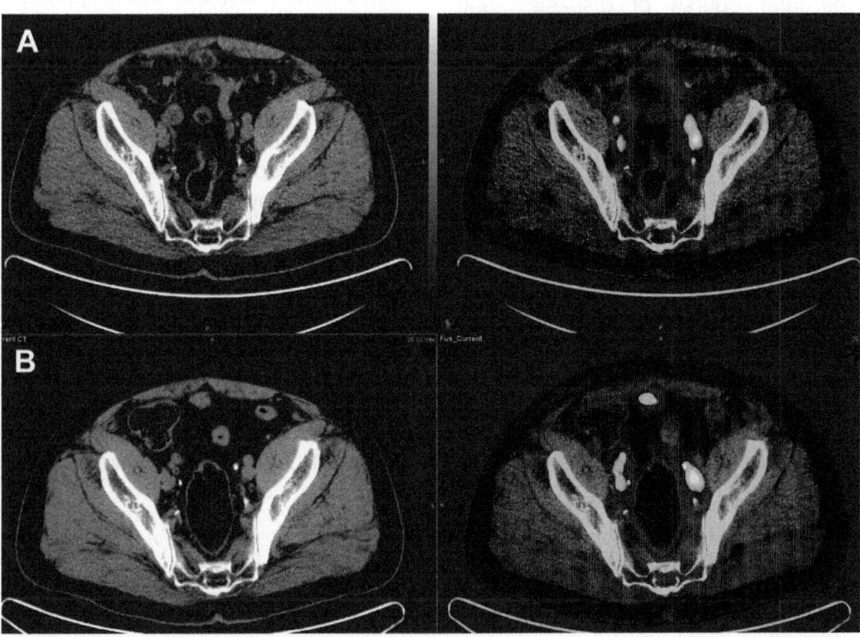

Fig. 6. Top row (*A*). PSMA PET/CT (*left*) and CT (*right*) in a patient with biochemical relapse of PCa demonstrates 2 foci of uptake in the left and one in the right side of pelvis. Bottom row (*B*). PSMA PET/CT urogram protocol (*left*) and CT urogram (*right*) in the same patient. Enhanced ureters/ureteric activity are easily differentiated from PSMA avid nodal disease.

compared with 86.7% to 89.3% and 60.8% to 96.1% for BS and of region-based analysis were 98.8% to 99.0% and 98.9% to 100% for PET compared with 82.4% to 86.6% and 91.6% to 97.9% for BS. The majority of these patients had only planar BS and only 30 patients underwent an additional single-photon emission CT. It seems, however, that BS in patients who have undergone PSMA PET only rarely offers additional information.[78]

Although moderate or intense focal uptake in bones usually indicate the presence of bone metastases, this should be interpreted in conjunction with findings on corresponding CT because PSMA uptake could be seen in other pathologies. In addition, faint uptake in various regions of the skeleton, especially in the ribs, can be found and, therefore, clinical caution needs to be taken because it remains unclear whether this uptake is really related to bone metastasis or might constitute false-positive findings. Artigas and colleagues[79] reported increased ^{68}Ga-PSMA uptake in a patient with Paget disease likely related to an overexpression of PSMA in areas with an abnormal bone remodeling and increased vascularity. In addition, healing fractures for example, ribs or pelvis, are known to potentially show faint increased PSMA ligand uptake.[80]

Visceral metastases

Visceral metastases are less common than lymph node or bone metastases and occur predominantly in the later course of disease[81] and have negative prognostic implications.[82] In a postmortem study, the predominant sites of visceral metastases in patient with distant metastases were lung (46%), liver (25%), pleura (21%), and adrenals (13%).[83] The differentiation between PCa metastases and lesions of different origin using conventional imaging may be challenging and, in many cases, warrants histologic clarification.

The differentiation between lung metastases for PCa and lesions of different origin, for example, primary lung cancer or even a non-neoplastic etiology, is a common clinical question. In study by Wang and colleagues,[84] immunohistochemistry analysis was performed to detect PSMA expression in a total of 150 lung specimens of patients with lung cancer. It was shown that PSMA is expressed not only in 85% of tumor neovasculature endothelial cells of non–small cell lung carcinomas (NSCLCs) and 70% of small cell lung carcinomas but also in 54% of tumor cells of NSCLC patients.[84] Pyka and colleagues[85] performed a study on lung lesions found on ^{68}Ga-PSMA PET/CT; 89 lesions in 45 patients were identified, 76 of which were classified as metastatic PCa (39 proved and 37 highly probable), 7 as primary lung cancer, and 2 as activated tuberculosis; 4 lesions remained unclear. On quantitative (standardized uptake value) analysis of ^{68}Ga-PSMA, PET was not able to discriminate between pulmonary metastases and primary lung cancer in PCa patients.[85] Therefore, morphologic characteristics of the lung lesions is of paramount importance in the interpretation of ^{68}Ga-PSMA PET because it is well known to be the case for FDG PET/CT studies (**Fig. 7**).

High background activity in the liver potentially can conceal liver metastases. In addition, in advanced disease, liver metastases especially tend to loose PSMA expression—most likely due to dedifferentiation. Therefore, in advanced disease, correlation with contrast-enhanced CT or MR imaging is required. Despite multimodality imaging, differentiation between PCa metastases and lesions of different origin, especially when PSMA negative, can be challenging and histologic clarification may be warranted.

Prostate-specific membrane antigen expression in other pathologies

Because ^{68}Ga-PSMA PET/CT imaging is a new imaging technique, it is important to be aware that ^{68}Ga-PSMA it is not completely specific for PCa to avoid scan misinterpretation. Intense staining for PSMA has been observed in endothelial cells of capillary vessels in peritumoral and endotumoral areas of some solid organ malignancies, which has been attributed to tumor angiogenesis. These tumors includes colon cancer, breast cancer, renal cell carcinoma, and transitional cell carcinoma. PSMA expression was also noted in subpopulation of neuroendocrine cells.[10] Other investigators have reported increased PSMA expression for other malignancies, such as glioblastoma, hepatocellular carcinoma, pancreatic cancer, and thyroid cancer.[85–89]

There have been increasing case reports of increased PSMA uptake in benign lesions, such as thyroid adenoma, Paget disease, schwannoma, tuberculosis, adrenal adenoma, and splenic sarcoidosis[90–92] (**Figs. 8** and **9**).

Finally, not all cases of PCa exhibit a significant PSMA overexpression. In a study of Maurer and colleagues,[93] approximately 8% of patients with primary PCa did not show PSMA overexpression—with currently no specific biological explanation.

Summary

Experience with ^{68}Ga-PSMA PET/CT has rapidly evolved since it was first described by the Heidelberg group in 2013. Although it was first used for detection of biochemical recurrence, it also has a role in staging high-risk patients prior to surgery

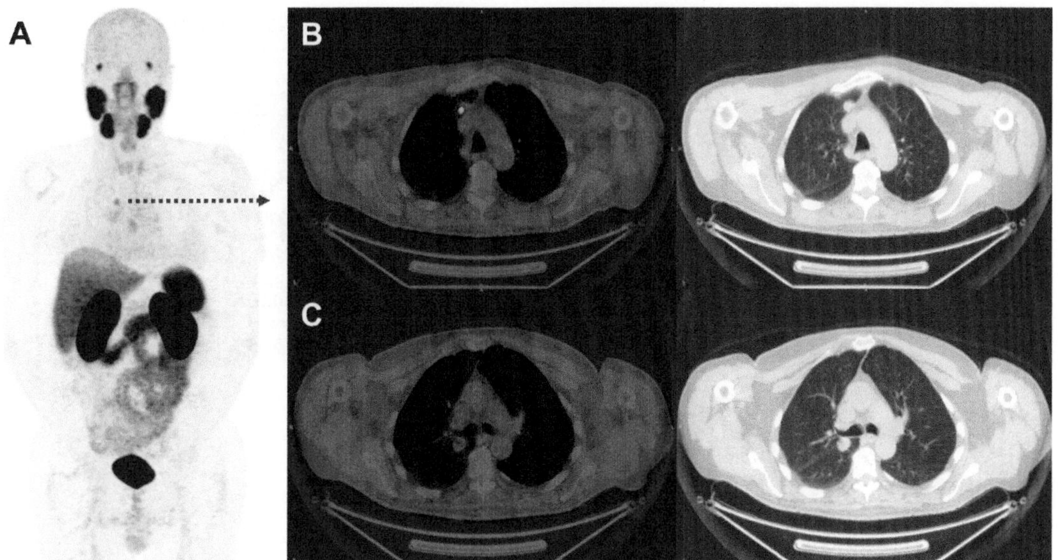

Fig. 7. PSMA PET MIP image (*A*) shows mild uptake in the lung (*dashed arrow*). Top row (*B*) PSMA PET/CT (*left*) and CT (*right*) images demonstrate low grade uptake in the lung metastases (histologically proved) from PCa. Bottom row (*C*). PET/CT (*left*) and CT (*right*) images show the other lung metastases with no increased PSMA uptake.

or radiotherapy and restaging patients with known metastases to assess response to systemic therapy. There is also an evolving role for using ^{68}Ga-PSMA PET/CT to select patients who may be suitable for ^{177}Lu-PSMA radionuclide therapy. Further research is needed to establish the indications where PSMA PET/CT may improve patient outcomes and whether it should be used in addition to or replace conventional imaging modalities (**Table 1**). Newer-generation PSMA ligands, including kit-based ^{68}Ga or ^{18}F

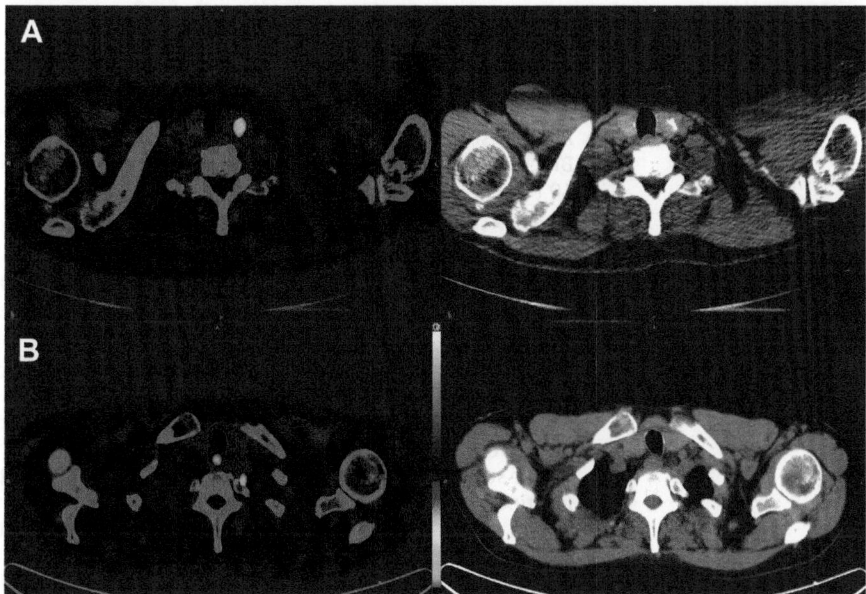

Fig. 8. Top row (*A*). PSMA PET/CT (*left*) and CT (*right*) images demonstrate focal activity corresponding to a partially calcified thyroid nodule. Bottom row (*B*). PSMA PET/CT (*left*) and CT (*right*) images show focal activity in the expected anatomic region of stellate ganglion.

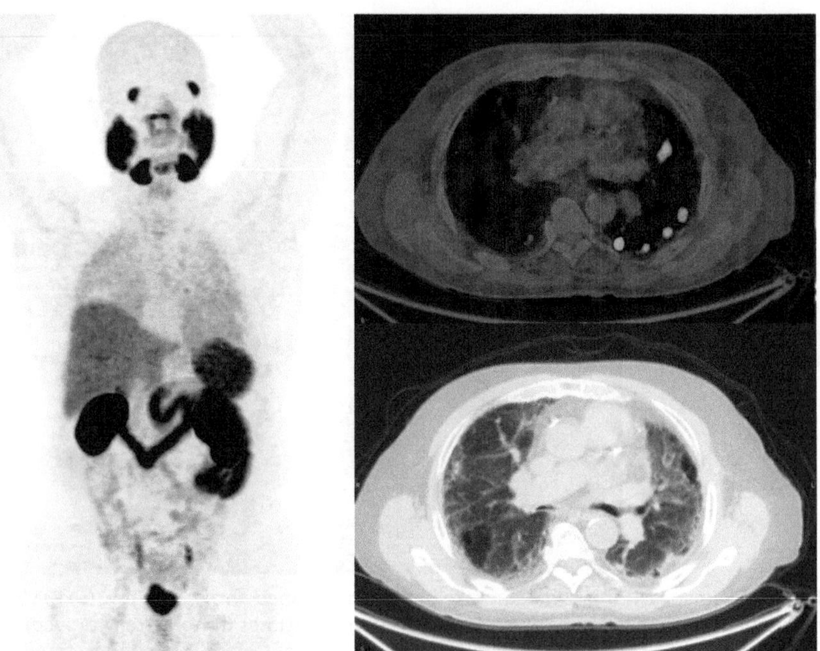

Fig. 9. PSMA PET of a 75-year-old man with biochemical relapse of PCa with PSA of 1.8 ng/L. MIP (*left*), PET/CT (*top right*) and CT (*bottom right*) images demonstrate diffuse uptake in the lungs consistent with the known history of interstitial lung disease.

Table 1
A summary of evolving clinical indications for prostate-specific membrane antigen PET/CT

Benefit Using ^{68}Ga-PSMA PET/CT	Patient Group
High clinical yield	• Primary staging in high-risk disease (D'Amico risk classification) • Biochemical recurrence with low PSA values (0.2 ng/mL to 10 ng/mL)
Low clinical yield	• Primary staging in low-risk and intermediate-risk disease (D'Amico risk classification)
Potential application with promising preliminary data	• Biopsy targeting after previous negative biopsy but high suspicion of PCa (especially in combination with multiparametric MR imaging using PET/MR imaging)
Potential application with current lack of published data	• Monitoring of systemic treatment in metastatic castration-resistant PCa • Monitoring of systemic treatment in metastatic castration-sensitive PCa • Active surveillance of the primary (especially in combination with multiparametric MR imaging using PET/MR imaging) • Active surveillance of the low-volume indolent metastatic PCa • Treatment monitoring in metastatic castration-resistant PCa undergoing radioligand therapy targeting PSMA (eg, ^{177}Lu-PSMA ligand)

Adapted from Rauscher I, Maurer T, Fendler WP, et al. (68)Ga-PSMA ligand PET/CT in patients with prostate cancer: how we review and report. Cancer Imaging 2016;16(1):14.

derivatives, may further improve accuracy and availability.

REFERENCES

1. Hovels AM, Heesakkers RA, Adang EM, et al. The diagnostic accuracy of CT and MRI in the staging of pelvic lymph nodes in patients with prostate cancer: a meta-analysis. Clin Radiol 2008;63(4):387–95.
2. Jadvar H. Molecular imaging of prostate cancer with PET. J Nucl Med 2013;54(10):1685–8.
3. Afshar-Oromieh A, Haberkorn U, Hadaschik B, et al. PET/MRI with a 68Ga-PSMA ligand for the detection of prostate cancer. Eur J Nucl Med Mol Imaging 2013;40(10):1629–30.
4. Afshar-Oromieh A, Malcher A, Eder M, et al. PET imaging with a [68Ga]gallium-labelled PSMA ligand for the diagnosis of prostate cancer: biodistribution in humans and first evaluation of tumour lesions. Eur J Nucl Med Mol Imaging 2013;40(4):486–95.
5. Roethke MC, Kuru TH, Afshar-Oromieh A, et al. Hybrid positron emission tomography-magnetic resonance imaging with gallium 68 prostate-specific membrane antigen tracer: a next step for imaging of recurrent prostate cancer-preliminary results. Eur Urol 2013;64(5):862–4.
6. Israeli RS, Powell CT, Fair WR, et al. Molecular cloning of a complementary DNA encoding a prostate-specific membrane antigen. Cancer Res 1993; 53(2):227–30.
7. Mease RC, Foss CA, Pomper MG. PET imaging in prostate cancer: focus on prostate-specific membrane antigen. Curr Top Med Chem 2013;13(8):951–62.
8. Demirkol MO, Acar Ö, Uçar B, et al. Prostate-specific membrane antigen-based imaging in prostate cancer: impact on clinical decision making process. Prostate 2015;75(7):748–57.
9. Sokoloff RL, Norton KC, Gasior CL, et al. A dual-monoclonal sandwich assay for prostate-specific membrane antigen: levels in tissues, seminal fluid and urine. Prostate 2000;43(2):150–7.
10. Silver DA, Pellicer I, Fair WR, et al. Prostate-specific membrane antigen expression in normal and malignant human tissues. Clin Cancer Res 1997;3(1):81–5.
11. Bouchelouche K, Choyke PL, Capala J. Prostate specific membrane antigen- a target for imaging and therapy with radionuclides. Discov Med 2010; 9(44):55–61.
12. Conway RE, Petrovic N, Li Z, et al. Prostate-specific membrane antigen regulates angiogenesis by modulating integrin signal transduction. Mol Cell Biol 2006;26(14):5310–24.
13. Ananias HJ, van den Heuvel MC, Helfrich W, et al. Expression of the gastrin-releasing peptide receptor, the prostate stem cell antigen and the prostate-specific membrane antigen in lymph node and bone metastases of prostate cancer. Prostate 2009;69(10):1101–8.
14. Minner S, van den Heuvel MC, Helfrich W, et al. High level PSMA expression is associated with early PSA recurrence in surgically treated prostate cancer. Prostate 2011;71(3):281–8.
15. Rybalov M, Ananias HJ, Hoving HD, et al. PSMA, EpCAM, VEGF and GRPR as imaging targets in locally recurrent prostate cancer after radiotherapy. Int J Mol Sci 2014;15(4):6046–61.
16. Bostwick DG, Pacelli A, Blute M, et al. Prostate specific membrane antigen expression in prostatic intraepithelial neoplasia and adenocarcinoma: a study of 184 cases. Cancer 1998;82(11):2256–61.
17. Graham K, Lesche R, Gromov AV, et al. Radiofluorinated derivatives of 2-(phosphonomethyl)pentanedioic acid as inhibitors of prostate specific membrane antigen (PSMA) for the imaging of prostate cancer. J Med Chem 2012;55(22):9510–20.
18. Kawakami M, Nakayama J. Enhanced expression of prostate-specific membrane antigen gene in prostate cancer as revealed by in situ hybridization. Cancer Res 1997;57(12):2321–4.
19. Troyer JK, Beckett ML, Wright GL Jr. Detection and characterization of the prostate-specific membrane antigen (PSMA) in tissue extracts and body fluids. Int J Cancer 1995;62(5):552–8.
20. Wright GL Jr, Grob BM, Haley C, et al. Upregulation of prostate-specific membrane antigen after androgen-deprivation therapy. Urology 1996;48(2): 326–34.
21. Ross JS, Sheehan CE, Fisher HA, et al. Correlation of primary tumor prostate-specific membrane antigen expression with disease recurrence in prostate cancer. Clin Cancer Res 2003;9(17):6357–62.
22. Horoszewicz JS, Kawinski E, Murphy GP. Monoclonal antibodies to a new antigenic marker in epithelial prostatic cells and serum of prostatic cancer patients. Anticancer Res 1987;7(5B):927–35.
23. Franc BL, Cho SY, Rosenthal SA, et al. Detection and localization of carcinoma within the prostate using high resolution transrectal gamma imaging (TRGI) of monoclonal antibody directed at prostate specific membrane antigen (PSMA)–proof of concept and initial imaging results. Eur J Radiol 2013;82(11):1877–84.
24. Ponsky LE, Cherullo EE, Starkey R, et al. Evaluation of preoperative ProstaScint scans in the prediction of nodal disease. Prostate Cancer Prostatic Dis 2002;5(2):132–5.
25. Liu H, Rajasekaran AK, Moy P, et al. Constitutive and antibody-induced internalization of prostate-specific membrane antigen. Cancer Res 1998;58(18): 4055–60.
26. Bander NH, Trabulsi EJ, Kostakoglu L, et al. Targeting metastatic prostate cancer with radiolabeled monoclonal antibody J591 to the extracellular

domain of prostate specific membrane antigen. J Urol 2003;170(5):1717–21.
27. Tagawa ST, Milowsky MI, Morris M, et al. Phase II study of Lutetium-177-labeled anti-prostate-specific membrane antigen monoclonal antibody J591 for metastatic castration-resistant prostate cancer. Clin Cancer Res 2013;19(18):5182–91.
28. Tsukamoto T, Wozniak KM, Slusher BS. Progress in the discovery and development of glutamate carboxypeptidase II inhibitors. Drug Discov Today 2007;12(17–18):767–76.
29. Foss CA, Mease RC, Fan H, et al. Radiolabeled small-molecule ligands for prostate-specific membrane antigen: in vivo imaging in experimental models of prostate cancer. Clin Cancer Res 2005; 11(11):4022–8.
30. Mease RC, Dusich CL, Foss CA, et al. N-[N-[(S)-1,3-Dicarboxypropyl]carbamoyl]-4-[18F]fluorobenzyl-L-cysteine, [18F]DCFBC: a new imaging probe for prostate cancer. Clin Cancer Res 2008;14(10): 3036–43.
31. Maresca KP, Hillier SM, Femia FJ, et al. A series of halogenated heterodimeric inhibitors of prostate specific membrane antigen (PSMA) as radiolabeled probes for targeting prostate cancer. J Med Chem 2009;52(2):347–57.
32. Banerjee SR, Foss CA, Castanares M, et al. Synthesis and evaluation of technetium-99m- and rhenium-labeled inhibitors of the prostate-specific membrane antigen (PSMA). J Med Chem 2008;51(15):4504–17.
33. Hillier SM, Maresca KP, Lu G, et al. 99mTc-labeled small-molecule inhibitors of prostate-specific membrane antigen for molecular imaging of prostate cancer. J Nucl Med 2013;54(8):1369–76.
34. Banerjee SR, Pullambhatla M, Byun Y, et al. 68Ga-labeled inhibitors of prostate-specific membrane antigen (PSMA) for imaging prostate cancer. J Med Chem 2010;53(14):5333–41.
35. Schafer M, Bauder-Wüst U, Leotta K, et al. A dimerized urea-based inhibitor of the prostate-specific membrane antigen for 68Ga-PET imaging of prostate cancer. EJNMMI Res 2012;2(1):23.
36. Chen Y, Pullambhatla M, Banerjee SR, et al. Synthesis and biological evaluation of low molecular weight fluorescent imaging agents for the prostate-specific membrane antigen. Bioconjug Chem 2012;23(12):2377–85.
37. Barrett JA, Coleman RE, Goldsmith SJ, et al. First-in-man evaluation of 2 high-affinity PSMA-avid small molecules for imaging prostate cancer. J Nucl Med 2013;54(3):380–7.
38. Vallabhajosula S, Nikolopoulou A, Babich JW, et al. 99mTc-labeled small-molecule inhibitors of prostate-specific membrane antigen: pharmacokinetics and biodistribution studies in healthy subjects and patients with metastatic prostate cancer. J Nucl Med 2014;55(11):1791–8.
39. Cho SY, Gage KL, Mease RC, et al. Biodistribution, tumor detection, and radiation dosimetry of 18F-DCFBC, a low-molecular-weight inhibitor of prostate-specific membrane antigen, in patients with metastatic prostate cancer. J Nucl Med 2012;53(12):1883–91.
40. Afshar-Oromieh A, Haberkorn U, Schlemmer HP, et al. Comparison of PET/CT and PET/MRI hybrid systems using a 68Ga-labelled PSMA ligand for the diagnosis of recurrent prostate cancer: initial experience. Eur J Nucl Med Mol Imaging 2014; 41(5):887–97.
41. Afshar-Oromieh A, Zechmann CM, Malcher A, et al. Comparison of PET imaging with a (68)Ga-labelled PSMA ligand and (18)F-choline-based PET/CT for the diagnosis of recurrent prostate cancer. Eur J Nucl Med Mol Imaging 2014;41(1):11–20.
42. Zechmann CM, Afshar-Oromieh A, Armor T, et al. Radiation dosimetry and first therapy results with a (124)I/(131)I-labeled small molecule (MIP-1095) targeting PSMA for prostate cancer therapy. Eur J Nucl Med Mol Imaging 2014;41(7):1280–92.
43. Reubi JC, Maecke HR. Peptide-based probes for cancer imaging. J Nucl Med 2008;49(11):1735–8.
44. Hofman MS, Kong G, Neels OC, et al. High management impact of Ga-68 DOTATATE (GaTate) PET/CT for imaging neuroendocrine and other somatostatin expressing tumours. J Med Imaging Radiat Oncol 2012;56(1):40–7.
45. Hofman MS, Lau WF, Hicks RJ. Somatostatin receptor imaging with 68Ga DOTATATE PET/CT: clinical utility, normal patterns, pearls, and pitfalls in interpretation. Radiographics 2015;35(2):500–16.
46. Eder M, Schäfer M, Bauder-Wüst U, et al. 68Ga-complex lipophilicity and the targeting property of a urea-based PSMA inhibitor for PET imaging. Bioconjug Chem 2012;23(4):688–97.
47. Roesch F, Riss PJ. The renaissance of the (6)(8)Ge/(6)(8)Ga radionuclide generator initiates new developments in (6)(8)Ga radiopharmaceutical chemistry. Curr Top Med Chem 2010;10(16):1633–68.
48. Afshar-Oromieh A, Hetzheim H, Kübler W, et al. Radiation dosimetry of (68)Ga-PSMA-11 (HBED-CC) and preliminary evaluation of optimal imaging timing. Eur J Nucl Med Mol Imaging 2016;43(9):1611–20.
49. Heidenreich A, Bastian PJ, Bellmunt J, et al. EAU guidelines on prostate cancer. Part II: treatment of advanced, relapsing, and castration-resistant prostate cancer. Eur Urol 2014;65(2):467–79.
50. Jereczek-Fossa BA, Beltramo G, Fariselli L, et al. Robotic image-guided stereotactic radiotherapy, for isolated recurrent primary, lymph node or metastatic prostate cancer. Int J Radiat Oncol Biol Phys 2012;82(2):889–97.
51. Afshar-Oromieh A, Avtzi E, Giesel FL, et al. The diagnostic value of PET/CT imaging with the (68)Ga-labelled PSMA ligand HBED-CC in the diagnosis of

recurrent prostate cancer. Eur J Nucl Med Mol Imaging 2015;42(2):197–209.

52. Eiber M, Maurer T, Souvatzoglou M, et al. Evaluation of hybrid (6)(8)Ga-PSMA ligand PET/CT in 248 patients with biochemical recurrence after radical prostatectomy. J Nucl Med 2015;56(5):668–74.
53. Perera M, Papa N, Christidis D, et al. Sensitivity, specificity, and predictors of positive 68Ga-Prostate-specific membrane antigen positron emission tomography in advanced prostate cancer: a systematic review and meta-analysis. Eur Urol 2016;70(6):926–37.
54. Brogsitter C, Zophel K, Kotzerke J. 18F-Choline, 11C-choline and 11C-acetate PET/CT: comparative analysis for imaging prostate cancer patients. Eur J Nucl Med Mol Imaging 2013;40(Suppl 1):S18–27.
55. Bluemel C, Krebs M, Polat B, et al. 68Ga-PSMA-PET/CT in patients with biochemical prostate cancer recurrence and negative 18F-choline-PET/CT. Clin Nucl Med 2016;41(7):515–21.
56. Rauscher I, Maurer T, Beer AJ, et al. Value of 68Ga-PSMA HBED-CC PET for the assessment of lymph node metastases in prostate cancer patients with biochemical recurrence: comparison with histopathology after salvage lymphadenectomy. J Nucl Med 2016;57(11):1713–9.
57. Giesel FL, Fiedler H, Stefanova M, et al. PSMA PET/CT with Glu-urea-Lys-(Ahx)-[(6)(8)Ga(HBED-CC)] versus 3D CT volumetric lymph node assessment in recurrent prostate cancer. Eur J Nucl Med Mol Imaging 2015;42(12):1794–800.
58. Ceci F, Uprimny C, Nilica B, et al. (68)Ga-PSMA PET/CT for restaging recurrent prostate cancer: which factors are associated with PET/CT detection rate? Eur J Nucl Med Mol Imaging 2015;42(8):1284–94.
59. Briganti A, Blute ML, Eastham JH, et al. Pelvic lymph node dissection in prostate cancer. Eur Urol 2009; 55(6):1251–65.
60. Eiber M, Maurer T, Beer AJ, et al. Prospective evaluation of PSMA-PET imaging for preoperative lymph node staging in prostate cancer. J Nucl Med 2014; 55(Suppl 1):20.
61. Budaus L, Leyh-Bannurah SR, Steuber T, et al. Initial experience of (68)Ga-PSMA PET/CT imaging in high-risk prostate cancer patients prior to radical prostatectomy. Eur Urol 2016;69(3):393–6.
62. Sonn GA, Chang E, Natarajan S, et al. Value of targeted prostate biopsy using magnetic resonance-ultrasound fusion in men with prior negative biopsy and elevated prostate-specific antigen. Eur Urol 2014;65(4):809–15.
63. Wu LM, Xu JR, Ye YQ, et al. The clinical value of diffusion-weighted imaging in combination with T2-weighted imaging in diagnosing prostate carcinoma: a systematic review and meta-analysis. AJR Am J Roentgenol 2012;199(1):103–10.
64. Muller BG, Shih JH, Sankineni S, et al. Prostate cancer: interobserver agreement and accuracy with the revised prostate imaging reporting and data system at multiparametric MR imaging. Radiology 2015; 277(3):741–50.
65. Heidenreich A, Bastian PJ, Bellmunt J, et al. EAU guidelines on prostate cancer. part 1: screening, diagnosis, and local treatment with curative intent-update 2013. Eur Urol 2014;65(1):124–37.
66. Maurer T, Beer AJ, Wester HJ, et al. Positron emission tomography/magnetic resonance imaging with 68Gallium-labeled ligand of prostate-specific membrane antigen: promising novel option in prostate cancer imaging? Int J Urol 2014;21(12):1286–8.
67. Fendler WP, Schmidt DF, Wenter V, et al. 68Ga-PSMA-HBED-CC PET/CT detects location and extent of primary prostate cancer. J Nucl Med 2016;57(11):1720–5.
68. Mowatt G, Scotland G, Boachie C, et al. The diagnostic accuracy and cost-effectiveness of magnetic resonance spectroscopy and enhanced magnetic resonance imaging techniques in aiding the localisation of prostate abnormalities for biopsy: a systematic review and economic evaluation. Health Technol Assess 2013;17(20):vii–xix, 1–281.
69. Scher HI, Halabi S, Tannock I, et al. Design and end points of clinical trials for patients with progressive prostate cancer and castrate levels of testosterone: recommendations of the Prostate Cancer Clinical Trials Working Group. J Clin Oncol 2008;26(7):1148–59.
70. Lecouvet FE, Talbot JN, Messiou C, et al. Monitoring the response of bone metastases to treatment with Magnetic Resonance Imaging and nuclear medicine techniques: a review and position statement by the European Organisation for Research and Treatment of Cancer imaging group. Eur J Cancer 2014;50(15): 2519–31.
71. De Giorgi U, Caroli P, Scarpi E, et al. (18)F-Fluorocholine PET/CT for early response assessment in patients with metastatic castration-resistant prostate cancer treated with enzalutamide. Eur J Nucl Med Mol Imaging 2015;42(8):1276–83.
72. Krohn T, Verburg FA, Pufe T, et al. [(68)Ga]PSMA-HBED uptake mimicking lymph node metastasis in coeliac ganglia: an important pitfall in clinical practice. Eur J Nucl Med Mol Imaging 2015;42(2):210–4.
73. Chang SS, Reuter VE, Heston WD, et al. Five different anti-prostate-specific membrane antigen (PSMA) antibodies confirm PSMA expression in tumor-associated neovasculature. Cancer Res 1999;59(13):3192–8.
74. Kabasakal L, Demirci E, Ocak M, et al. Evaluation of PSMA PET/CT imaging using a 68Ga-HBED-CC ligand in patients with prostate cancer and the value of early pelvic imaging. Nucl Med Commun 2015; 36(6):582–7.
75. Rauscher I, Maurer T, Fendler WP, et al. (68)Ga-PSMA ligand PET/CT in patients with prostate cancer: How we review and report. Cancer Imaging 2016;16(1):14.

76. Iravani A, Mulcahy T, Hofman M, et al. The diagnostic value of 68Ga PSMA-HBED PET with CT urogram protocol in the initial staging and biochemical relapse of prostate cancer. Intern Med J 2016;46(Suppl 1):6.
77. Eiber M, Pyka T, Okamoto S, et al. 68Gallium-HBED-CC-PSMA PET compared to conventional bone scintigraphy for evaluation of bone metastases in prostate cancer patients. European Urology Supplements 2016;15(3):e566.
78. Pyka T, Okamoto S, Dahlbender M, et al. Comparison of bone scintigraphy and 68Ga-PSMA PET for skeletal staging in prostate cancer. Eur J Nucl Med Mol Imaging 2016;43(12):2114–21.
79. Artigas C, Alexiou J, Garcia C, et al. Paget bone disease demonstrated on (68)Ga-PSMA ligand PET/CT. Eur J Nucl Med Mol Imaging 2016;43(1):195–6.
80. Gykiere P, Goethals L, Everaert H. Healing sacral fracture masquerading as metastatic bone disease on a 68Ga-PSMA PET/CT. Clin Nucl Med 2016; 41(7):e346–7.
81. Moschini M, Sharma V, Zattoni F, et al. Natural history of clinical recurrence patterns of lymph node-positive prostate cancer after radical prostatectomy. Eur Urol 2016;69(1):135–42.
82. Goodman OB Jr, Flaig TW, Molina A, et al. Exploratory analysis of the visceral disease subgroup in a phase III study of abiraterone acetate in metastatic castration-resistant prostate cancer. Prostate Cancer Prostatic Dis 2014;17(1):34–9.
83. Bubendorf L, Schöpfer A, Wagner U, et al. Metastatic patterns of prostate cancer: an autopsy study of 1,589 patients. Hum Pathol 2000;31(5):578–83.
84. Wang HL, Wang SS, Song WH, et al. Expression of prostate-specific membrane antigen in lung cancer cells and tumor neovasculature endothelial cells and its clinical significance. PLoS One 2015;10(5): e0125924.
85. Pyka T, Weirich G, Einspieler I, et al. 68Ga-PSMA-HBED-CC PET for differential diagnosis of suggestive lung lesions in patients with prostate cancer. J Nucl Med 2016;57(3):367–71.
86. Rowe SP, Gorin MA, Hammers HJ, et al. Imaging of metastatic clear cell renal cell carcinoma with PSMA-targeted (1)(8)F-DCFPyL PET/CT. Ann Nucl Med 2015;29(10):877–82.
87. Sasikumar A, Joy A, Nanabala R, et al. (68)Ga-PSMA PET/CT imaging in primary hepatocellular carcinoma. Eur J Nucl Med Mol Imaging 2016; 43(4):795–6.
88. Schwenck J, Tabatabai G, Skardelly M, et al. In vivo visualization of prostate-specific membrane antigen in glioblastoma. Eur J Nucl Med Mol Imaging 2015; 42(1):170–1.
89. Verburg FA, Krohn T, Heinzel A, et al. First evidence of PSMA expression in differentiated thyroid cancer using [(6)(8)Ga]PSMA-HBED-CC PET/CT. Eur J Nucl Med Mol Imaging 2015;42(10):1622–3.
90. Kanthan GL, Drummond J, Schembri GP, et al. Follicular thyroid adenoma showing avid uptake on 68Ga PSMA-HBED-CC PET/CT. Clin Nucl Med 2016;41(4):331–2.
91. Kobe C, Maintz D, Fischer T, et al. Prostate-specific membrane antigen PET/CT in splenic sarcoidosis. Clin Nucl Med 2015;40(11):897–8.
92. Rischpler C, Maurer T, Schwaiger M, et al. Intense PSMA-expression using (68)Ga-PSMA PET/CT in a paravertebral schwannoma mimicking prostate cancer metastasis. Eur J Nucl Med Mol Imaging 2016; 43(1):193–4.
93. Maurer T, Gschwend JE, Rauscher I, et al. Diagnostic efficacy of (68)Gallium-PSMA positron emission tomography compared to conventional imaging for lymph node staging of 130 consecutive patients with intermediate to high risk prostate cancer. J Urol 2016;195(5):1436–43.

Clinical Experience with ^{18}F-Labeled Small Molecule Inhibitors of Prostate-Specific Membrane Antigen

CrossMark

Steven P. Rowe, MD, PhD[a,*], Michael A. Gorin, MD[b], Roberto A. Salas Fragomeni, MD[a], Alexander Drzezga, MD[c], Martin G. Pomper, MD, PhD[a]

KEYWORDS

• DCFBC • DCFPyL • BAY 1075553 • Prostate cancer • Radiopharmaceutical

KEY POINTS

- Prostate cancer (PCa) is the most common noncutaneous malignancy diagnosed in men.
- Despite the large number of men who will suffer from PCa at some point during their lives, conventional imaging modalities for this important disease have provided only marginal to moderate success in appropriately guiding patient management in certain clinical contexts.
- The development of molecular imaging probes for improved in vivo visualization of sites of PCa offers the possibility of altering the paradigm of how certain types of PCa are treated.
- As prostate-specific membrane antigen–based imaging becomes more widely available, the intrinsic advantages of ^{18}F-labeled compounds will become of increasing importance.

INTRODUCTION

Prostate-specific membrane antigen (PSMA) is a type II transmembrane glycoprotein that is currently being extensively investigated as a target for prostate cancer (PCa) molecular imaging.[1–3] Much of the interest in PSMA derives from the high percentage of PCa specimens in which it is expressed (>95%) as well as the apparent direct correlation that exists between PSMA expression levels and measures of tumor aggressiveness.[4–6]

Several potential clinical applications for PSMA-targeted imaging have been postulated and recently reviewed.[2,3] Among these applications are (1) the noninvasive detection and characterization of primary PCa, including pretreatment risk stratification; (2) preoperative staging in patients with high-risk

Disclosures: Dr Pomper is a coinventor on a US Patent covering [^{18}F]DCFPyL and as such is entitled to a portion of any licensing fees and royalties generated by this technology. This arrangement has been reviewed and approved by the Johns Hopkins University in accordance with its conflict-of-interest policies. Dr Gorin has served as a consultant to Progenics Pharmaceuticals, the licensee of [^{18}F]DCFPyL. Drs Rowe, Fragomeni, and Drzezga have nothing to disclose.

[a] The Russell H. Morgan Department of Radiology and Radiological Science, Johns Hopkins University School of Medicine, Baltimore, MD, USA; [b] The James Buchanan Brady Urological Institute and Department of Urology, Johns Hopkins University School of Medicine, Baltimore, MD, USA; [c] Department of Nuclear Medicine, University Hospital of Cologne, Cologne, Germany

* Corresponding author: Johns Hopkins University School of Medicine, 600 North Wolfe Street, Baltimore, MD 21287.

E-mail address: srowe8@jhmi.edu

PET Clin 12 (2017) 235–241

http://dx.doi.org/10.1016/j.cpet.2016.12.006

primary PCa; (3) evaluation of androgen signaling and response to neoadjuvant androgen deprivation therapy in locally advanced PCa; (4) early detection of sites of disease and guidance of therapy in biochemical recurrence; (5) guidance of therapy in oligometastatic disease; (6) evaluation of patients with widespread metastatic PCa; and (7) selection of patients for theranostic radionuclide therapy using PSMA-targeted ligands (see Gorin and colleagues' article, "Clinical Applications of Molecular Imaging in the Management of Prostate Cancer," in this issue for a more in-depth discussion of the clinical spaces within which PCa molecular imaging may have an important role).

Most of the available clinical data has focused on the use of radiotracers for PET imaging. Indeed, the largest body of data from a single class of compounds for PSMA are the ^{68}Ga-labeled small molecule inhibitors of PSMA ([^{68}Ga]Ga-PSMA, [^{68}Ga]Ga-PSMA-11, [^{68}Ga]Ga-PSMA-617, [^{68}Ga]Ga-PSMA-I&T, and so forth). Such compounds have in recent years been rapidly adopted across Europe and Australia, and several large, important retrospective studies have been carried out (see, for example, Refs.[7,8] and please also see meta-analysis).[9] As the demand for PSMA-based imaging continues to expand, there are compelling reasons for the field to embrace ^{18}F-labeled agents, including: (1) a longer physical half-life of the radionuclide (109 minutes vs 68 minutes) providing the opportunity to centrally produce and distribute radiofluorinated PSMA agents as well as to incorporate delayed imaging time points into imaging protocols that might improve target-to-background ratios and increase sensitivity for subtle disease; (2) the ability to produce very large quantities of radiofluoride using a cyclotron, which would also aid in central production and distribution and markedly increase the number of patients that can be imaged relative to a generator-produced radionuclide; and (3) the lower ^{18}F positron energy leading to intrinsically shorter path length in tissue and improved spatial resolution.[10,11] As a result of these advantages, the authors have focused on the development of radiofluorinated PSMA-targeted small molecules. Herein, the authors summarize the clinical experience with such agents from their group and others.

PRECLINICAL DEVELOPMENT OF ^{18}F-LABELED PSMA INHIBITORS

Arising out of synthetic efforts toward a variety of radiolabeled, urea-based small molecule inhibitors of PSMA,[12,13] the authors have developed a series of ^{18}F-labeled small molecule inhibitors of PSMA that have subsequently seen clinical application. The first of these was [^{18}F]DCFBC (N-[N-[(*S*)-1,3-dicarboxypropyl]carbamoyl]-4-[^{18}F]fluorobenzyl-L-cysteine; **Fig. 1**), which in preclinical mouse imaging studies demonstrated high uptake within PSMA-expressing PC3 prolactin-inducible protein (PIP) tumor xenografts while having low nontarget background with the exception of uptake and excretion by the kidneys and excretion into the urinary bladder.[14] This promising uptake within tumor as well as the favorable biodistribution properties of the compound led to clinical translation of this agent, as discussed later.

A subsequent, second-generation urea-based small molecule from the same group termed [^{18}F]DCFPyL (2-(3-{1-carboxy-5-[(6-[^{18}F]fluoro-pyridine-3-carbonyl)-amino]-pentyl}-ureido)-pentanedioic acid; see **Fig. 1**) was found during

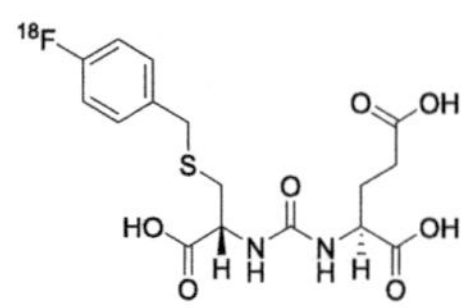

[^{18}F]DCFBC

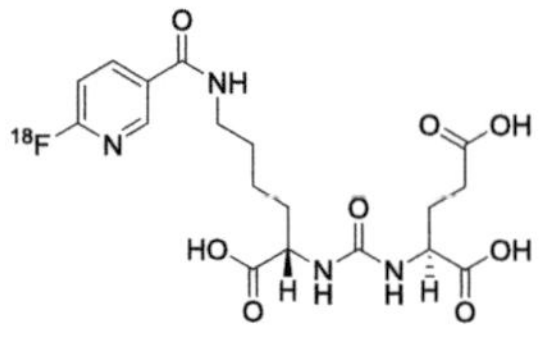

[^{18}F]DCFPyL

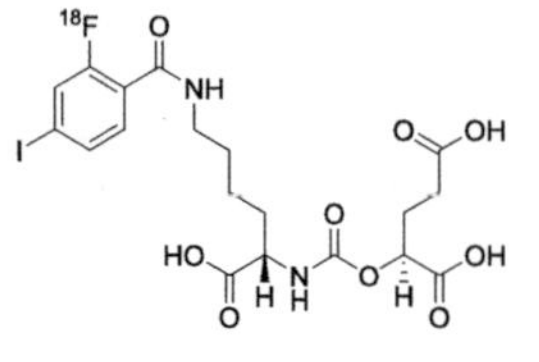

4-iodo-2-[^{18}F]fluorobenzoyllysine OPA

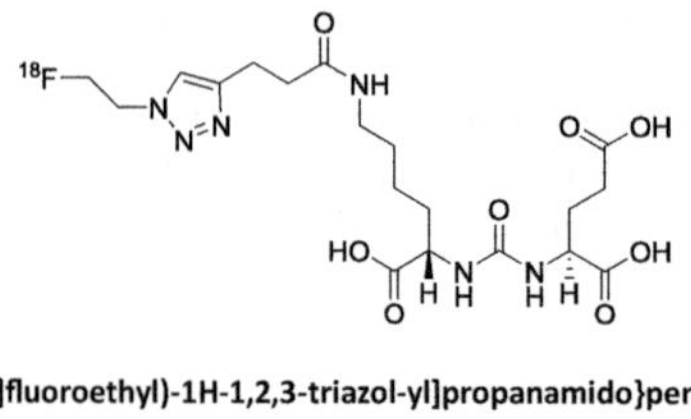

2-[3-(1-carboxy-5-{3-[1-(2-[^{18}F]fluoroethyl)-1H-1,2,3-triazol-yl]propanamido}pentyl)ureido]pentanedioic acid

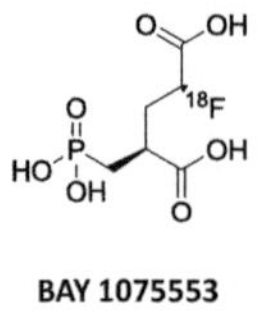

BAY 1075553

Fig. 1. Selected radiofluorinated small molecules that target PSMA and allow for PET imaging of PSMA-expressing tumors. OPA, oxypentanedioic acid.

preclinical development to improve upon many characteristics of [^{18}F]DCFBC.[15] For example, the reported radiochemical yield for the initial published synthesis of [^{18}F]DCFPyL was significantly higher (36%–53%, decay corrected vs 16% ± 6% for [^{18}F]DCFBC). Furthermore, [^{18}F]DCFPyL was superior to [^{18}F]DCFBC in mouse experiments, with higher uptake in tumor tissue (39.4% ± 5.4% injected dose in PSMA-expressing PC3 PIP tumor xenografts, vs 8.2% ± 2.6% for [^{18}F]DCFBC in the same tumor model) and a better tumor-to-background ratio (358:1 ratio of uptake between PSMA-expressing PC3 PIP tumor xenografts and PSMA-negative PC3 flu xenografts, vs 20:1 ratio of PSMA-expressing PC3 PIP tumor xenografts to muscle for [^{18}F]DCFBC). For these reasons, soon after the clinical translation of [^{18}F]DCFBC, [^{18}F]DCFPyL was also brought into the clinic.

The authors continue to work on new generations of ^{18}F-labeled agents, primarily with the goal of improving the diagnostic utility and theranostic/therapeutic potential of PSMA-targeted compounds. Recent examples include multiple compounds based around a novel carbamate scaffold (4-bromo-2-[^{18}F]fluorobenzoyllysineoxypentanedioic acid carbamate and 4-iodo-2-[^{18}F]fluorobenzoyllysineoxypentanedioic acid carbamate; **Fig. 1**)[16] as well as a urea-based small molecule synthesized through click chemistry (2-[3-(1-carboxy-5-{3-[1-(2-[^{18}F]fluoroethyl)-1H-1,2,3-triazolyl]propanamido}pentyl)ureido]pentanedioic acid; see **Fig. 1**).[17] These new agents have shown either high tumor uptake, slow tumor clearance, or low nontarget organ uptake in preclinical models. Although none of these agents have yet been clinically translated, their imaging properties in mice suggest that they may be able to improve on the already impressive diagnostic yield of PSMA agents in detecting PCa in humans or they may point to less toxic PSMA-targeted therapeutic compounds.

Several other urea-based ^{18}F-labeled agents have also been synthesized and have previously been reviewed.[1] Outside of urea-based compounds, other scaffolds that have been investigated are phosphoramidates[18] and phosphonomethyl derivatives,[19] with both classes of radiotracers demonstrating promising preclinical findings in mouse tumor xenograft models. Recently, the ^{18}F-labeled phosphonomethyl compound BAY 1075553 ((2*S*, 4*S*)-2-[^{18}F]fluoro-4-phosphonomethyl-pentanedioic acid [major stereoisomer]; **Fig. 1**) has been translated for human studies with good initial results from a first-in-human trial,[20] as will be discussed further later.

EVALUATION OF [^{18}F]DCFBC IN PROSTATE CANCER

A group of small, published, prospective studies has been performed with [^{18}F]DCFBC. The first-in-man study of [^{18}F]DCFBC appeared in 2012 and included biodistribution, safety, and feasibility data on the compound.[21] Five patients with radiographic evidence of metastatic PCa were imaged with [^{18}F]DCFBC PET/computed tomography (CT). In those 5 patients, 32 sites of definitive abnormal radiotracer uptake were identified, 21 (66%) of which corresponded to findings of metastatic PCa on conventional imaging (CT and/or bone scan). The remaining 11 (34%) discordant sites were considered suggestive of early metastatic lesions, although pathologic proof was not available to confirm that supposition. Nonetheless, this study constituted early evidence that the sensitivity of PSMA-targeted PET for lesions in metastatic PCa patients might be higher than conventional imaging.

Following the first-in-man trial, a prospective study evaluating the ability of [^{18}F]DCFBC to identify and characterize primary PCa was undertaken. Thirteen patients were imaged with [^{18}F]DCFBC PET/CT using a protocol that included 2-dimensional (to attempt to decrease scatter from the urinary bladder) and 3-dimensional (3D) single bed position imaging of the pelvis as well as a 3D whole-body acquisition.[22] Ultimately, the 3D whole-body images were used for analysis because they provided the highest tumor-to-blood pool ratios. Twelve of the 13 patients in the study also underwent prostate MR imaging. The relatively high persistent blood pool activity of [^{18}F]DCFBC and relatively low tumor uptake levels with this agent limited the sensitivity of [^{18}F]DCFBC PET/CT for detection of primary PCa. MR imaging had superior sensitivity to [^{18}F]DCFBC PET/CT both on a segment-based analysis (12-segment model) and on the basis of dominant lesion detection.

However, [^{18}F]DCFBC was able to reliably detect high-volume, high Gleason score disease with higher specificity than MR imaging. A positive correlation between uptake and Gleason score was observed, although the small number of patients led to wide confidence intervals associated with that correlation. Furthermore, [^{18}F]DCFBC uptake in benign prostatic hyperplasia was statistically significantly less than in radiotracer-avid foci of PCa, again demonstrating specificity and implying a role for PSMA-targeted radiotracers in being able to differentiate PCa from other hypermetabolic processes such as inflammatory lesions. Ultimately, these promising findings would need to be borne out in larger prospective trials in order to inform clinical decision making in primary PCa patients.

Although the results of the first-in-man trial with [^{18}F]DCFBC provided preliminary evidence that PSMA-based imaging could have improved sensitivity for metastatic PCa relative to conventional imaging, this point was more extensively explored in a follow-up prospective study of [^{18}F]DCFBC PET/CT in metastatic PCa that included 17 patients (9 who were naive to treatment with androgen deprivation and 8 with castration-resistant disease).[23] Lesion-by-lesion analysis in these patients demonstrated an increased detection rate for [^{18}F]DCFBC PET/CT relative to CT and bone scan for sites suspicious for metastatic disease (592 definitive lesions with an additional 63 equivocal lesions with [^{18}F]DCFBC PET/CT vs 520 definitive lesions with another 61 equivocal lesions with conventional imaging). This increased lesion detection rate held true in both androgen-deprivation-naive and castration-resistant patients. For those lesions that could be assessed with follow-up imaging, the putative sensitivity for [^{18}F]DCFBC PET/CT was 0.92 versus 0.71 for conventional imaging.

Despite the promising results of the [^{18}F]DCFBC primary and metastatic PCa studies, the preclinical advantages that were apparent with [^{18}F]DCFPyL have led the authors to primarily focus on this latter compound. However, [^{18}F]DCFBC continues to be used in imaging trials of PCa patients by the National Cancer Institute at the National Institutes of Health in Bethesda, Maryland (ClinicalTrials.gov identifier NCT02190279).

STUDIES OF [^{18}F]DCFPYL IN PROSTATE CANCER

Given the improved characteristics of [^{18}F]DCFPyL relative to [^{18}F]DCFBC in the preclinical setting, [^{18}F]DCFPyL PET/CT was expected to improve significantly on the advances already achieved with [^{18}F]DCFBC PET/CT (compare **Fig. 2**). The first-in-man evaluation of [^{18}F]DCFPyL including 9 patients was published in 2015 and found that the compound was safe and produced very high uptake in presumed sites of primary and

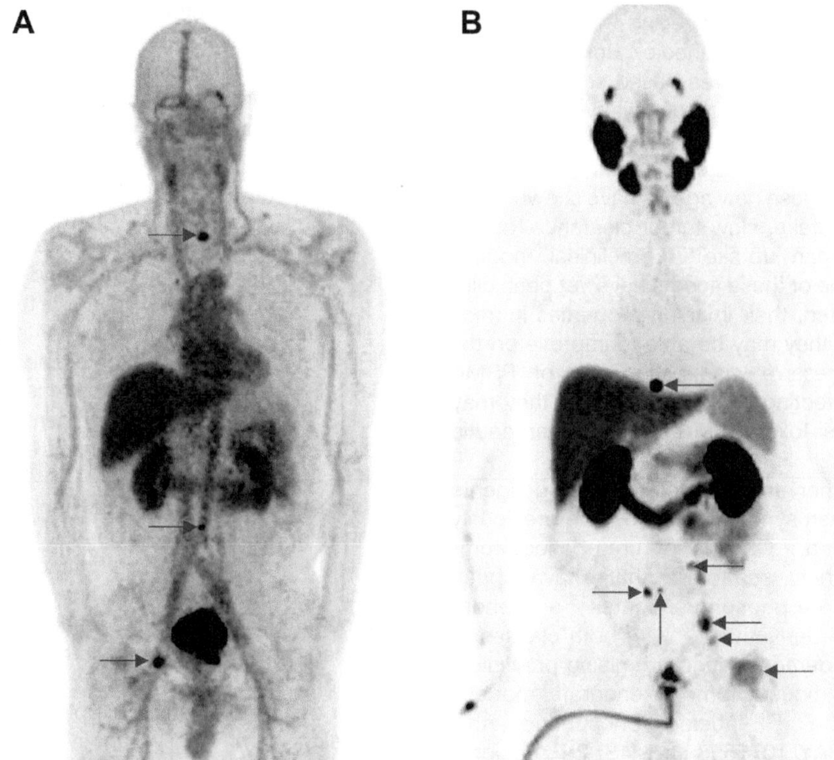

Fig. 2. Maximum intensity projection images of (*A*) [^{18}F]DCFBC and (*B*) [^{18}F]DCFPyL in 2 different patients with metastatic PCa with windowing adjusted to display the same relative liver uptake. Although putative bone and lymph node metastases are clearly visible in both patients (*arrows*), [^{18}F]DCFPyL demonstrates significantly lower blood pool and overall background levels of uptake, allowing even small and relatively low uptake lesions to be visible (*upwards pointing arrow* in [*B*]).

metastatic PCa.[24] A secondary analysis of the lesion detection efficiency in 8 of those 9 patients noted a significant superiority of [^{18}F]DCFPyL PET/CT to conventional imaging with CT and bone scan that appeared to be far in excess of the improved detection rate previously described with [^{18}F]DCFBC[25] (**Fig. 3**). Indeed, 138 definitively positive lesions with one equivocal lesion were visible with [^{18}F]DCFPyL PET/CT, whereas CT and bone scan were only able to identify 30 definitively positive and 15 equivocal lesions. Not only did [^{18}F]DCFPyL PET/CT identify more lesions but also the very low rate of equivocal lesions is demonstrative of the high tumor-to-background ratios typical of this radiotracer. A subsequent report comparing [^{18}F]DCFPyL PET/CT to Na^{18}F PET/CT and bone scan also suggested a very high sensitivity of [^{18}F]DCFPyL for identifying sites of putative bone metastases.[26]

With the rapid expansion of the utilization of ^{68}Ga-labeled PSMA radiotracers during the time leading up to the first-in-man report of [^{18}F] DCFPyL, it is perhaps not surprising that a head-to-head comparison would be carried out. Dietlein and colleagues[27] compared the most commonly used ^{68}Ga-labeled agent (variously known in the literature as [^{68}Ga]Ga-PSMA, [^{68}Ga]Ga-PSMA-11, and [^{68}Ga]Ga-PSMA-HBED-CC) to [^{18}F]DCFPyL in a group of 14 patients with recurrent PCa. Both radiotracers were able to identify sites of suspected PCa in 10/14 (71%) patients, although [^{18}F] DCFPyL found additional lesions that were not visible with [^{68}Ga]Ga-PSMA-HBED-CC in 3 patients, implying an improved sensitivity for the ^{18}F-labeled compound.

The authors, and other groups, have continued to study [^{18}F]DCFPyL clinically. Recently, the authors completed accrual of a prospective study evaluating the utility of this radiotracer to aid in the preoperative staging of patients with clinically localized high-risk to very high-risk PCa. In addition, they are actively studying this agent in men with elevated prostate-specific antigen (PSA) values following radical prostatectomy (ie, patients with PSA persistence or biochemical recurrence). They expect to report the findings from these prospective studies in a timely manner.

Recently, 2 new publications have appeared describing improved radiosynthetic approaches to [^{18}F]DCFPyL.[28,29] These important studies describe high-yield, automated methods for the potential production of large quantities of [^{18}F] DCFPyL, a necessary step toward the eventual goal of central production and widespread distribution of this promising agent for PSMA-targeted PET imaging. These new synthetic methods should also allow easier implementation of multicenter trials to prospectively validate the utility of PSMA imaging in PCa patients.

USE OF BAY 1075553 IN PROSTATE CANCER

As noted previously, BAY 1075553 is an example of a non–urea-based radiofluorinated PSMA inhibitor that has now been investigated in human subjects. In a recent study, 9 patients with primary PCa undergoing preoperative evaluation and 3 patients with recurrent PCa were prospectively accrued and imaged with both BAY 1075553 and [^{18}F]fluorocholine PET/CT.[20] BAY 1075553 was found to be a safe compound with no reported adverse events. BAY 1075553 PET/CT was able to identify sites of primary and metastatic PCa, although the established comparison radiotracer [^{18}F]fluorocholine demonstrated better detection efficiency for sites of lymph node and bone lesions. It is worth noting that although the sensitivity of [^{18}F]fluorocholine for detecting lymph node involvement in the preoperative cohort was higher than the sensitivity of BAY 1075553 (81.2% vs

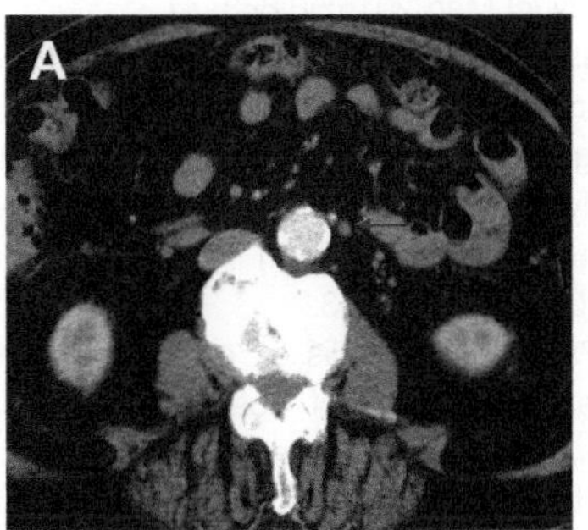

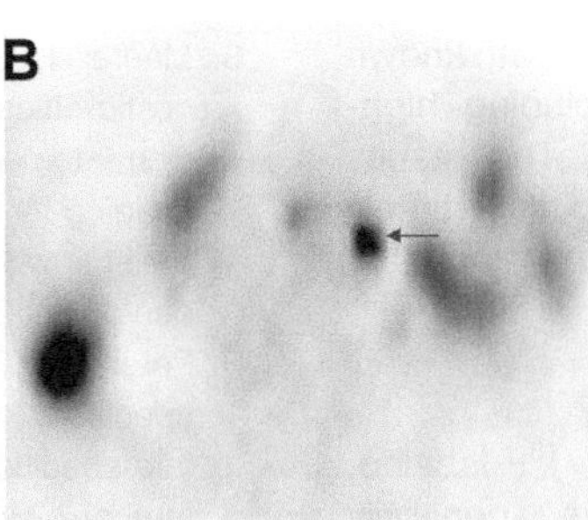

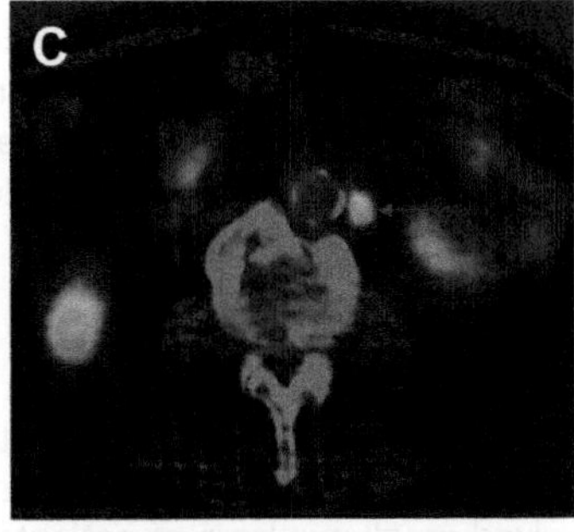

Fig. 3. (*A*) Axial contrast-enhanced CT, (*B*) axial [^{18}F]DCFPyL PET, and (*C*) axial [^{18}F]DCFPyL PET/CT images from a patient with known metastatic PCa demonstrating a 0.5-cm short-axis diameter retroperitoneal lymph node with intense focal [^{18}F]DCFPyL uptake (*arrows*). Although this lymph node is not pathologically enlarged, the radiotracer uptake is distinctly abnormal. This is indicative of the ability of PSMA-targeted imaging agents to identify lesions that are otherwise occult on conventional imaging.

43.8%, respectively), the specificity of BAY 1075553 was perfect in this group of patients (100.0%, in comparison to only 50.0% for [^{18}F]fluorocholine). The high specificity of BAY 1075553 in this pilot study suggests the need to further evaluate this promising radiotracer in larger studies.

EVALUATION OF [^{18}F]DCFPYL IN NONPROSTATE CANCERS

Although the vast majority of published data with PSMA-targeted agents remains focused on PCa, an expanding volume of case reports and case series has suggested the utility of imaging PSMA in other cancers. For most non-PCas, the distribution of PSMA expression is primarily within the tumor neovasculature,[30,31] as opposed to the predominantly epithelial expression of PSMA in PCa. To date, the authors have successfully applied [^{18}F] DCFPyL PET/CT imaging to clear cell renal cell carcinoma (ccRCC),[32–34] which represents a highly neovascularized tumor type with known PSMA expression.[35,36] A pilot study of 5 patients identified multiple sites of abnormal uptake that were suspicious for metastatic disease but were occult on contrast-enhanced CT and MR imaging, suggesting a higher sensitivity for putative metastases than conventional imaging (94.7% vs 78.9%).[32] Early results also indicated a potentially higher sensitivity for ccRCC metastatic lesions and higher tumor radiotracer uptake than are achievable with [^{18}F]FDG PET.[33] More recently, a patient with widely metastatic ccRCC was imaged with [^{18}F] DCFPyL PET/CT shortly before death and undergoing a rapid autopsy.[34] Twelve foci of increased radiotracer uptake that were suspicious for metastases were visible only with PET and were occult on CT; of those, 8 were accessible during the rapid autopsy and 7 were found to be definitively positive for metastatic deposits.

The authors continue to explore the role of [^{18}F] DCFPyL in ccRCC and have also begun to image patients with a variety of other cancers with known PSMA neovascular expression, including high-grade gliomas and breast cancer. The results from those studies will be reported in a timely manner.

SUMMARY

Although the published trials with ^{18}F-labeled, PSMA-targeted radiotracers have generally involved small numbers of patients, the prospective nature of many of these studies and the promising results so far obtained indicate the need to continue to evaluate these agents in larger trials that can definitively establish clinical utility. As PSMA-based imaging becomes more widely available, the intrinsic advantages of ^{18}F-labeled compounds will become of increasing importance.

ACKNOWLEDGMENTS

The authors' work in this field has been supported, in part, by NIH CA124675, CA184228, and CA183031 and the Prostate Cancer Foundation Young Investigator Award.

REFERENCES

1. Kiess AP, Banerjee SR, Mease RC, et al. Prostate-specific membrane antigen as a target for cancer imaging and therapy. Q J Nucl Med Mol Imaging 2015;59:241–68.
2. Maurer T, Eiber M, Schwaiger M, et al. Current use of PSMA-PET in prostate cancer management. Nat Rev Urol 2016;13:226–35.
3. Rowe SP, Gorin MA, Allaf ME, et al. PET imaging of prostate-specific membrane antigen in prostate cancer: current state of the art and future challenges. Prostate Cancer Prostatic Dis 2016;19(3): 223–30.
4. Sweat SD, Pacelli A, Murphy GP, et al. Prostate-specific membrane antigen expression is greatest in prostate adenocarcinoma and lymph node metastases. Urology 1998;52:637–40.
5. Perner S, Hofer MD, Kim R, et al. Prostate-specific membrane antigen expression as a predictor of prostate cancer progression. Hum Pathol 2007;38: 696–701.
6. Ross JS, Sheehan CE, Fisher HA, et al. Correlation of primary tumor prostate-specific membrane antigen expression with disease recurrence in prostate cancer. Clin Cancer Res 2003;9:6357–62.
7. Eiber M, Maurer T, Souvatzoglou M, et al. Evaluation of hybrid (6)(8)Ga-PSMA ligand PET/CT in 248 patients with biochemical recurrence after radical prostatectomy. J Nucl Med 2015;56:668–74.
8. Maurer T, Gschwend JE, Rauscher I, et al. Diagnostic efficacy of (68)Gallium-PSMA positron emission tomography compared to conventional imaging for lymph node staging of 130 consecutive patients with intermediate to high risk prostate cancer. J Urol 2016;195:1436–43.
9. Perera M, Papa N, Christidis D, et al. Sensitivity, specificity, and predictors of positive 68Ga-prostate-specific membrane antigen positron emission tomography in advanced prostate cancer: a systematic review and meta-analysis. Eur Urol 2016;70: 926–37.
10. Sanchez-Crespo A. Comparison of Gallium-68 and Fluorine-18 imaging characteristics in positron emission tomography. Appl Radiat Isot 2013;76:55–62.

11. Gorin MA, Pomper MG, Rowe SP. PSMA-targeted imaging of prostate cancer: the best is yet to come. BJU Int 2016;117:715–6.
12. Pomper MG, Musachio JL, Zhang J, et al. 11C-MCG: synthesis, uptake selectivity, and primate PET of a probe for glutamate carboxypeptidase II (NAALADase). Mol Imaging 2002;1:96–101.
13. Foss CA, Mease RC, Fan H, et al. Radiolabeled small-molecule ligands for prostate-specific membrane antigen: in vivo imaging in experimental models of prostate cancer. Clin Cancer Res 2005; 11:4022–8.
14. Mease RC, Dusich CL, Foss CA, et al. N-[N-[(S)-1,3-dicarboxypropyl]carbamoyl]-4-[18F]fluorobenzyl-L-cysteine, [18F]DCFBC: a new imaging probe for prostate cancer. Clin Cancer Res 2008;14:3036–43.
15. Chen Y, Pullambhatla M, Foss CA, et al. 2-(3-{1-Carboxy-5-[(6-[18F]fluoro-pyridine-3-carbonyl)-amino]-pentyl}-ureido)-pen tanedioic acid, [18F]DCFPyL, a PSMA-based PET imaging agent for prostate cancer. Clin Cancer Res 2011;17:7645–53.
16. Yang X, Mease RC, Pullambhatla M, et al. [(18)F]Fluorobenzoyllysinepentanedioic acid carbamates: new scaffolds for positron emission tomography (PET) imaging of prostate-specific membrane antigen (PSMA). J Med Chem 2016;59:206–18.
17. Chen Y, Lisok A, Chatterjee S, et al. [(18)F]Fluoroethyl triazole substituted PSMA inhibitor exhibiting rapid normal organ clearance. Bioconjug Chem 2016;27:1655–62.
18. Lapi SE, Wahnishe H, Pham D, et al. Assessment of an 18F-labeled phosphoramidate peptidomimetic as a new prostate-specific membrane antigen-targeted imaging agent for prostate cancer. J Nucl Med 2009;50:2042–8.
19. Graham K, Lesche R, Gromov AV, et al. Radiofluorinated derivatives of 2-(phosphonomethyl)pentanedioic acid as inhibitors of prostate specific membrane antigen (PSMA) for the imaging of prostate cancer. J Med Chem 2012;55:9510–20.
20. Beheshti M, Kunit T, Haim S, et al. BAY 1075553 PET-CT for staging and restaging prostate cancer patients: comparison with [18F] fluorocholine PET-CT (phase I study). Mol Imaging Biol 2015;17:424–33.
21. Cho SY, Gage KL, Mease RC, et al. Biodistribution, tumor detection, and radiation dosimetry of 18F-DCFBC, a low-molecular-weight inhibitor of prostate-specific membrane antigen, in patients with metastatic prostate cancer. J Nucl Med 2012; 53:1883–91.
22. Rowe SP, Gage KL, Faraj SF, et al. (1)(8)F-DCFBC PET/CT for PSMA-based detection and characterization of primary prostate cancer. J Nucl Med 2015;56:1003–10.
23. Rowe SP, Macura KJ, Ciarallo A, et al. Comparison of prostate-specific membrane antigen-based 18F-DCFBC PET/CT to conventional imaging modalities for detection of hormone-naive and castration-resistant metastatic prostate cancer. J Nucl Med 2016;57:46–53.
24. Szabo Z, Mena E, Rowe SP, et al. Initial evaluation of [(18)F]DCFPyL for prostate-specific membrane antigen (PSMA)-targeted PET imaging of prostate cancer. Mol Imaging Biol 2015;17:565–74.
25. Rowe SP, Macura KJ, Mena E, et al. PSMA-Based [(18)F]DCFPyL PET/CT is superior to conventional imaging for lesion detection in patients with metastatic prostate cancer. Mol Imaging Biol 2016;18: 411–9.
26. Rowe SP, Mana-Ay M, Javadi MS, et al. PSMA-based detection of prostate cancer bone lesions with (1)(8)F-DCFPyL PET/CT: a sensitive alternative to ((9)(9)m)Tc-MDP Bone Scan and Na(1)(8)F PET/CT? Clin Genitourin Cancer 2016;14:e115–8.
27. Dietlein M, Kobe C, Kuhnert G, et al. Comparison of [(18)F]DCFPyL and [(68)Ga]Ga-PSMA-HBED-CC for PSMA-PET imaging in patients with relapsed prostate cancer. Mol Imaging Biol 2015;17:575–84.
28. Bouvet V, Wuest M, Jans HS, et al. Automated synthesis of [(18)F]DCFPyL via direct radiofluorination and validation in preclinical prostate cancer models. EJNMMI Res 2016;6:40.
29. Ravert HT, Holt DP, Chen Y, et al. An improved synthesis of the radiolabeled prostate-specific membrane antigen inhibitor, [18 F]DCFPyL. J Labelled Comp Radiopharm 2016;59(11):439–50.
30. Chang SS, O'Keefe DS, Bacich DJ, et al. Prostate-specific membrane antigen is produced in tumor-associated neovasculature. Clin Cancer Res 1999; 5:2674–81.
31. Chang SS, Reuter VE, Heston WD, et al. Comparison of anti-prostate-specific membrane antigen antibodies and other immunomarkers in metastatic prostate carcinoma. Urology 2001;57:1179–83.
32. Rowe SP, Gorin MA, Hammers HJ, et al. Imaging of metastatic clear cell renal cell carcinoma with PSMA-targeted (18)F-DCFPyL PET/CT. Ann Nucl Med 2015;29:877–82.
33. Rowe SP, Gorin MA, Hammers HJ, et al. Detection of 18F-FDG PET/CT occult lesions with 18F-DCFPyL PET/CT in a patient with metastatic renal cell carcinoma. Clin Nucl Med 2016;41:83–5.
34. Gorin MA, Rowe SP, Hooper JE, et al. PSMA-targeted 18F-DCFPyL PET/CT imaging of clear cell renal cell carcinoma: results from a rapid autopsy. Eur Urol 2016;71(1):145–6.
35. Chang SS, Reuter VE, Heston WD, et al. Metastatic renal cell carcinoma neovasculature expresses prostate-specific membrane antigen. Urology 2001;57:801–5.
36. Baccala A, Sercia L, Li J, et al. Expression of prostate-specific membrane antigen in tumor-associated neovasculature of renal neoplasms. Urology 2007;70:385–90.

Imaging of Prostate Cancer Using Urokinase-Type Plasminogen Activator Receptor PET

Dorthe Skovgaard, MD, PhD[a], Morten Persson, MSc, PhD[b], Andreas Kjaer, MD, PhD, DMSc[a,*]

KEYWORDS

• uPAR • PET • Prostate cancer • Radionuclide imaging • Theranostics • Molecular imaging

KEY POINTS

- Urokinase plasminogen activator receptor (uPAR) is a key component in proteolysis and extracellular matrix degradation during cancer invasion and metastasis.
- uPAR expression in prostate cancer provides independent prognostic information in addition to that contributed by PSA, Gleason score, and other clinicopathologic parameters.
- PET imaging of uPAR in prostate cancer is a new and clinically relevant diagnostic and prognostic biomarker.
- Two recent phase I uPAR PET studies including patients with prostate cancer have shown encouraging data and support large-scale clinical trials.

INTRODUCTION

The most commonly diagnosed malignancy among men in Western countries is prostate cancer (PC).[1] PC has a highly variable prognosis with some PCs remaining indolent and not causing any clinical symptoms or morbidity, whereas other PCs are or become aggressive and are associated with fast progression and high mortality.[1,2] Conventional anatomic imaging methods in PC—including MR imaging for primary disease and contrast-enhanced computed tomography (CT) and ^{99m}Tc-methylene diphosphonate–bone scintigraphy for metastatic disease—have several significant limitations, especially considering sensitivity and specificity.[3] These limitations and an increasing understanding of the complex nature and the underlying heterogeneity of PC have stimulated the development of new imaging approaches that allow direct visualization of the molecular pathology in malignant prostate tissue. These methods include multiparametric MR imaging and PET using radioligands, such as choline, gastrin-releasing peptide receptor, and prostate-specific membrane antigen-targeting ligands.[1] Indeed, functional and metabolic imaging techniques are gaining importance as the therapeutic paradigm has shifted from structural tumor detection alone

Disclosure Statement: Dr A. Kjaer and Dr M. Persson are inventors of the composition of matter of uPAR PET with a filed patent application: Positron Emitting Radionuclides Labeled Peptides for Human uPAR PET Imaging (WO 2014/086364 A1). Dr M. Perrson and Dr A. Kjaer are cofounders of Curasight, which has licensed the uPAR PET patent to commercialize uPAR PET technology. Dr D. Skovgaard has received financial research support from Curasight.

[a] Department of Clinical Physiology, Nuclear Medicine & PET and Cluster for Molecular Imaging, Rigshospitalet and University of Copenhagen, Blegdamsvej 9, 4011, Copenhagen, DK-2100, Denmark; [b] Curasight Aps, Ole Maaloesvej 3, Copenhagen, DK-2200, Denmark

* Corresponding author.

E-mail address: akjaer@sund.ku.dk

PET Clin 12 (2017) 243–255

http://dx.doi.org/10.1016/j.cpet.2016.12.005

to distinguishing patients with indolent tumors that are managed conservatively from patients with more aggressive tumors, which may require immediate treatment with surgery or radiation therapy. This has led to a search for upregulated tumor-specific markers that can serve as candidates for tumor imaging with the potential of identifying the aggressive tumor phenotype. Urokinase-type plasminogen activator receptor (uPAR) has recently been identified as a promising imaging target candidate for PC.[4] Several strategies to develop uPAR-targeting radiopharmaceuticals have been explored, using peptides, proteins, small molecules, antibodies, and nanoparticles.[5] We have recently successfully translated two of these radioligands, both based on the uPAR-targeting small linear peptide AE105, into the clinic with the first ever human studies of uPAR PET imaging in PC.[6,7]

This article focuses on PET imaging of uPAR in PC as a new and clinically relevant diagnostic and prognostic imaging biomarker technique. The potential use of uPAR PET to evaluate uPAR-directed anticancer therapy and the applicability of a uPAR-ligand for targeted radionuclide therapy are also discussed.

UROKINASE PLASMINOGEN ACTIVATOR RECEPTOR IN PROSTATE CANCER

PC metastasizes from the prostate gland through pelvic lymphatic drainage and hematogenous routes resulting in a high prevalence of metastases to regional nodes and bones, particularly the spine. The exact mechanisms involved in PC progression remain unclear. A key requirement in the complex process of tumor invasion and metastasis is the ability of tumor cells to produce and recruit growth factors and proteolytic enzymes within the tumor cell environment to promote neovascularization, tumor growth, and extracellular matrix degradation to facilitate tumor metastasis.[8] A central player in this process is the uPAR system (**Fig. 1**). The plasminogen activator system consists of a serine protease urokinase-type plasminogen (uPA), its glycosylphosphatidylinositol-anchored cell membrane receptor (uPAR), and two specific inhibitors PAI-1 and PAI-2. uPA binds with high affinity to uPAR and subsequently converts plasminogen to active plasmin, which in turn activates several proteases related to the degradation of extracellular matrix proteins and basal membranes, thereby facilitating cancer cell invasion and metastasis.[2,5,9–13] In addition, uPA/uPAR binding affects multiple other aspects of the tumor progression and development by eliciting tumor-associated processes including cell proliferation, cell adhesion, and migration, through interactions with coreceptors, such as integrins, G-protein-coupled receptors, and growth factor receptors activating intracellular signaling pathways.[14,15] A particular high uPAR expression in cancer cells is found at the invasive

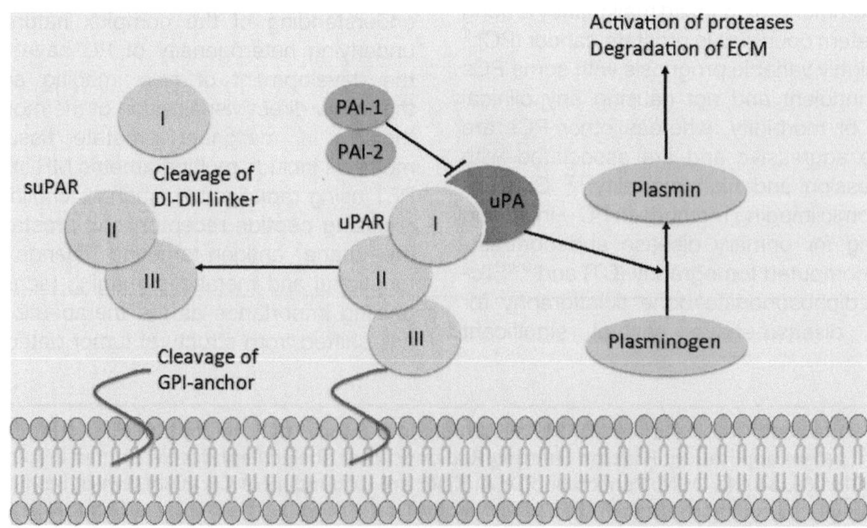

Fig. 1. Overview of the urokinase-type plasminogen (uPA)/uPAR system. uPAR consists of three domains (I, II, III) and is attached to the cell surface by a glycosyl phosphatidylinositol (GPI) anchor. uPA bound to uPAR cleaves plasminogen, generating the active protease plasmin. Plasmin activates matrix metalloproteases. Both plasmin and matrix metalloproteases degrade extracellular matrix (ECM) and thereby promote cancer invasion and metastasis. The proteolytic activities of uPA and plasmin are inhibited by PAI-1 and PAI-2. Soluble uPAR (suPAR) is released from the plasma membrane by cleavage of the GPI anchor. Both uPAR and suPAR can be cleaved in the region that links domains DI to DII to yield a DI and DIIDIII fragment.

front of the tumor and in tumor-associated stromal cells, such as fibroblasts and macrophages.[15–17] Using various biochemical assays, immunohistochemistry, tissue microarrays, and reverse-transcriptase polymerase chain reactions on PC tissue (biopsies or surgical specimens), several studies have demonstrated overexpression of uPAR in PC cells, surrounding tumor-associated stromal cells and lymph node metastases compared with normal prostate tissue.[10,18–22] High uPAR expression is associated with relevant pathologic and clinical parameters, such as high Gleason score, advanced tumor stage, lymph node metastases, and shorter recurrence-free survival and overall survival.[20] However, a few studies have not been able to confirm these associations, and these contradictories can possibly be related to differences in methodologic approaches, such as antibody specificity, incomparable patient populations, and limited follow-up periods with only a few patients experiencing biochemical progression[21,23,24] (**Table 1**).

Others have investigated circulating uPAR forms in blood samples (serum/plasma) of PC patients. uPAR can be cleaved from the membrane, and high levels of soluble uPAR and/or various uPAR forms in the blood have been reported in several cancers.[13] Intact uPAR (I–III) can be cleaved by uPA, releasing domain I (uPAR [I]), while leaving uPAR (II–III) on the cell surface. Both of the glycolipid-anchored uPAR forms (uPAR [II–III] and uPAR [I–III]) can be shed from the cell membrane, resulting in three soluble uPAR forms (uPAR [I–III], uPAR [II–III], and uPAR [I]) detectable in the blood.[25] The levels of the cleaved forms may reflect the catalytic activity of uPA.[26] The cleaved soluble uPAR forms have been demonstrated to be independent prognostic markers in PC and various other types of cancer,[27] such as colorectal,[28,29] breast,[30] and lung.[26] In line with this, serum from patients with PC contains elevated levels of soluble uPAR compared with patients with benign prostatic hypertrophy and healthy control subjects.[31] Also, preoperative circulating total uPAR levels were found to be higher among patients with increasing biopsy Gleason score, extraprostatic extension, and lymph node metastatic disease after radical prostatectomy, and especially patients with PC with bone metastasis exhibited significantly higher uPAR levels compared with patients with localized disease or patients with only regional lymph node metastasis.[32] Furthermore, studies have found significantly lowered overall survival rate of patients with PC with high plasma levels of uPAR compared with low serum uPAR levels.[24,31] In the most recently published study, the plasma levels of the cleaved uPAR forms uPAR (I–III) plus uPAR (II–III) and uPAR (I) levels were significantly higher, whereas the level of intact uPAR (I–III) did not differ, in hormone-naive and castrate-resistant patients compared with patients with localized disease.[33]

The measurement of soluble uPAR from blood has obvious advantages compared with tissue-derived uPAR and could therefore be performed before therapy and during follow-up. However, measurement of plasma levels of uPAR (intact/cleaved domains) will always only be an indirect indicator for the expression level in the tumor. Moreover, the lack of correlation between tumor tissue uPAR expression and the level of secreted different forms of uPAR,[27] together with the fact the most cancer patients have uPAR levels within the reference interval of healthy individuals,[34] further complicate the information achievable. This is perhaps the main reason for the lack of routine clinical use of plasma uPAR measurements. It seems that localized measurements, encompassing the heterogeneity of the tumor and local microenvironment, are necessary for optimal uPAR-based diagnostic and prognostic information.

Although no definite conclusion can be drawn, most studies find uPAR expression, either assessed directly in the malignant PC tissue or in plasma (intact/cleaved forms), to be a largely independent analytical variable, conceivably offering clinical information that is different from and additive to that contributed by prostate-specific antigen, Gleason score, and other relevant pathologic/clinical parameters. These observations highlight and support that noninvasive imaging of uPAR in PC, with the possibility of distinguishing indolent tumors from the invasive phenotype, could become a widely applicable, clinically relevant diagnostic and prognostic imaging biomarker, as also identified by different authors.[4,11]

PRECLINICAL UROKINASE PLASMINOGEN ACTIVATOR RECEPTOR PET IMAGING

A major advantage of noninvasive molecular imaging of uPAR by PET is that information on the global expression profile of uPAR is obtained noninvasively and without the risk of missing the target because of tumor heterogeneity. This is of special importance in PC, which is characterized as a multifocal, heterogeneous disease with a broad spectrum of clinical, pathologic, and molecular characteristics, emphasized by the routinely used 12-core biopsy protocol for diagnosis of PC.[35]

Table 1
Overview of literature on association of tissue and blood RNA/protein levels of urokinase plasminogen activator system family with clinicopathologic parameters in prostate cancer

Target	Method	Study Population	Results	Association with Clinical Parameters	Reference
Tissue					
uPA, uPAR	mRNA: in situ hybridization Protein: IHC	25 PC, 4 BPH	mRNA and protein: Expression of uPA, uPAR in PC; weak/no expression of uPA, uPAR in BPH	NA	Gavrilov et al,[19] 2001
uPA, uPAR, PAI-1	mRNA: in situ hybridization Protein: IHC	16 PC, 6 BPH	mRNA and protein: Expression of uPA, uPA, PAI-1 in PC + BPH	No association with GS	Usher et al,[18] 2005
uPA, uPAR, PAI-1	mRNA: qPCR	44 PC, 23 BPH	uPAR, PAI-1 mRNA increased in PC compared with BPH, uPA not increased	NA	Riddick et al,[22] 2005
uPA, uPAR	Protein: IHC	120 PC, 40 control subjects, 15 BPH, 10 LN mets	Expression of uPA, uPAR in PC and LN Weak/no expression BPH and normal control subjects	uPA and uPAR associated with GS, tumor stage, surgical margin; uPA associated with LN metastases	Cozzi et al,[21] 2006
uPA, uPAR, PAI-1	Protein: IHC	230 PC Follow-up 63 mo	Expression of UPA (39%), PAI-1 (34%), uPAR (55%) in PC	uPA and uPAI-1 associated with biochemical RFS	Gupta et al,[23] 2009
uPA, uPAR, PAI-1	Protein: IHC	153 PC Follow-up 61 mo	Expression of uPA, uPAR, PAI-1 in PC	uPA, uPAR associated with tumor stage, GS, surgical margin status, LN metastases; PAI-1 associated with tumor stage, surgical margin status; uPA, uPAR, and PAI-1 associated with biochemical RFS	Kumano et al,[20] 2009
uPA, uPAR, PAI-1	mRNA: qPCR	132 PC	uPA, uPAR, PAI-1 mRNA not elevated in PC biopsies compared with nonmalignant biopsies	uPA associated with GS	Al-Janabi et al,[24] 2014

Blood					
uPA, suPAR	Serum (ELISA)	72 PC, 62 BPH, 52 control subjects Follow-up 50 mo	Increased uPA, suPAR PC compared with BPH and control	uPA and suPAR associated with tumor stage, metastasis, and OS	Miyake et al,[31] 1999
uPA, uPAR, suPAR (I), suPAR (II–III) + suPAR (I–III)	Serum (ELISA)	355 referred for prostate biopsy	All forms higher in PC	NA	Steuber et al,[36] 2007
uPA, suPAR	Plasma (ELISA)	429 PC, 19 PC with LN metastases, 10 PC with bone metastases 44 control subjects	uPA, uPAR > PC with bone metastases > PC with LN metastases > localized PC > control subjects	uPA and suPAR associated with GS, LN metastases, biochemical RFS, and aggressive disease	Shariat et al,[32] 2007
uPA, suPAR	Serum (ELISA)	423 PC	NA	uPA and uPAR associated with biochemical RFS	Shariat & Roehrborn[58] 2008
uPA, suPAR, suPAR (II–III), suPAR (I–III)	Serum (TR-FIA)	312 men in screening trial for PC, follow-up 15 y, 64 with PC	No difference in suPAR from men with PC compared with non-PC	suPAR associated with OS	Kjellmann et al,[37] 2011
uPA, suPAR, suPAR (I), suPAR (II–III) + uPAR (I–III)	Serum (TR-FIA)	132 PC Follow-up 4.9 y	NA	All uPAR form associated with OS	Almasi et al,[2] 2011
uPA, suPAR, PAI-1	Serum (ELISA)	81 PC 36 BPH	NA	uPAR associated with OS	Al-Janabi et al,[24] 2014
suPAR	Serum (ELISA)	146 PC, 35 BPH, 19 control subjects	suPAR increased in PC	suPAR associated with GS, OS, and disease-specific survival	Wach et al,[38] 2015
uPA, suPAR, suPAR (I), suPAR (II–III) + uPAR (I–III)	Plasma (TR-FIA)	397 PC	suPAR (I-III) + suPAR, suPAR (I) higher in hormone-naive and castration-resistant PC compared with localized PC	NA	Lippert et al,[33] 2016

Abbreviations: BPH, benign prostatic hyperplasia; ELISA, enzyme-linked immunosorbent assay; GS, Gleason score; IHC, immunohistochemistry; LN, lymph node; NA, not applicable; OS, overall survival; qPCR, quantitative polymerase chain reaction; RFS, recurrence-free survival; suPAR; soluble PAR; TR-FIA, time-resolved fluorescence immunoassay.

Knowledge of the molecular basis behind the interactions between uPAR and its ligand uPA obtained by radiograph crystallography and surface plasmon resonance studies have promoted the development of a series of small peptides applicable for noninvasive molecular imaging of uPAR expression in vivo by PET.[5,12] Peptides is regarded an attractive class of molecular imaging ligands because of many favorable characteristics including fast clearance; rapid tissue penetration; low antigenicity; and relatively simple, automated means of synthesizing.[39]

To date, most uPAR-targeted imaging and therapy studies are based on the high-affinity peptide AE105 and its corresponding derivatives. The peptide has the following sequence: Asp^1-Cha^2-Phe^3-ser^4-arg^5-Tyr^6-Leu^7-Trp^8-Ser.[9] Because of the presence of Cha, cyclohexyl-(L)-alanine, which is an unnatural amino acid, the peptide is remarkably stable in serum, an important characteristic for a successful use of the peptide for PET imaging.[5,40]

The first uPAR PET proof-of-concept study[41] conjugated AE105 with the metal chelator DOTA in the N-terminal and labeled with 64Cu and performed micro-PET imaging of mice bearing uPAR-positive U87 MG human glioblastoma and uPAR negative MDA-MB-435 human breast cancer xenograft. The study demonstrated the ability of ^{64}Cu-DOTA-AE105 to specifically detect human uPAR. A high accumulation in the uPAR-positive U87 MG xenograft tumor compared with the uPAR-negative MDA-MB-435 xenograft tumor was found. Tracer specificity was further demonstrated by comparing the uptake of a nonbinding variant of the peptide in the uPAR-positive U87 MG xenograft and by performing a blocking experiment using excessive predosing of nonlabelled peptide.[38]

Our research group has used AE105 for development of uPAR-targeting PET ligands. We have investigated the use of different metal-binding chelators and isotopes, including ^{64}Cu, ^{68}Ga, and ^{18}F[9,42–45] (**Table 2**). In our initial experiments, we found a significant correlation between tumor uptake of ^{64}Cu-DOTA-AE105 on micro-PET images of human tumor xenografts and uPAR expression level in the tumor tissue[39] (**Fig. 2**). However, our results also revealed a high accumulation of ^{64}Cu in the liver. This was not surprising because the liver is a known site for ^{64}Cu accumulation and a well-established indirect marker of instability of ^{64}Cu-based ligands in rodents.[46,47] Accordingly, two improved metal chelators (^{64}Cu-CB-TE2A-AE105 and ^{64}Cu-CB-TE2A-PA-AE105) based on cross-bridge cyclam N-conjugated to the AE105 were

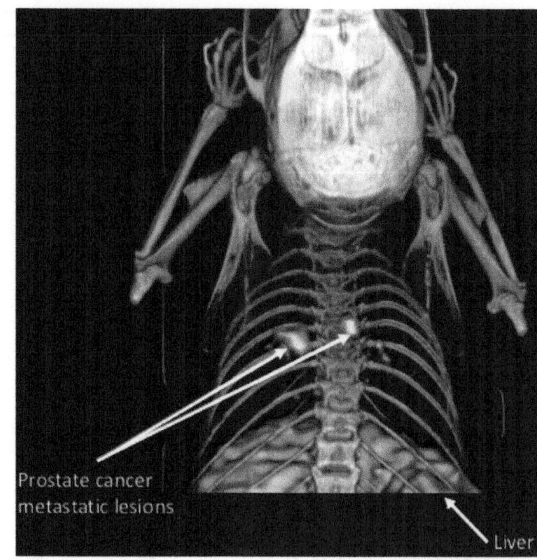

Fig. 2. ^{64}Cu-DOTA-AE105 uPAR PET imaging of metastatic lesions in a mouse model of disseminated human prostate cancer. Human prostate cancer C-3M-LUC2 cells were inoculated by intracardiac injection to mimic intravascular dissemination and subsequent systemic establishment of metastatic disease. The PC-3M-LUC2 cell-line was stably transfected with luciferase, and formation of small metastatic lesions could be followed with bioluminescence imaging (BLI). All tumor lesions identified on BLI were also identified on uPAR PET 31 days after injection. Arrows indicate metastatic lesions with high uptake of ^{64}Cu-DOTA-AE105. Also shown is the unspecific liver uptake of ^{64}Cu. (*From* Persson M, Juhl K, Rasmussen P, et al. uPAR targeted radionuclide therapy with (177) Lu-DOTA-AE105 inhibits dissemination of metastatic prostate cancer. Mol Pharm 2014;11:2803; © the American Chemical Society, with permission.)

Table 2
Overview of current PET-ligands based on the peptide AE105

^{64}Cu	^{68}Ga	^{18}F
^{64}Cu-DOTA-AE105	^{68}Ga-DOTA-AE105	^{18}F-AlF-NOTA-AE105
^{64}Cu-CB-TE2A-AE105	^{68}Ga-NODAGA-AE105	^{18}F-FB-AE105
^{64}Cu-CB-TE2A-PPA-AE105	^{68}Ga-NOTA-AE105	^{18}F-Click-AE105
^{64}Cu-NOTA-AE105		

developed and tested both in vitro and in vivo in preclinical mouse cancer models.[44] In particular, ^{64}Cu-CB-TE2A-PA-AE105 exhibited an improved tumor-to-liver ratio. In accordance with this, and based on the fast tumor uptake observed in our study, we hypothesized that the use of ^{68}Ga instead of ^{64}Cu could maintain tumor uptake and reduce the nonspecific uptake in nontarget tissue, in particular in the liver. Using ^{68}Ga in preclinical xenograft tumor mouse models did indeed show a significant reduction in liver uptake for ^{68}Ga-DOTA-AE105 and ^{68}Ga-NODAGA-AE105.[43] Unfortunately, also a reduction in tumor uptake and a lower tumor-to-kidney ratio, compared with ^{64}Cu-DOTA-AE105, were seen. Next we tested ^{18}F-labeled uPAR PET ligand, ^{18}F-AlF-NOTA-AE105, and effectively visualized noninvasively uPAR-positive PC in mouse models with high tumor-to-background ratios.[9] Ex vivo uPAR expression measured on extracted tumors confirmed that tumor uptake of ^{18}F-AlF-NOTA-AE105 correlated strongly with human uPAR expression. Most recently our efforts to develop clinical translatable uPAR PET ligands, ^{64}Cu-NOTA-AE105 and ^{68}Ga-NOTA-AE105, were produced and investigated in a human orthotopic glioblastoma model in mice.[45] Also here, uPAR expression levels correlated well with uPAR PET ligand uptake in tumors.

Other categories of uPAR-targeting PET ligands are obtainable based, for example, on uPA fragments, small molecules, anti-uPAR antibodies, or nanoparticles,[40] but to our knowledge such ligands specific for PET imaging have not been described in the literature, except in a recent proof-of-concept study, where a small-molecule-based multimodal and multifunctional PET and optical imaging probe was prepared and successfully integrated with AE105 providing the uPAR binding property.[48] However, imaging and uPAR targeting ability of this ^{64}Cu-labelled dual-modality (PET/optical imaging) ligand was investigated in mouse models with glioblastoma tumor xenografts (U87 MG) and has yet to be applied in PC.

Not included in this review is a variety of non-PET uPAR-targeting ligands for other modalities. These include optical imaging,[49] MR imaging,[50,51] single-photon emission CT,[52,53] and even probes targeting uPA,[54] the natural agonist of uPAR, currently under investigation in preclinical models and with possible future prospects within PC.

CLINICAL EXPERIENCES

^{64}Cu-DOTA-AE105

Our first step toward clinical translation of uPAR PET imaging was to undertake a first-in-humans phase I clinical trial of ^{64}Cu-DOTA-AE105 (ClinicalTrials.gov: NCT02139371) where the results were recently published.[6] By definition, the primary end points of a phase I clinical study are safety, biodistribution, and dosimetry assessment. In our phase I study we included a total of 10 patients with urinary bladder cancer (three patients), breast cancer (three patients), and PC (four patients). No adverse events or clinically detectable pharmacologic effects were found. Radiation dosimetry analysis estimated an effective dose of 0.0276 mSv/MBq, which was close to the predicted effective dose projected from our previous mouse study.[55] The radiation dose equals 5.5 mSv for the planned 200-MBq dose, which is lower or comparable with the dose received from a standard fluorodeoxyglucose-PET.[56] Secondary objectives were to investigate the uptake in primary tumor lesions and potential metastases. A total of four patients with newly diagnosed and biopsy-proven PC were uPAR PET/CT scanned before surgical pelvic lymphadenectomy for staging and prostatectomy if indicated. In all patients with PC a high and specific uptake in the primary intraprostatic lesion was found. Histopathology performed on the three available surgical specimens confirmed a uPAR expression in the primary tumor, supporting target-specific uptake of ^{64}Cu-DOTA-AE105. One patient had several visible uPAR PET-positive lymph nodes in the pelvic region, which were confirmed during the open surgical staging procedure with pelvic lymph node dissection followed by histopathologic assessment. In this patient, three out of six removed lymph nodes showed histologically prostate adenocarcinoma (**Fig. 3**). Two patients had no signs of metastases on uPAR PET or perioperative staging, whereas the last patient was found to have a metastasis in 1 out of 17 regional lymph nodes that was not visualized on uPAR PET or CT.

The results of this phase I study were encouraging with uPAR PET being able to identify primary tumors and lymph node metastases in PC thereby providing preliminary evidence for uPAR PET imaging in patients with cancer.

^{68}Ga-NOTA-AE105

Clinical translation of ^{64}Cu-based radioligands is hampered by limited availability and the necessity of a cyclotron facility to produce the PET isotopes. In line with this, the generator-based PET isotope ^{68}Ga has gained special attention because of its independence of an onsite cyclotron and a physical half-life of 68 minutes, which matches well with the pharmacokinetics of

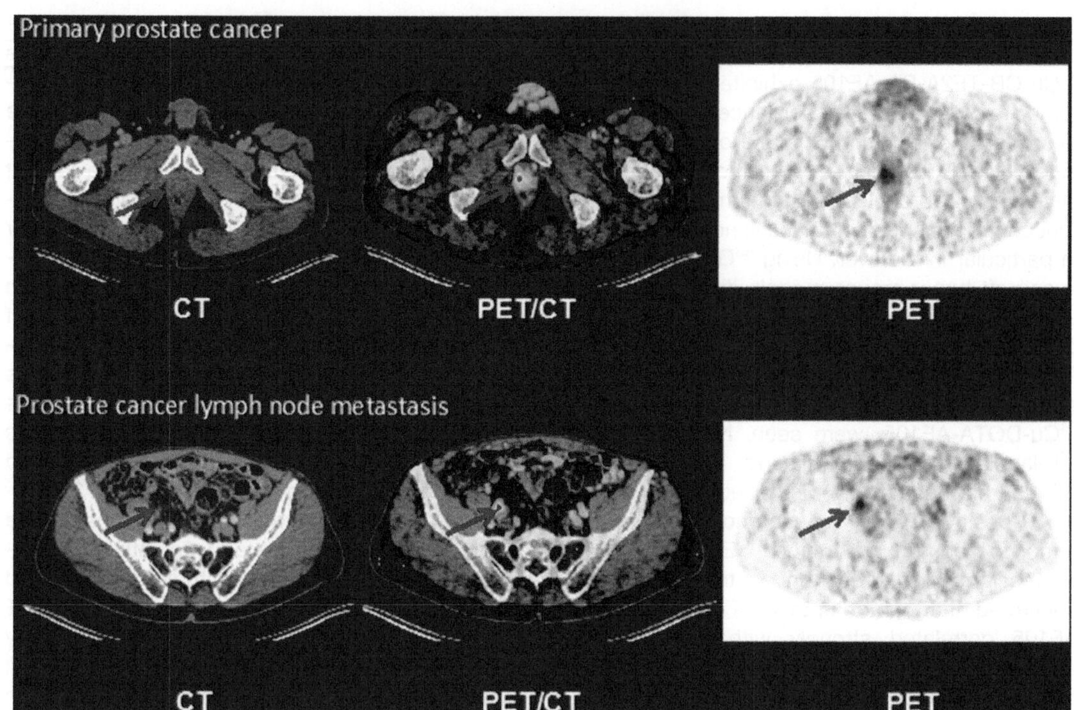

Fig. 3. ^{64}Cu-DOTA-AE105 uPAR PET imaging of patients with prostate cancer. Typical transverse CT, PET, and fused PET/CT images from the first-ever human uPAR PET study. Top shows high uptake of ^{64}Cu-DOTA-AE105 in primary prostate cancer (*arrows*). uPAR immunohistochemistry on removed cancer tissue confirmed uPAR expression. Bottom shows a regional lymph node metastasis (*arrows*) with high ^{64}Cu-DOTA-AE105 uptake. The subsequent staging operation and histopathologic assessment confirmed prostate adenocarcinoma in several lymph nodes.

peptides, such as the AE105.[57] Therefore, we recently conducted another phase I study (ClinicalTrials.gov: NCT02437539) where the results were recently published (**Fig. 4**).[7] The goal of the study was to investigate the feasibility of the ^{68}Ga-labeled version of our uPAR-targeting ligand (^{68}Ga-NOTA-AE105) for tumor imaging in humans. Again, the primary aim was to evaluate the safety, pharmacokinetics and internal radiation dosimetry of a single-dose injection of the ^{68}Ga-NOTA-AE105 in patients with cancer using PET/CT imaging.

Four patients with newly diagnosed locally advanced PC were included in the study before a planned open staging procedure with pelvic lymph node dissection. In these patients a low, heterogeneous intraprostatic distribution of the radioligand was found with no distinct tumor uptake and no detectable tracer uptake in regional lymph nodes. The latter was in line with the findings following staging because pathologic examinations of the removed pelvic lymph nodes showed no lymph node involvement. In addition, two patients with disseminated PC and bone metastases were included and evaluated during a chemotherapy regime. Both patients had multiple bone metastases with significant ^{68}Ga-NOTA-AE105 uptake concurrent with heterogeneous uptake at the site of the primary tumor within the prostate gland.

The two first ever uPAR PET clinical imaging studies in patients with PC show perceivable, heterogeneous uptake of the uPAR targeting radioligands in primary PC tissue and metastases (lymph node and bone) possibly reflecting relevant disparate uPAR expression patterns. Future phase II studies in larger patient populations with PC will investigate the application and utility of uPAR PET in relevant clinical PC settings.

POSSIBLE APPLICATION OF UROKINASE PLASMINOGEN ACTIVATOR RECEPTOR PET

uPAR PET visualizing uPAR expression noninvasively seems to be highly promising. Within PC, an array of important clinical questions in primary and metastatic PC can potentially be addressed with the use of uPAR PET.

In diagnostic work-up of patients suspected of PC, several imaging modalities have been suggested to improve detection and localization of intraprostatic tumors.[1] Following current guidelines, transrectal/perineal core needle biopsies carry a false-negative rate of 20% to 25%[58] and it is suggested that use of specific molecular imaging could be helpful in obtaining image-guided biopsies, in particular in patients with prior negative findings.[59] However, because overtreatment is a major challenge in localized PC, the main clinical potential lies in the possibility of distinguishing indolent tumors from the invasive phenotype. uPAR expression correlates with PC aggressiveness. As such, it could be expected that with a quantitative imaging modality, such as PET, the degree of tracer uptake will correlate with pathologic and clinical parameters, such as Gleason score and prognosis. Clinically significant disease that would benefit from aggressive therapy with prostatectomy or radiotherapy rather than watchful-waiting could thereby potentially be identified noninvasively by uPAR PET imaging.

Another important clinical implication of uPAR PET is preoperative staging. However, the ability of uPAR PET to preoperatively identify pelvic lymph node involvement in high-risk primary PC will have to be investigated in future, thoroughly designed prospective studies. In addition, uPAR PET can be applied in the context of biochemical recurrence, usually detected as a rise in serum prostate-specific antigen levels, following failed local therapy. In these patients a sensitive and reliable imaging assessment for localization of the site of recurrent disease would potentially provide better guidance of treatment and possibly support use of new salvage treatment options by identifying patients with limited oligometastatic disease that are suitable for surgery.[60]

In addition to imaging, uPAR is a promising candidate as a molecular target for cancer therapy.[61] In the last decade, academia and industry have sought to develop new and specific pharmaceuticals targeting uPAR, which could ideally enter a translational pipeline as new treatment modalities in management of patients with cancer. These endeavors include the assessment of inhibitory recombinant proteins, monoclonal antibodies, protease-activated prodrugs, synthetic antagonist peptides, low-molecular-weight compounds, and various means of gene silencing.[61] Targeting of uPAR with a monoclonal antibody blocking the biologic functions of uPAR was recently shown to have a potent and encouraging therapeutic effect in murine PC models, including bone metastases formation,[62] but has still to move into clinical

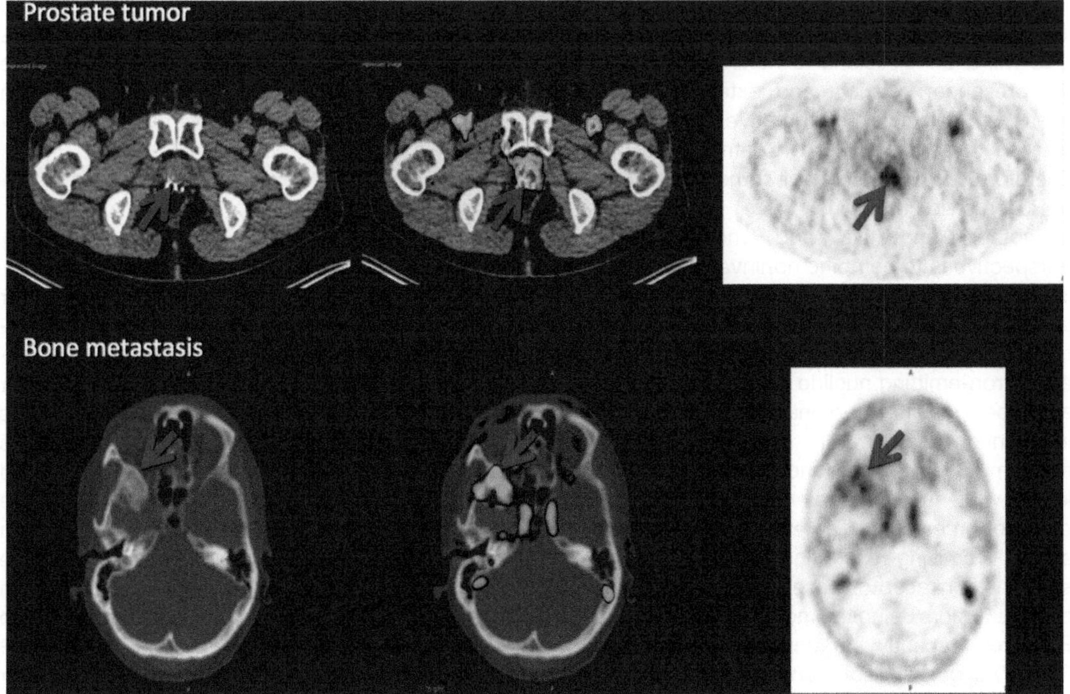

Fig. 4. uPAR PET imaging in prostate cancer with ^{68}Ga-NOTA-AE105. (*Top*) Representative transverse CT, PET, and coregistered PET/CT images with uptake of ^{68}Ga-NOTA-AE105 at the site of the primary tumor (*arrows*). (*Bottom*) Images show a uPAR-positive metastasis in the sphenoid bone (*arrows*) with significant uptake in the same patient. (*From* Skovgaard D, Persson M, Brandt-Larsen M, et al. Safety, dosimetry and tumor detection ability of 68Ga-NOTA-AE105—a novel radioligand for uPAR PET imaging: first-in-humans study. J Nucl Med 2016 [Epub ahead of print]; with permission.)

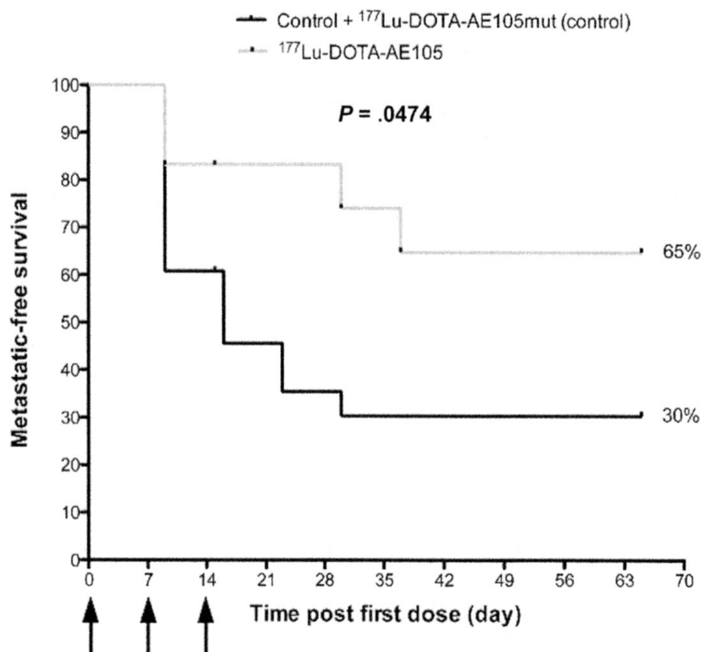

Fig. 5. uPAR targeted radionuclide therapy with 177Lu-DOTA-AE105 inhibits dissemination of metastatic prostate cancer. In a mouse model of disseminated prostate cancer, formation of metastatic lesions was followed with bioluminescence imaging. The study investigated three groups: (1) vehicle-treated controls, (2) control group treated with ^{177}Lu-labeled nonbinding control peptide, and (3) treatment group receiving ^{177}Lu-DOTA-A5015. Kaplan-Meier plot shows a significantly longer metastatic-free survival, when comparing the treatment group with a pool of the two control groups. The median metastatic-free survival was 12.5 days, 16 days, and greater than 65 days in vehicle, ^{177}Lu-DOTA-AE105mut, and ^{177}Lu-DOTA-AE105 treatment groups, respectively. Arrows indicate dosing days. (*From* Persson M, Juhl K, Rasmussen P, et al. uPAR targeted radionuclide therapy with (177) Lu-DOTA-AE105 inhibits dissemination of metastatic prostate cancer. Mol Pharm 2014;11:2801; © the American Chemical Society, with permission.)

trials. In this context uPAR PET can serve as a "companion diagnostics" to identifying patients likely to respond to a uPAR-targeted treatment. This will allow clinicians to noninvasively assess the presence, location, and extent of PC, and even for objective, quantitative monitoring of disease progression and treatment response. Therefore, uPAR PET may become key in practice of PC precision medicine.

Another innovative and most interesting perspective is to combine noninvasive PET imaging and targeted radionuclide therapy in the management of metastatic PC. The concept of using the same targeting ligand radiolabeled with either a positron-emitting nuclide for PET imaging or an alpha/beta emitter radionuclide for therapeutic intervention is currently gaining clinical momentum. Such a dual functionality aligns excellently with the concept of personalized and precision medicine. Targeted radiotherapy has shown promising results in several cancers, with somatostatin receptor-based targeting of neuroendocrine tumors being the most successful so far.[63] However, recently radionuclide therapy using ^{223}Ra (Xofigo), an alpha-emitter, for treatment of bone-related pain in castration-resistant PC with bone metastases was proven most successful.[64] In line with the theranostic concept, we have recently conducted two preclinical proof-of-concept studies using DOTA-AE105 conjugated with the beta-emitter ^{177}Lu for uPAR-targeted radionuclide therapy in colorectal cancer[65] and in metastatic PC.[66] In metastatic PC (**Fig. 5**), we found a significant reduction in metastatic lesions and longer overall metastatic-free survival in mice treated with ^{177}Lu-DOTA-AE105 compared with control animals, thus paving the way for a uPAR-mediated theranostic approach.[66]

SUMMARY

uPAR is a key player in and predictor of cancer invasion and metastatic spread in many cancer forms including PC. Accordingly, uPAR is an interesting molecular target for noninvasive PET imaging in cancer. In particular in PC, a better diagnostic and prognostic imaging biomarker is currently needed and uPAR PET may serve as such. Several uPAR-targeting PET ligands based on the high-affinity peptide ligand AE105 have been synthesized and evaluated successfully in human xenograft mouse models. Recently, we conducted a study of clinical uPAR PET in humans. In the first study in humans that also included patients with PC, we used ^{64}Cu-DOTA-AE105. Shortly thereafter, we performed another first-in-humans study again including patients with PC, a ^{68}Ga-labelled version of AE105 (^{68}Ga-NOTA-AE105). The clinical results so far are most promising and support continuation with large-scale clinical trials to determine the utility of uPAR PET in the management of patients with

PC, with the ultimate goal of improving outcome for the patients.

REFERENCES

1. Evangelista L, Briganti A, Fanti S, et al. New clinical indications for F/C-choline, new tracers for positron emission tomography and a promising hybrid device for prostate cancer staging: a systematic review of the literature. Eur Urol 2016;70(1):161–75.
2. Almasi CE, Brasso K, Iversen P, et al. Prognostic and predictive value of intact and cleaved forms of the urokinase plasminogen activator receptor in metastatic prostate cancer. Prostate 2011;71(8):899–907.
3. Rowe SP, Gorin MA, Allaf ME, et al. PET imaging of prostate-specific membrane antigen in prostate cancer: current state of the art and future challenges. Prostate Cancer Prostatic Dis 2016;19(3): 223–30.
4. Yang Y, Adelstein SJ, Kassis AI. General approach to identifying potential targets for cancer imaging by integrated bioinformatics analysis of publicly available genomic profiles. Mol Imaging 2011; 10(2):123–34.
5. Persson M, Kjaer A. Urokinase-type plasminogen activator receptor (uPAR) as a promising new imaging target: potential clinical applications. Clin Physiol Funct Imaging 2013;33(5):329–37.
6. Persson M, Skovgaard D, Brandt-Larsen M, et al. First-in-human uPAR PET: imaging of cancer aggressiveness. Theranostics 2015;5(12):1303–16.
7. Skovgaard D, Persson M, Brandt-Larsen M, et al. Safety, dosimetry and tumor detection ability of 68Ga-NOTA-AE105 - a novel radioligand for uPAR PET imaging: first-in-humans study. J Nucl Med 2016. [Epub ahead of print].
8. Jin JK, Dayyani F, Gallick GE. Steps in prostate cancer progression that lead to bone metastasis. Int J Cancer 2011;128(11):2545–61.
9. Persson M, Liu H, Madsen J, et al. First (18)F-labeled ligand for PET imaging of uPAR: in vivo studies in human prostate cancer xenografts. Nucl Med Biol 2013;40(5):618–24.
10. Duffy MJ. The urokinase plasminogen activator system: role in malignancy. Curr Pharm Des 2004;10(1): 39–49.
11. Boonstra MC, Verspaget HW, Ganesh S, et al. Clinical applications of the urokinase receptor (uPAR) for cancer patients. Curr Pharm Des 2011;17(19): 1890–910.
12. Ploug M. Structure-driven design of radionuclide tracers for non-invasive imaging of uPAR: the tale of a synthetic peptide antagonist. Theranostics 2012; 3(7):467–76.
13. Dano K, Behrendt N, Hoyer-Hansen G, et al. Plasminogen activation and cancer. Thromb Haemost 2005;93(4):676–81.
14. Noh H, Hong S, Huang S. Role of urokinase receptor in tumor progression and development. Theranostics 2013;3(7):487–95.
15. Mekkawy AH, Pourgholami MH, Morris DL. Involvement of urokinase-type plasminogen activator system in cancer: an overview. Med Res Rev 2014; 34(5):918–56.
16. Jacobsen B, Ploug M. The urokinase receptor and its structural homologue C4.4A in human cancer: expression, prognosis and pharmacological inhibition. Curr Med Chem 2008;15(25):2559–73.
17. Alpizar-Alpizar W, Christensen IJ, Santoni-Rugiu E, et al. Urokinase plasminogen activator receptor on invasive cancer cells: a prognostic factor in distal gastric adenocarcinoma. Int J Cancer 2012;131(4): E329–36.
18. Usher PA, Thomsen OF, Iversen P, et al. Expression of urokinase plasminogen activator, its receptor and type-1 inhibitor in malignant and benign prostate tissue. Int J Cancer 2005;113(6):870–80.
19. Gavrilov V, Kenzior O, Evans M, et al. Expression of urokinase plasminogen activator and receptor in conjunction with the ets family and AP-1 complex transcription factors in high grade prostate cancers. Eur J Cancer 2001;37:1033–40.
20. Kumano M, Miyake H, Muramaki M, et al. Expression of urokinase-type plasminogen activator system in prostate cancer: correlation with clinicopathological outcomes in patients undergoing radical prostatectomy. Urol Oncol 2009;27(2):180–6.
21. Cozzi PJ, Wang J, Delprado W, et al. Evaluation of urokinase plasminogen activator and its receptor in different grades of human prostate cancer. Hum Pathol 2006;37(11):1442–51.
22. Riddick AC, Shukla CJ, Pennington CJ, et al. Identification of degradome components associated with prostate cancer progression by expression analysis of human prostatic tissues. Br J Cancer 2005;92(12): 2171–80.
23. Gupta A, Lotan Y, Ashfaq R, et al. Predictive value of the differential expression of the urokinase plasminogen activation axis in radical prostatectomy patients. Eur Urol 2009;55(5):1124–33.
24. Al-Janabi O, Taubert H, Lohse-Fischer A, et al. Association of tissue mRNA and serum antigen levels of members of the urokinase-type plasminogen activator system with clinical and prognostic parameters in prostate cancer. Biomed Res Int 2014;2014: 972587.
25. Hoyer-Hansen G, Ronne E, Solberg H, et al. Urokinase plasminogen activator cleaves its cell surface receptor releasing the ligand-binding domain. J Biol Chem 1992;267(25):18224–9.
26. Almasi CE, Drivsholm L, Pappot H, et al. The liberated domain I of urokinase plasminogen activator receptor: a new tumour marker in small cell lung cancer. APMIS 2013;121(3):189–96.

27. Rasch MG, Lund IK, Almasi CE, et al. Intact and cleaved uPAR forms: diagnostic and prognostic value in cancer. Front Biosci 2008;13:6752–62.
28. Ganesh S, Sier CF, Griffioen G, et al. Prognostic relevance of plasminogen activators and their inhibitors in colorectal cancer. Cancer Res 1994;54(15): 4065–71.
29. Stephens RW, Nielsen HJ, Christensen IJ, et al. Plasma urokinase receptor levels in patients with colorectal cancer: relationship to prognosis. J Natl Cancer Inst 1999;91(10):869–74.
30. Riisbro R, Christensen IJ, Piironen T, et al. Prognostic significance of soluble urokinase plasminogen activator receptor in serum and cytosol of tumor tissue from patients with primary breast cancer. Clin Cancer Res 2002;8(5):1132–41.
31. Miyake H, Hara I, Yamanaka K, et al. Elevation of serum levels of urokinase-type plasminogen activator and its receptor is associated with disease progression and prognosis in patients with prostate cancer. Prostate 1999;39(2):123–9.
32. Shariat SF, Roehrborn CG, McConnell JD, et al. Association of the circulating levels of the urokinase system of plasminogen activation with the presence of prostate cancer and invasion, progression, and metastasis. J Clin Oncol 2007; 25(4):349–55.
33. Lippert B, Berg K, Hoejer-Hansen G, et al. Copenhagen uPAR prostate cancer (CuPCa) database: protocol and early results. Biomark Med 2016;10(2):209–16.
34. Ganesh S, Cornelius F. Urokinase receptor and colorectal cancer survival. Lancet 1994;344(8919): 401–2.
35. Shah RB, Bentley J, Jeffery Z, et al. Heterogeneity of PTEN and ERG expression in prostate cancer on core needle biopsies: implications for cancer risk stratification and biomarker sampling. Hum Pathol 2015;46(5):698–706.
36. Steuber T, Vickers A, Haese A, et al. Free PSA isoforms and intact and cleaved forms of urokinase plasminogen activator receptor in serum improve selection of patients for prostate cancer biopsy. Int J Cancer 2007;120(7):1499–504.
37. Kjellman A, Akre O, Gustafsson O, et al. Soluble urokinase plasminogen activator receptor as a prognostic marker in men participating in prostate cancer screening. J Intern Med 2011;269(3):299–305.
38. Wach S, Al-Janabi O, Weigelt K, et al. The combined serum levels of miR-375 and urokinase plasminogen activator receptor are suggested as diagnostic and prognostic biomarkers in prostate cancer. Int J Cancer 2015;137(6):1406–16.
39. James ML, Gambhir SS. A molecular imaging primer: modalities, imaging agents, and applications. Physiol Rev 2012;92(2):897–965.
40. Li D, Liu S, Shan H, et al. Urokinase plasminogen activator receptor (uPAR) targeted nuclear imaging and radionuclide therapy. Theranostics 2013;3(7): 507–15.
41. Li ZB, Niu G, Wang H, et al. Imaging of urokinase-type plasminogen activator receptor expression using a 64Cu-labeled linear peptide antagonist by microPET. Clin Cancer Res 2008;14(15):4758–66.
42. Persson M, Madsen J, Ostergaard S, et al. Quantitative PET of human urokinase-type plasminogen activator receptor with 64Cu-DOTA-AE105: implications for visualizing cancer invasion. J Nucl Med 2012; 53(1):138–45.
43. Persson M, Madsen J, Ostergaard S, et al. (68)Ga-labeling and in vivo evaluation of a uPAR binding DOTA- and NODAGA-conjugated peptide for PET imaging of invasive cancers. Nucl Med Biol 2012; 39(4):560–9.
44. Persson M, Hosseini M, Madsen J, et al. Improved PET imaging of uPAR expression using new (64) Cu-labeled cross-bridged peptide ligands: comparative in vitro and in vivo studies. Theranostics 2013; 3(9):618–32.
45. Persson M, Nedergaard MK, Brandt-Larsen M, et al. Urokinase-type plasminogen activator receptor as a potential PET biomarker in glioblastoma. J Nucl Med 2016;57(2):272–8.
46. Boswell CA, Regino CA, Baidoo KE, et al. Synthesis of a cross-bridged cyclam derivative for peptide conjugation and 64Cu radiolabeling. Bioconjug Chem 2008;19(7):1476–84.
47. Bass LA, Wang M, Welch MJ, et al. In vivo transchelation of copper-64 from TETA-octreotide to superoxide dismutase in rat liver. Bioconjug Chem 2000; 11(4):527–32.
48. Sun Y, Ma X, Cheng K, et al. Strained cyclooctyne as a molecular platform for construction of multimodal imaging probes. Angew Chem Int Ed Engl 2015; 54(20):5981–4.
49. Juhl K, Christensen A, Persson M, et al. Peptide-based optical uPAR imaging for surgery: in vivo testing of ICG-Glu-Glu-AE105. PLoS One 2016; 11(2):e0147428.
50. Yang L, Peng XH, Wang YA, et al. Receptor-targeted nanoparticles for in vivo imaging of breast cancer. Clin Cancer Res 2009;15(14):4722–32.
51. Yang L, Mao H, Cao Z, et al. Molecular imaging of pancreatic cancer in an animal model using targeted multifunctional nanoparticles. Gastroenterology 2009;136(5):1514–25.e2.
52. Liu D, Overbey D, Watkinson L, et al. Synthesis and characterization of an (111)in-labeled peptide for the in vivo localization of human cancers expressing the urokinase-type plasminogen activator receptor (uPAR). Bioconjug Chem 2009;20(5):888–94.
53. LeBeau AM, Sevillano N, King ML, et al. Imaging the urokinase plasminongen activator receptor in preclinical breast cancer models of acquired drug resistance. Theranostics 2014;4(3):267–79.

54. Ides J, Thomae D, Wyffels L, et al. Synthesis and in vivo preclinical evaluation of an (18)F labeled uPA inhibitor as a potential PET imaging agent. Nucl Med Biol 2014;41(6):477–87.
55. Persson M, El Ali HH, Binderup T, et al. Dosimetry of 64Cu-DOTA-AE105, a PET tracer for uPAR imaging. Nucl Med Biol 2014;41(3):290–5.
56. Deloar HM, Fujiwara T, Shidahara M, et al. Estimation of absorbed dose for 2-[F-18]fluoro-2-deoxy-D-glucose using whole-body positron emission tomography and magnetic resonance imaging. Eur J Nucl Med 1998;25(6):565–74.
57. Velikyan I. Prospective of (6)(8)Ga-radiopharmaceutical development. Theranostics 2013;4(1):47–80.
58. Shariat S, Roehrborn CG. Using biopsy to detect prostate cancer. Rev Urol 2008;10(4):262–80.
59. Maurer T, Eiber M, Schwaiger M, et al. Current use of PSMA-PET in prostate cancer management. Nat Rev Urol 2016;13(4):226–35.
60. Leiblich A, Stevens D, Sooriakumaran P. The utility of molecular imaging in prostate cancer. Curr Urol Rep 2016;17(3):26.
61. Mazar AP, Ahn RW, O'Halloran TV. Development of novel therapeutics targeting the Urokinase Plasminogen Activator Receptor (uPAR) and their translation toward the clinic. Curr Pharm Des 2011;17(19):1970–8.
62. Rabbani SA, Ateeq B, Arakelian A, et al. An anti-urokinase plasminogen activator receptor antibody (ATN-658) blocks prostate cancer invasion, migration, growth, and experimental skeletal metastasis in vitro and in vivo. Neoplasia 2010;12(10):778–88.
63. Brabander T, Teunissen JJ, Van Eijck CH, et al. Peptide receptor radionuclide therapy of neuroendocrine tumours. Best Pract Res Clin Endocrinol Metab 2016;30(1):103–14.
64. Humm JL, Sartor O, Parker C, et al. Radium-223 in the treatment of osteoblastic metastases: a critical clinical review. Int J Radiat Oncol Biol Phys 2015;91(5):898–906.
65. Persson M, Rasmussen P, Madsen J, et al. New peptide receptor radionuclide therapy of invasive cancer cells: in vivo studies using 177Lu-DOTA-AE105 targeting uPAR in human colorectal cancer xenografts. Nucl Med Biol 2012;39(7):962–9.
66. Persson M, Juhl K, Rasmussen P, et al. uPAR targeted radionuclide therapy with (177)Lu-DOTA-AE105 inhibits dissemination of metastatic prostate cancer. Mol Pharm 2014;11(8):2796–806.

PET/Computed Tomography for Radiation Therapy Planning of Prostate Cancer

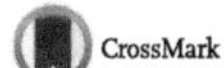

Kalevi J.A. Kairemo, MD, PhD, MSc (Eng)[a,b,c,*]

KEYWORDS

• Prostate cancer • PET • External beam radiation therapy • Dose planning • Biological target volume • PET radiopharmaceuticals

KEY POINTS

- Biological target volume (BTV) definition for external beam radiation therapy (EBRT) can be made by several PET tracers in prostate cancer.
- Preliminary research supports PET techniques in clinical decision making.
- Due to a lack of prospective and randomized trials, and single-institution experiences, the PET dose planning method cannot yet be recommended as clinical routine.

Radical prostatectomy (RP) and definite radiotherapy are 2 main treatments for locoregional prostate cancer. RP may include limited and extended pelvic lymph node dissection (PLND). Radiotherapy involves EBRT or brachytherapy or their combinations. Brachytherapy gives little radiation to surrounding normal organs.

EBRT is developed from conventional 2-D EBRT to 3-D conformal radiotherapy, image-guided radiotherapy, intensity-modulated radiotherapy (IMRT), and volumetric-modulated arch therapy (VMAT). High-risk patients are often treated with combinatory therapies in addition to RP and EBRT, such as androgen deprivation therapy (ADT).

BRIEF INTRODUCTION TO EXTERNAL BEAM RADIATION THERAPY METHODS IN PROSTATE CANCER

External Beam Radiation Therapy

Definitive EBRT is radiotherapy with a curative intention. EBRT for intermediate-risk patients mainly involves image-guided radiotherapy, IMRT, ADT, and a high radiation dose of 75 Gy to 86 Gy.[1] EBRT mainly uses a conventional fractionation schedule, a dose of 1.8 Gy to 2.0 Gy for each fraction, and 5 fractions each week. Patients with low-risk and intermediate-risk had a better prostate-specific antigen (PSA) recurrence-free survival after high-dose IMRT than high-risk patients,[2] and controlled trials of EBRT showed that a high radiation dose for localized prostate cancer increased PSA recurrence-free survival.

EBRT may be given as an adjuvant after surgery (RP and PLND). Previously, patients with node-negative disease were given adjuvant EBRT after RP if the risk of occult metastases in regional lymph nodes were estimated to be higher than 15% based on clinical findings.[3–5]

Staging with PET/computed tomography (CT) is a noninvasive alternative to PLND. Retrospective studies indicated that survival increased if adjuvant EBRT was added to the treatment of patients with pelvic lymph node metastases given

Disclosure Statement: The author has nothing to disclose.

[a] Department of Molecular Radiotherapy, Docrates Cancer Center, Saukonpaadenranta 2, Helsinki FI-00180, Finland; [b] Department of Nuclear Medicine, Docrates Cancer Center, Saukonpaadenranta 2, Helsinki FI-00180, Finland; [c] Department of Nuclear Medicine, The University of Texas MD Anderson Cancer Center, 1400 Pressler Street, Houston, TX 77030, USA
* Docrates Cancer Center, Saukonpaadenranta 2, Helsinki FI-00180, Finland.
E-mail address: kalevi.kairemo@docrates.fi

PET Clin 12 (2017) 257–267
http://dx.doi.org/10.1016/j.cpet.2016.12.003
1556-8598/17/

RP, PLND, and ADT[6]; adjuvant EBRT after RP improved survival in a controlled trial of patients with localized prostate cancer.

Intensity-Modulated Radiotherapy or Volumetric-Modulated Arch Therapy with RapidArc

VMAT (such as RapidArc [Varian, Palo Alto, CA]) needs shorter treatment time than IMRT (such as ThomoTherapy [Accuray, Sunnyvale, CA]) for each fraction. A short treatment time reduces the risk for organ movements during treatment, allowing smaller margins around the gross tumor volume (GTV). Plans for IMRT and VMAT give similar dose-volume histograms. **Fig. 1** shows the differences in the dose distribution between IMRT and VMAT. In this example, the dose to urinary bladder differs marginally, and these methods have been compared in the literature for treating prostate cancer.[7] Another article[8] compared EBRT planning for IMRT, intensity-modulated proton therapy, and RapidArc, and the investigators preferred RapidArc. CyberKnife, and RapidArc[9] and did not find advantages between choosing Cyberknife or RapidArc. TomoTherapy and RapidArc have also been compared in the management of prostate cancer.[10,11] Ost and colleagues[12] compared IMRT and VMAT as a boost for GTV_{PET}; VMAT allowed an increased median dose boost for GTV_{PET} of 93 Gy with better sparing of radiation to the rectum. CT data from PET/CT scans could be transferred directly to CT planning systems for radiotherapy.

External Beam Radiation Therapy and Brachytherapy

The new radiotherapy technologies allowed a high radiation dose to the planned target volume (PTV) and a low radiation dose to surrounding normal organs.[13] Radiotherapy may also be improved otherwise: 2 randomized trials showed a better PSA recurrence-free survival from combined IMRT and brachytherapy.[14,15] Also, intermediate-risk patients could benefit from combining IMRT and brachytherapy increased radiation dose and combination improved PSA recurrence-free survival compared with IMRT as monotherapy.[16] The bimodal radiotherapy added little toxicity. Brachytherapy as monotherapy also has less toxicity than EBRT. Toxicity may be reduced by installing a gel to increase the distance between gross intraprostatic tumor volume and rectum during the radiotherapy.

PET/COMPUTED TOMOGRAPHY FOR RADIATION THERAPY PLANNING OF PROSTATE CANCER

Molecular imaging is the only way of defining BTV for EBRT and may be used for advanced targeting in dose planning and dose painting.[17,18] In the literature, there are only a few reports about the EBRT response when dose planning is based on BTV target definition in prostate cancer.

PET Tracers

Centers with departments for nuclear medicine and access to a cyclotron increasingly use PET/CT for imaging of prostate cancer. The United States uses mainly sodium ^{18}F-fluoride (NaF) and ^{18}F-fluorodeoxyglucose (FDG).

FDG PET/CT, and now maybe *trans*-1-amino-3-^{18}F-fluorocyclobutanecarboxylic acid (^{18}F-FACBC), which received Food and Drug Administration approval in June 2016. Europe prefers ^{11}C-choline and ^{18}F-choline(FCH) PET/CT,[19] because FCH is a registered radiopharmaceutical in more than 15 European Union countries. Radiolabeled choline PET/CT scans provide whole-body staging and delineate GTVs in a single test. Previous meta-analyses summarized the clinical use of radiolabeled choline PET/CT for prostate cancer.[19] A summary of PET tracers is presented in **Table 1**.

Target Delineation and Biological Target Volume

At present, there is no consensus on irradiation treatment volumes for high-risk primary or

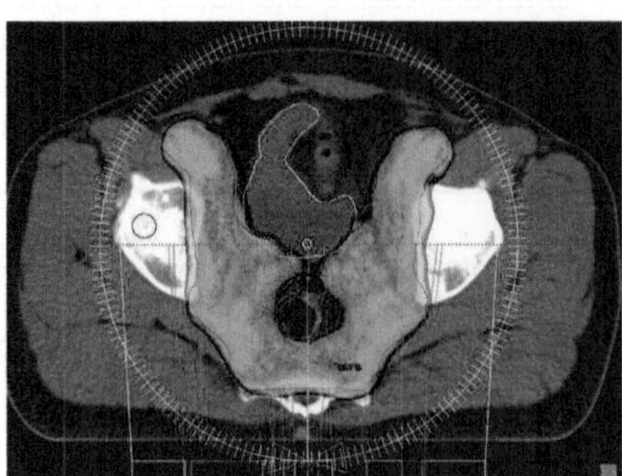
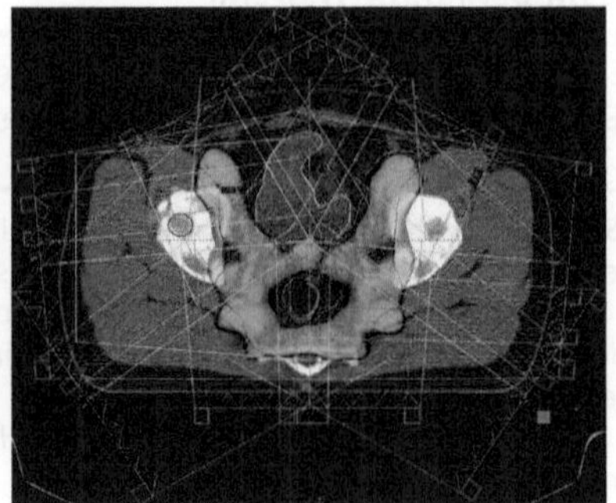

Fig. 1. Dose color wash presentation, 85%, demonstrates the difference between VMAT and IMRT.

Table 1
PET tracers in prostate cancer

Target	Event	Tracer	Significance
glut1, *glut3*, hexokinase	Glycolysis	FDG	Prognostic, aggressive disease
Choline kinase	Membrane synthesis	FCH; ^{11}C-CHO	(T)NM staging
L-amino acid transporter	Amino acid transport	FACBC; ^{11}C-Met	(T)N(M) staging
Androgen receptor	Hormone receptor	FDHT	AR-status
PSMA	Transmembrane protein	^{68}Ga-PSMA; DCFBC; ^{89}Zr-PSMA-MAb; ^{18}F-DCFPyL	TNM staging
Acetyl CoA	Lipid synthesis	^{11}C-acetate	(T)NM-staging
DNA	Cell proliferation	FLT	proliferation activity, response evaluation
Hydroxyapatite	Bone formation	Na ^{18}F	skeletal disease localization

Abbreviations: ^{11}C-CHO, ^{11}C-choline; ^{11}C-Met, ^{11}C-methione; ^{18}F-DCFBC, N-[N-[(S)-1,3-dicarboxypropyl]carbamoyl]-4-^{18}F-fluorobenzyl-L-cysteine; ^{18}F-FDHT, $^{16}\beta$-[^{18}F-]fluoro-5α-dihydrotestosterone; ^{18}F-DCFPyL, (S)-2-[3-((S)-1-carboxy-5-[3-(6-^{18}F-fluoropyridine)carbonyl)amino)pentyl)ureido]-pentanedioic acid; ^{89}Zr-PSMA-Mab, ^{89}Zr-labeled monoclonal antibodies against prostate-specific membrane antigen; Na^{18}F, sodium ^{18}F-fluoride; AR, androgen receptor; FCH, ^{18}F-choline or ^{18}F-methylcholine.

advanced prostate cancer. Conventional imaging modalities, such as CT, MR imaging, and transrectal ultrasound, are considered suboptimal for treatment decisions.[20] Molecular imaging is the only possibility in defining BTV for EBRT. Some investigators suggest that choline PET/CT should be used for the selection and delineation of clinical target volumes (CTVs), when the BTVs protrude outside the prostate gland or locate in the prostate fossa.[18] The volumes GTV, CTV, and PTV are defined in detail in the International Commission on Radiation Units and Measurements report.[21]

CLINICAL EXAMPLES

In the literature, there is only 1 retrospective study where dose delineation, performed either with metabolic PET/CT or with conventional morphologic dose planning based on CT and/or MR imaging, has been compared.[17] Both groups were treated with VMAT based on target definition by PET/CT (first group) or conventional imaging (second group). The median prescribed EBRT doses (grays) to primary tumors, seminal vesicles, local lymph nodes, and bone metastases were similar in both groups and a total of 64 lesions were treated. Biochemical relapse occurred in 16.6% (1 of 6) of the patients in the first group and 50% (3 of 6) patients in the second group during the follow-up period. Clinical manifestation of disease occurred in 33% (2 of 6) patients of the first group and in 83.3% (5 of 6) patients in the second; 4 patients in the first group had no biochemical relapse and no clinical manifestation during the follow-up period. The difference in the duration of progression-free period was statistically significant between the groups (P<.010), 16.5 $\pm$ 5.4 (10–24) months in the first group and 4.6 $\pm$ 2.9 (2–10) months in the second.[17]

Because patients with PET/CT-based VMAT had lower incidence of biochemical relapse, fewer clinical manifestations, and longer, statistically significant duration of progression-free period compared with patients treated with VMAT based on conventional imaging, preliminary results suggested introducing BTV definition based on PET imaging for VMAT in the EBRT of prostate cancer.

METHOD EXAMPLE

External Bean Radiation Therapy Contouring

The rectum was contoured with its contents, as recommended by quantitative analysis of normal tissue effects in the clinic (QUANTEC),[22] and the bladder using a single CT simulation image. To minimize bladder volume variation, patients emptied the bladder and drank 200 mL of water 30 minutes prior to all imaging and treatment sessions.

PTVprost was contoured using the MR (T2-weighted) image (CTV) with a 5-mm margin. PTVsv was most often painted according to the CT image (CTV) with a 5-mm margin. PTVln was based on the CT image and was contoured according to the Radiation Therapy Oncology Group consensus.[23] PTVln covered all visible lymph node metastases in CT, MR imaging, or PET-CT. Bone metastases were most often drawn using the PET images, fused with dose planning CT and MR imaging. PTVbone had a 5-mm margin for GTVbone.

Eaxmple of External Bean Radiation Therapy Technique

The RapidArc VMAT technique was applied in all patients individually to provide best possible treatment; 2 full arcs were typically used, but for some patients with complex PTVs a complementary arc was introduced. Treatment planning was done using the Eclipse dose calculation analytical anisotropic algorithm (Varian). Radiation therapy course began with large fields, including lymph nodes, metastases, seminal vesicles, and prostate. After 50 Gy to 56 Gy (25–28 fractions), $PTV_{prostate}$ was the only target. The total dose to prostate ranged between 76 Gy and 80 Gy with 2 Gy/d fractionation. PTVsv was similarly fractionated as the prostate, whereas PTVln fractionation was 1.8 Gy/d. For bone metastases, the fractionation varied: typically, PTVbone was as lymph nodes during the first 5 weeks (45 Gy/25 fractions) and then boosted to higher doses, with variable fractions (1.8 Gy–3.5 Gy) for bone metastases ranging from 39 Gy to 76 Gy depending on the number and location of metastases. Typical doses are summarized in **Box 1**. Patients were treated with a linear accelerator equipped with on-board imaging. Orthogonal x-ray imaging was used daily to match prostate markers with the digitally reconstructed radiograph image. Cone-beam CT imaging was used in first 3 fractions to check bladder and rectum filling and its influence on the PTVs. Even large (>5-mm) table corrections based on the fiducial markers were routinely accepted, if target coverage was confirmed with cone-beam CT imaging. If there was a difference between the bones and the markers, the PTVbone margin was increased in concordance with the daily prostate movement.

Box 1
Summary of target delineation principle and planned doses in high-risk prostate cancer

- High-risk prostate cancer
  - GTV = prostate + visible metastases
    - Prostate based on fusion MR imaging
    - Metastases based on PET, MR imaging, and CT
  - CTV = prostate + SV + regional LN
    - Based on CT
  - PTV = CTV + treatment margin (5–10 mm)
- PTV_prostate: 78–80 Gy
- PTV_SV: 50–56 Gy
- PTV_LN: 45–50 Gy
- PTV_metastases: 45–78 Gy

Volumes of GTV, CTV, and PTV are presented and typical doses to prostate, SN, LN, and distant metastases are given.
Abbreviations: LN, lymph nodes; SN, seminal vesicles.

CASE ILLUSTRATIONS

Some practical cases are presented, where PET has been applied in dose delineation.

Case 1

^{18}F-choline or ^{18}F-methylcholine (FCH)/sodium fluoride (NaF)-PET studies in for VMAT EBRT planning (RapidArc). On the left of **Fig. 2**, FCH-PET demonstrates pelvic soft tissue disease (prostate), oligometastatic skeletal disease, and NaF-PET skeletal disease in the same locations. On the right of **Fig. 2**, examples of treatment plans are shown. This patient was originally treated with EBRT combined with ADT. A biochemical relapse was observed. Salvage treatment with VMAT was given to oligometastatic disease with response (see **Fig. 2**).

Case 2

FCH/NaF-PET studies in for VMAT EBRT planning (RapidArc). On the left of **Fig. 3**, FCH-PET demonstrates cerebral (meningeal) soft tissue disease, oligometastatic skeletal disease, and NaF-PET skeletal disease in the same locations. On the right of **Fig. 3**, examples of treatment plans are shown. This patient was treated RP, with EBRT combined with ADT. A biochemical relapse was observed in the skeleton. Palliation treatment with VMAT was given to oligometastatic disease with response (see **Fig. 3**).

Case 3

NaF-PET studies in for VMAT EBRT planning (RapidArc). On the left of **Fig. 4**, NaF-PET demonstrates pelvic skeletal disease in multiple locations. On the right of **Fig. 4**, examples of treatment plans are shown. This patient was treated with EBRT combined with ADT. A biochemical relapse was observed in the skeleton. Palliation treatment with VMAT was given to oligometastatic disease with response (see **Fig. 4**).

Case 4

FACBC-PET studies in for VMAT EBRT planning (RapidArc). On the left of **Fig. 5**, FACBC-PET demonstrates soft tissue disease (lymph node). On the right of **Fig. 5**, examples of treatment plans are shown.

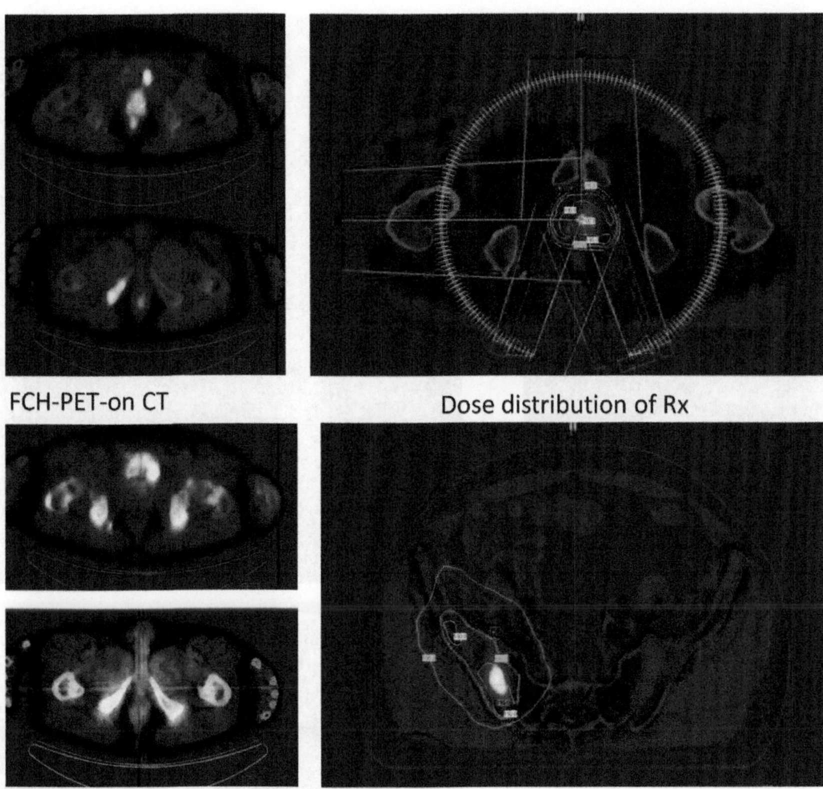

Fig. 2. FCH/NaF-PET studies in for VMAT EBRT planning (RapidArc). On the left, FCH-PET demonstrates pelvic soft tissue disease (prostate), oligometastatic skeletal disease, and NaF-PET skeletal disease in the same location. On the right, examples of treatment plans are shown. This patient was originally treated with EBRT combined with ADT. A biochemical relapse was observed. Salvage treatment with VMAT was given to oligometastatic disease with response.

This patient was treated with RP. A biochemical relapse was observed in soft tissue. Treatment with VMAT was given with response (see **Fig. 5**).

Case 5

Gallium-68 (^{68}Ga)–prostate-specific membrane antigen (PSMA)–PET studies in for VMAT EBRT planning (RapidArc). On the left of **Fig. 6**, ^{68}Ga-PSMA–PET demonstrates oligometastatic skeletal disease. On the right of **Fig. 6**, examples of treatment plans are shown. This patient was treated earlier with EBRT and chemotherapy. A biochemical relapse was observed mainly in the skeleton. Palliative treatment with VMAT was given with response (see **Fig. 6**).

REVIEW OF THE LITERATURE

Change of Treatment Plans After PET/Computed Tomography

PET/CT changed treatment plans for many patients.[18,19] In an article by Souvatzoglou and colleagues,[24] 5 of 11 (46%) patients with biochemical recurrence and positive choline PET/CT had lesions outside the prostate bed. So the team extended the PTV for salvage EBRT. After EBRT, 56% of the patients had PSA recurrence-free survival for a follow-up of median 51 months. Jereczeck-Fossa and colleagues[25] undertook 82 PET/CT scans and changed treatment due to findings on 22 (27%) scans. Moussaid and colleagues[26] changed planned salvage EBRT for 6 of 11 (54%) PET/CT-positive patients.

Experience in External Beam Radiation Therapy Guided by PET/Computed Tomography

Of articles that reported PET/CT-guided planning of EBRT, most used radiolabeled choline PET/CT.[18] Six articles evaluated localized prostate cancer and reported 178 patients with PET/CT-guided planning of a boost to GTV_{PET}.[18] In 3 articles, Pinkawa and colleagues[27–29] simultaneously integrated a boost with 80 Gy for the GTV_{PET} with a dose of 76 Gy for the whole prostate. The small boost did not increase toxicity for normal organs at risk. The small boost did not increase toxicity

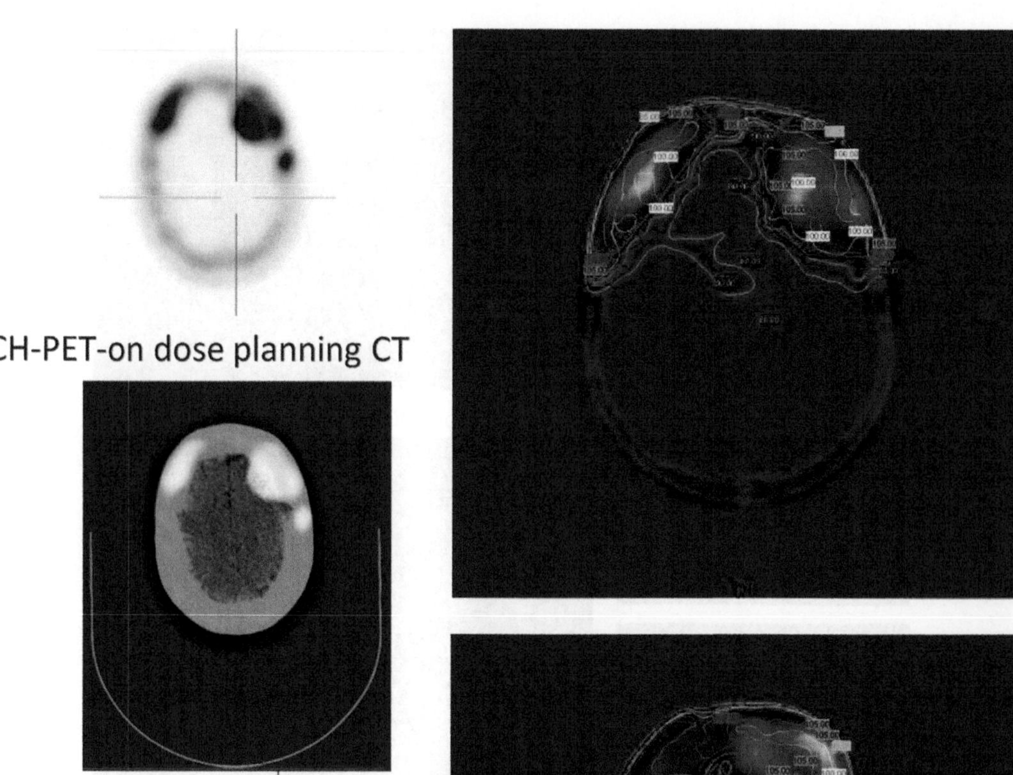

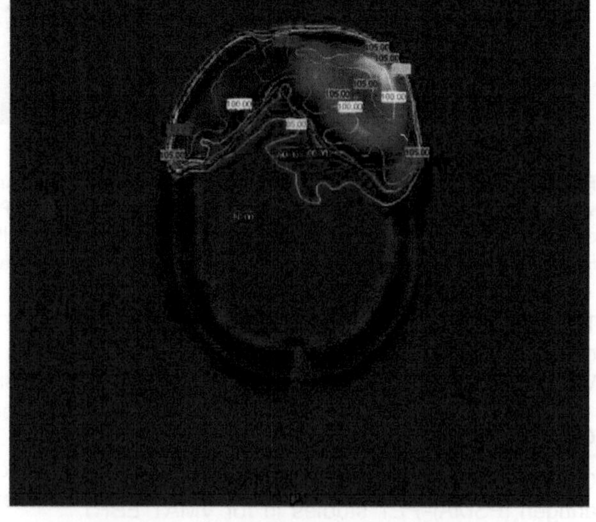

Fig. 3. FCH/NaF-PET studies in for VMAT EBRT planning (RapidArc). On the left, FCH-PET demonstrates cerebral (meningeal) soft tissue disease, oligometastatic skeletal disease, and NaF-PET skeletal disease in the same locations. On the right, examples of treatment plans are shown. This patient was treated RP with EBRT combined with ADT. A biochemical relapse was observed in the skeleton. Palliation treatment with VMAT was given to oligometastatic disease with response.

for normal organs at risk. Seppälä and colleagues[30] gave a simultaneously integrated boost of 90 Gy to the GTV_{PET} combined with 78 Gy to the prostate.

Four articles evaluated pelvic lymph node metastases and reported 254 patients with PET/CT-guided planning of EBRT for the pelvic lymph nodes.[18] Two articles followed patients for median 28 months (range 14–50 months): Casamassima and colleagues[31] found that 13 of 25 patients with lymph node lesions remained in remission to end of follow-up; Wurschmidt and colleagues[32] found that 2 of 4 patients with node-positive lesions remained in remission during follow-up. In a study by Picchio and colleagues,[33] 66 of 94 (70%) treatments gave a greater than 50% PSA reduction for 83 patients after helical TomoTherapy for recurrent prostate cancer with lymph node metastases; 36 of the 83 patients (47%) did

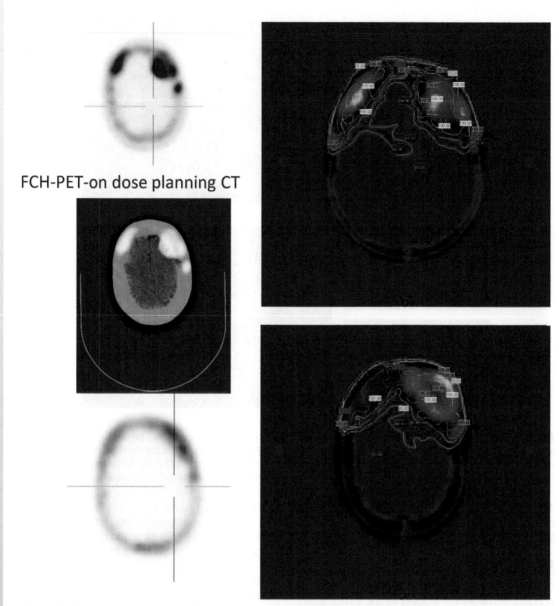

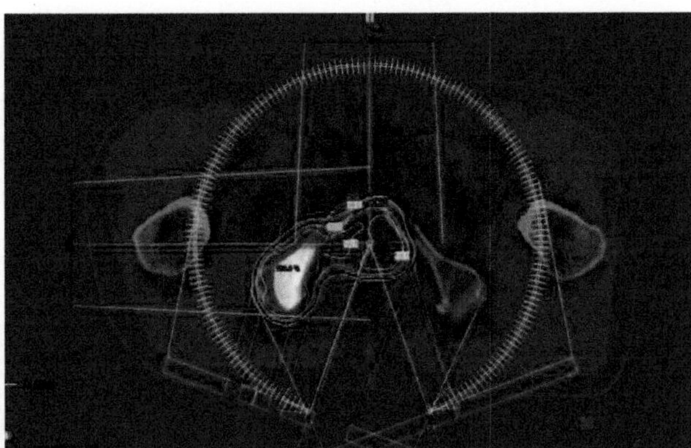

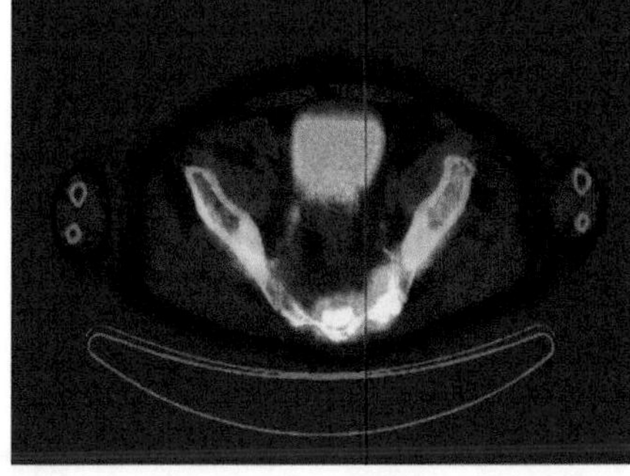

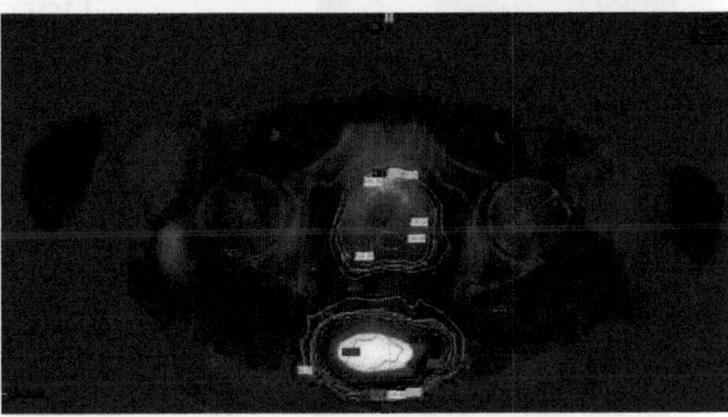

NaF-PET-on CT

Dose distribution of Rx

Fig. 4. NaF-PET studies in for VMAT EBRT planning (RapidArc). On the left, NaF-PET demonstrates pelvic skeletal disease in multiple locations. On the right, examples of treatment plans are shown. This patient was treated with EBRT combined with ADT. A biochemical relapse was observed in the skeleton. Palliation treatment with VMAT was given to oligometastatic disease with response.

not develop a second recurrence during the first short phase of follow-up; and 4 of 12 patients remained in partial PSA remission for 1 year.

Salvage External Beam Radiation Therapy Guided by Restaging with PET/Computed Tomography

Patients with biochemical recurrence after radiation therapy and a local site of recurrence had long-lasting response after salvage RP.[34] For other patients, radiolabeled choline PET/CT detected only a site of recurrence in pelvic lymph nodes.[35] A study undertook salvage lymph node dissection for sites of recurrence in pelvic and retroperitoneal lymph nodes[36]; 25 of 36 (69%) patients had a partial biochemical remission. Pelvic lymph node metastases have also been treated with pelvic radiotherapy. Radiation oncologists gave a simultaneously integrated boost to the site of recurrence together with the EBRT for the PTV.[37] In a study of 93 patients with sites of recurrence in lymph nodes, patients had a better biochemical recurrence-free survival if they had been treated with salvage lymph node dissection combined with radiotherapy than if they had been treated with only salvage lymph node dissection.[38] In 1 study, 4 of 11 (36%) patients underwent a change of treatment decisions after a PET/CT.[24] In a second study, choline F 18 PET/CT detected a site of recurrence in the prostate bed.[39] The detected site of recurrence was treated with a boost up to 80 Gy.

A study reported PET/CT as a prognostic factor.[36] In a study of salvage EBRT for abdominal lymph nodes, patients with recurrence in pelvic lymph nodes had a better disease-free survival than patients with recurrence in retroperitoneal lymph nodes.[37] In an Italian study of salvage radiation therapy, the patients who had a site in a pelvic lymph node and a small tumor volume less than 0.64 cm^3 had 100% biochemical recurrence-free survival for 5 years.[36] In contrast, all patients who had sites of recurrence in lymph nodes outside the pelvic region and a tumor volume greater than 0.64 cm^3 developed biochemical recurrence within 4 years.

There is an ongoing randomized phase II trial, Surveillance or metastasis-directed Therapy for

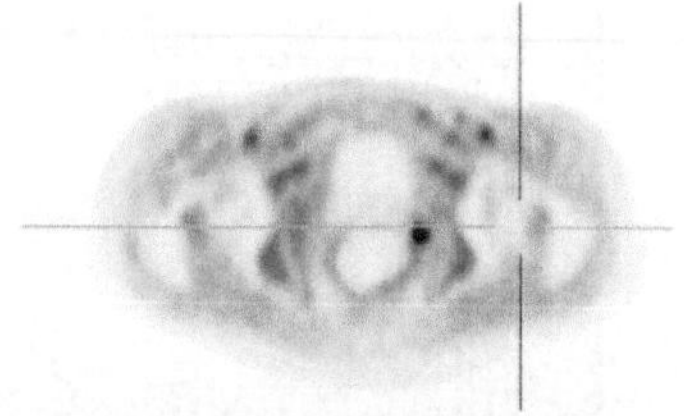

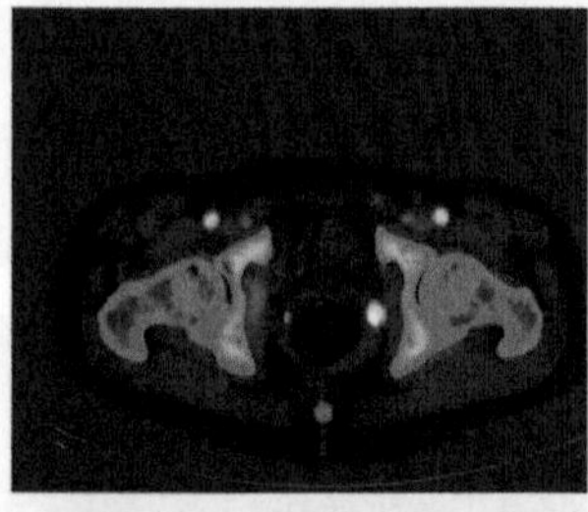

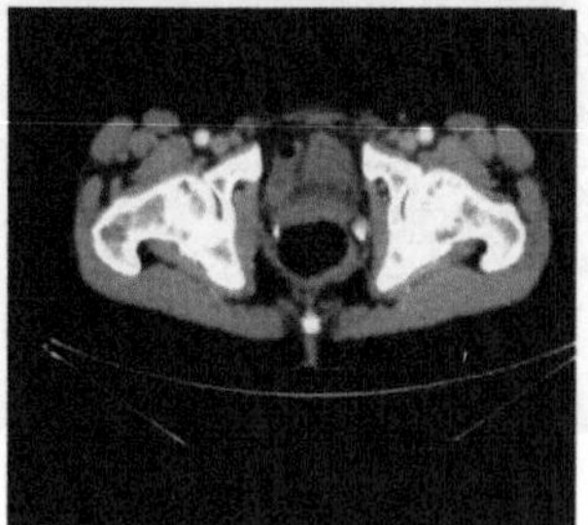

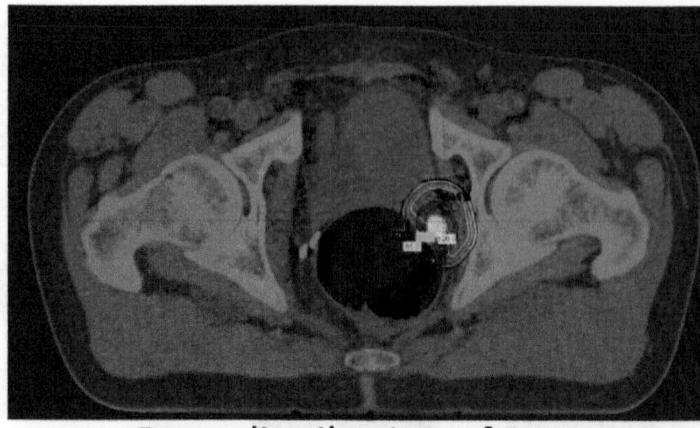

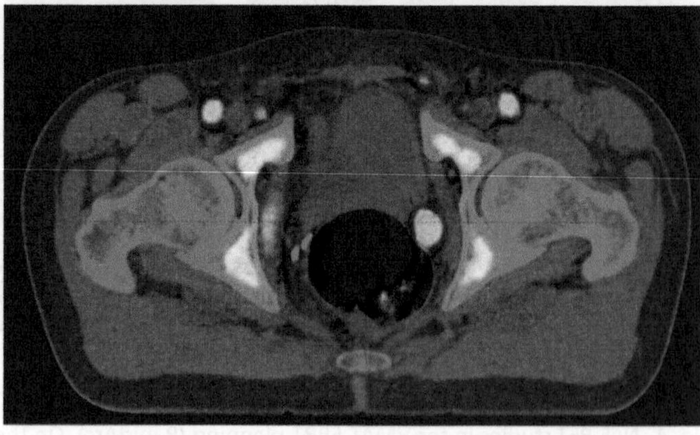

Fig. 5. FACBC-PET studies in for VMAT EBRT planning (RapidArc). On the left, FACBC-PET demonstrates soft tissue disease (lymph node). On the right, examples of treatment plans are shown. This patient was treated with RP. A biochemical relapse was observed in soft tissue. Treatment with VMAT was given with response.

OligoMetastatic Prostate cancer recurrence (STOMP).[40] The trial includes patients with biochemical recurrence after RP and radiation therapy and investigates whether salvage treatment of metastatic sites of recurrence guided by radiolabeled choline PET/CT may prolong disease progression-free survival.

FUTURE DIRECTIONS

Although PET/CTs using novel tracers hold great potential, the widespread availability of them is still limited and their value and impact on management and survival of men with advanced prostate cancer has not been proved. Almost all of the studies using PET/CT with new tracers are single-center protocols, neither prospective nor randomized, with questionable definition of reference standard, thus leading to lack of evidence to allow recommending such procedures for everyday practice.

With regard to the management of men with oligometastatic castration-naïve prostate cancer, this is an area where research should be conducted to define optimal management strategies. The available data on treatment of men with oligometastatic prostate cancer are sparse and heterogeneous with regard to definitions, patient populations, imaging methods, and treatment approaches applied. Therefore, for daily clinical practice, which is what, for example, Advanced Prostate Cancer Consensus Conference recommendations aim for, there is no consensus for a specific therapeutic approach due to insufficient data.[41]

VMAT is a new radiation treatment technique that can create highly conformal dose distribution in a short time. Despite wide use of this technique, a majority of published data on VMAT are dosimetric planning studies with limited clinical outcome data.[20] VMAT enables optimization and delivery of a complex dose painting treatment plans.[42]

In clinical practice, when VMAT is applied for the treatment of prostate cancer, the prostate or both the prostate and the seminal vesicles[43,44] are defined as a primary target volume by some investigators, but other investigators have also included the pelvic lymph nodes.[45]

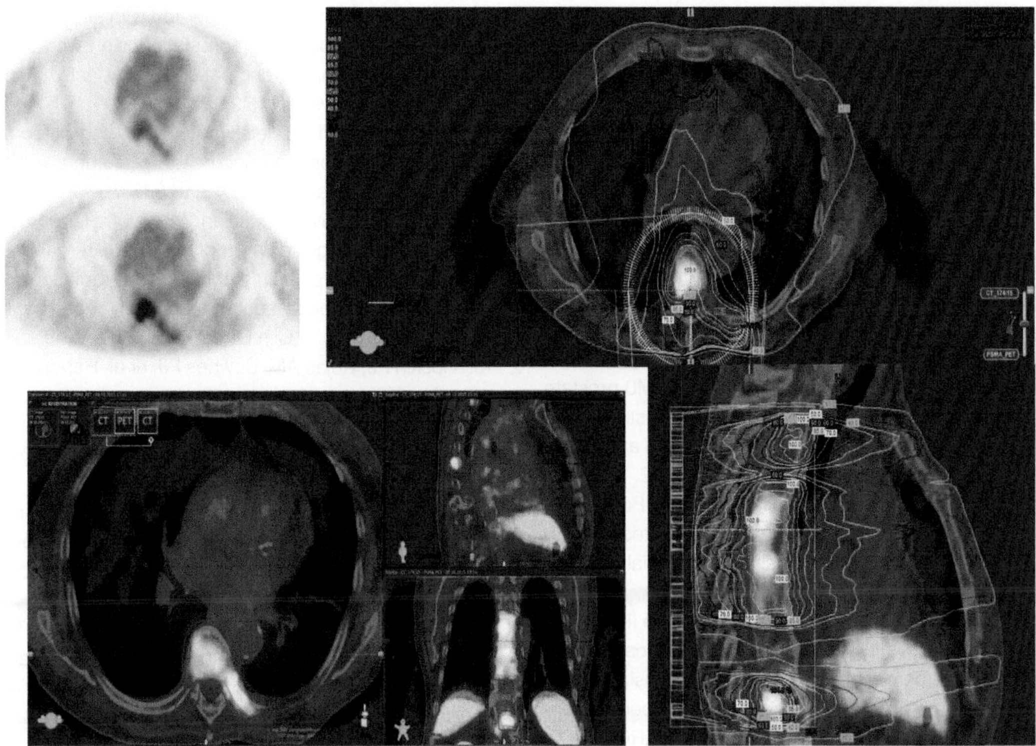

Fig. 6. ^{68}Ga-PSMA–PET studies in for VMAT EBRT planning (RapidArc). On the left, ^{68}Ga-PSMA–PET demonstrates thoracic skeletal disease in multiple locations (*upper left corner*). Fusion images are shown in the lower left corner (transaxial, sagittal, and coronal projections). These demonstrate disease in the transverse process besides vertebral body. On the right, examples of treatment plans are shown (transaxial view [*upper panel*]; sagittal view, [*lower panel*]). This patient was treated with EBRT because of back pain. Palliation treatment with VMAT was given to this oligometastatic disease with excellent response to tumor burden and pain.

The author's own retrospective analysis[19] found that the patients with advanced prostate cancer using PET/CT-based EBRT dose planning had lower incidence for biochemical relapse, fewer clinical manifestations of disease, and longer duration of disease-free period and biochemical stability compared with patients whose dose planning was based on conventional imaging.

The conventional radiologic images primarily provide anatomic information, whereas biological images reveal metabolic, functional, physiologic, genotypic, and phenotypic data. In contrast to morphologic imaging, the new metabolic and noninvasive imaging methods may offer 3-D radiobiological information.[46] This might be important for understanding the difference between the dose delineation methods and how they influence the outcome of radiotherapy. As is already known, theranostic imaging for radiation oncology is the use of molecular and functional imaging to define the distribution of radiation in 4-D—3-D plus time—of radiotherapy alone or combined with other treatments. Target changes can be monitored during EBRT, because several new imaging targets for PET, single-photon emission CT, and MR spectroscopy allow variations in microenvironmental or cellular phenotypes that modulate the effect of radiation to be mapped in 3-D. This is, however, complex and almost impossible during a clinical routine EBRT course.

Dose painting by numbers is a strategy by which the dose distribution delivered by EBRT is prescribed in 4-D. This approach may change the way that radiotherapy is prescribed and planned and, at least in theory, improve the therapeutic outcome in terms of local tumor control and side effects to unaffected tissue.[47] Preliminarily, patients who received PET/CT-based radiotherapy had more favorite clinical outcome than patients whose dose planning was not based on molecular and functional imaging.

However, the clinical outcome of the effect of PET dose delineation on EBRT has not yet been analyzed in a randomized and prospective clinical trial. Retrospective findings strongly support prospective randomized clinical trials, where GTV definition is based on PET imaging in the EBRT of prostate cancer.

REFERENCES

1. Zelefsky MJ, Lee WR, Zietman A, et al. Evaluation of adherence to quality measures for prostate cancer radiotherapy in the United States: results from the quality research in radiation oncology (QRRO) survey. Pract Radiat Oncol 2013;3:2–8.
2. Spratt DE, Pei X, Yamada J, et al. Long-term survival and toxicity in patients treated with high-dose intensity modulated radiation therapy for localized prostate cancer. Int J Radiat Oncol Biol Phys 2013;85:686–92.
3. Thompson IM, Tangen CM, Paradelo J, et al. Adjuvant radiotherapy for pathological T3N0M0 prostate cancer significantly reduces risk of metastases and improves survival: long-term follow up of a randomized clinical trial. J Urol 2009;181:956–62.
4. Bolla M, van Poppel H, Collette L, et al. Postoperative radiotherapy after radical prostatectomy: a randomised controlled trial (EORTC trial 22911). Lancet 2005;366:572–8.
5. Wiegel T, Bottke D, Steiner U, et al. Phase III postoperative adjuvant radiotherapy after radical prostatectomy compared with radical prostatectomy alone in pT3 prostate cancer with postoperative undetectable prostate-specific antigen: ARO 96-02/AUO AP 09/95. J Clin Oncol 2009;27:2924–30.
6. Abdollah F, Karnes RJ, Suardi N, et al. Predicting survival of patients with node-positive prostate cancer following multimodal treatment. Eur Urol 2014;65:554–62.
7. Hall WA, Fox TH, Jiang X, et al. Treatment efficiency of volumetric modulated arc therapy in comparison with intensity-modulated radiotherapy in the treatment of prostate cancer. J Am Coll Radiol 2013;10:128–34.
8. Weber DC, Wang H, Cozzi L, et al. RapidArc, intensity modulated photon and proton techniques for recurrent prostate cancer in previously irradiated patients: a treatment planning comparison study. Radiat Oncol 2009;4:34.
9. Macdougall ND, Dean C, Muirhead R. Stereotactic body radiotherapy in prostate cancer: is rapidarc a better solution than cyberknife? Clin Oncol (R Coll Radiol) 2014;26:4–9.
10. Jacob V, Bayer W, Astner ST, et al. A planning comparison of dynamic IMRT for different collimator leaf thicknesses with helical tomotherapy and RapidArc for prostate and head and neck tumors. Strahlenther Onkol 2010;186:502–10.
11. Rong Y, Tang G, Welsh JS, et al. Helical tomotherapy versus single-arc intensity modulated arc therapy: a collaborative dosimetric comparison between two institutions. Int J Radiat Oncol Biol Phys 2011;81:284–96.
12. Ost P, Speleers B, De Meerleer G, et al. Volumetric arc therapy and intensity modulated radiotherapy for primary prostate radiotherapy with simultaneous integrated boost to intraprostatic lesion with 6 and 18 MV: a planning comparison study. Int J Radiat Oncol Biol Phys 2011;79:920–6.
13. Polkinghorn WR, Zelefsky MJ. Improving outcomes in highrisk prostate cancer with radiotherapy. Rep Pract Oncol Radiother 2013;18:333–7.
14. Sathya JR, Davis IR, Julian JA, et al. Randomized trial comparing iridium implant plus external-beam radiation therapy with external-beam radiation therapy alone in node-negative locally advanced cancer of the prostate. J Clin Oncol 2005;23:1192–9.
15. Hoskin PJ, Rojas AM, Bownes PJ, et al. Randomised trial of external beam radiotherapy alone or combined with high-dose-rate brachytherapy boost for localized prostate cancer. Radiother Oncol 2012;103:217–22.
16. Spratt DE, Zumsteg ZS, Ghadjar P, et al. Comparison of high-dose (86.4 Gy) IMRT vs combined brachytherapy plus IMRT for intermediate-risk prostate cancer. BJU Int 2014;114:360–7.
17. Kairemo K, Rasulova N, Kiljunen T, et al. PET/CT dose planning for volumetric modulated arc radiation therapy (VMAT)- comparison with conventional approach in prostate cancer patients. Curr Radiopharm 2015;8(1):32–7.
18. von Eyben FE, Kairemo K, Kiljunen T, et al. Planning of external-beam radiation therapy for prostate cancer guided by PET/CT. Curr Radiopharm 2015;8(1):19–31.
19. von Eyben FE, Kairemo K. Meta-analysis of (11)C-choline and (18)F-choline PET/CT for management of patients with prostate cancer. Nucl Med Commun 2014;35:221–30.
20. Teoh M, Clark C, Wood K, et al. Volumetric modulated arc therapy: a review of current literature and clinical use in practice. Br J Radiol 2011;84(1007):967–96.
21. International Commission on Radiation Units and Measurements. ICRU Report 83: prescribing, Recording, and reporting photon-beam intensity-modulated radiation therapy (IMRT). J ICRU 2010;10(1). Report 83. Available at: http://www.fnkv.cz/soubory/216/icru-83.pdf.
22. Michalski J, Gay H, Jackson A, et al. Radiation dose–volume effects in radiation-induced rectal injury. Int J Radiat Oncol Biol Phys 2010;76(Suppl 3):S123–9.
23. Lawton C, Michalski J, El-Naqa I, et al. Radiation oncology specialists reach consensus on pelvic lymph node volumes for high-risk prostate cancer. Int J Radiat Oncol Biol Phys 2009;74(2):383–7.
24. Souvatzoglou M, Krause BJ, Purschel A, et al. Influence of (11)C-choline PET/CT on the treatment planning for salvage radiation therapy in patients with biochemical recurrence of prostate cancer. Radiother Oncol 2011;99:193–200.

25. Jereczek-Fossa BA, Rodari M, Bonora M, et al. [11C] choline PET/CT impacts treatment decision making in patients with prostate cancer referred for radiotherapy. Clin Genitourin Cancer 2014;12:155–9.
26. Moussaid Y, Bonardel G, Jacob J, et al. Single center experience of (18F)-fluorocholine positron emission tomography: analysis of its impact on salvage local therapy in patients with prostate adenocarcinoma. Cancer Radiother 2013;17:259–64.
27. Pinkawa M, Holy R, Piroth MD, et al. Intensity-modulated radiotherapy for prostate cancer implementing molecular imaging with 18F-choline PET-CT to define a simultaneous integrated boost. Strahlenther Onkol 2010;186:600–6.
28. Pinkawa M, Attieh C, Piroth MD, et al. Dose-escalation using intensity-modulated radiotherapy for prostate cancer–evaluation of the dose distribution with and without 18F-choline PET-CT detected simultaneous integrated boost. Radiother Oncol 2009;93: 213–9.
29. Pinkawa M, Piroth MD, Holy R, et al. Dose-escalation using intensity-modulated radiotherapy forprostate cancer - evaluation of quality of life with and without (18)F-choline PET-CT detected simultaneous integrated boost. Radiat Oncol 2012;7:14.
30. Seppälä J, Seppänen M, Arponen E, et al. Carbon-11 acetate PET/CT based dose escalated IMRT in prostate cancer. Radiother Oncol 2009;93:234–40.
31. Casamassima F, Masi L, Menichelli C, et al. Efficacy of eradicative radiotherapy for limited nodal metastases detected with choline PET scan in prostate cancer patients. Tumori 2011;97:49–55.
32. Wurschmidt F, Petersen C, Wahl A, et al. [18F]fluoroethylcholine-PET/CT imaging for radiation treatmentplanning of recurrent and primary prostate cancer with doseescalation to PET/CT-positive lymph nodes. Radiat Oncol 2011;6:44.
33. Picchio M, Berardi G, Fodor A, et al. (11)C-Choline PET/CT as a guide toradiation treatment planning of lymph-node relapses in prostate cancer patients. Eur J Nucl Med Mol Imaging 2014;41:1270–9.
34. Matei DV, Ferro M, Jereczek-Fossa BA, et al. Salvage radical prostatectomy after external beam radiation therapy: a systematic review of current approaches. Urol Int 2015;94:373–82.
35. Suardi N, Gandaglia G, Gallina A, et al. Long-term outcomes of salvage lymph node dissection for clinically recurrent prostate cancer: results of a single-institution series with a minimum follow-up of 5 years. Eur Urol 2015;67:299–309.
36. Rigatti P, Suardi N, Briganti A, et al. Pelvic/retroperitoneal salvage lymph node dissection for patients treated with radical prostatectomy with biochemical recurrence and nodal recurrence detected by [11C] choline positron emission tomography/computed tomography. Eur Urol 2011;60:935–43.
37. Incerti E, Fodor A, Mapelli P, et al. Radiation treatment of lymph node recurrence from prostate cancer: is 11C-choline PET/CT predictive of survival outcomes? J Nucl Med 2015;56(12):1836–42.
38. Rischke HC, Schultze-Seemann W, Wieser G, et al. Adjuvant radiotherapy after salvage lymph node dissection because of nodal relapse of prostate cancer versus salvage lymph node dissection only. Strahlenther Onkol 2015;191:310–20.
39. D'Angelillo RM, Sciuto R, Ramella S, et al. (1)(8) F-choline positron emission tomography/computed tomography-driven high-dose salvage radiation therapy in patients with biochemical progression after radical prostatectomy: feasibility study in 60 patients. Int J Radiat Oncol Biol Phys 2014;90: 296–302.
40. Decaestecker K, De Meerleer G, Ameye F, et al. Surveillance or metastasis-directed Therapy for Oligo-Metastatic Prostate cancer recurrence (STOMP): study protocol for a randomized phase II trial. BMC Cancer 2014;14:671.
41. Heidenreich A, Bastian PJ, Bellmunt J, et al. European Association of, U. EAU guidelines on prostate cancer. part 1: screening, diagnosis, and local treatment with curative intent-update 2013. Eur Urol 2014;65:124–37.
42. Korreman S, Ulrich S, Bowen S, et al. Feasibility of dose painting using volumetric modulated arc optimization and delivery. Acta Oncol 2010;49(7): 964–71.
43. Zhang P, Happersett L, Hunt M, et al. Volumetric modulated arc therapy: planning and evaluation for prostate cancer cases. Int J Radiat Oncol Biol Phys 2010;76:1456–62.
44. Wolff D, Stieler F, Welzel G, et al. Volumetric modulated arc therapy (VMAT) vs. serial tomotherapy, step-and-shoot IMRT and 3D-conformal RT for treatment of prostate cancer. Radiother Oncol 2009;93: 226–33.
45. Yoo S, Wu QJ, Lee WR, et al. Radiotherapy treatment plans with RapidArc for prostate cancer involving seminal vesicles and lymph nodes. Int J Radiat Oncol Biol Phys 2010;76:935–42.
46. Ling CC, Humm J, Larson S, et al. Towards multidimensional radiotherapy (MDCRT): biological imaging and biological conformality. Int J Radiat Oncol Biol Phys 2000;47(3):551–60.
47. Bentzen SM. Theragnostic imaging for radiation oncology: dose painting by numbers. Lancet Oncol 2005;6(2):112–7.

Printed and bound by CPI Group (UK) Ltd, Croydon, CR0 4YY

03/10/2024

01040304-0005